CUNNINGHAM'S MANUAL OF PRACTICAL ANATOMY

Volume 2

Cunningham's Manual of Practical Anatomy

CUNNINGHAM'S MANUAL OF PRACTICAL ANATOMY

Sixteenth edition

Volume 2 Thorax and abdomen

Dr Rachel Koshi MBBS, MS, PhD

Professor of Anatomy
Apollo Institute of Medical Sciences and Research
Chittoor, India

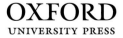

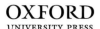
UNIVERSITY PRESS

Great Clarendon Street, Oxford, OX2 6DP,
United Kingdom

Oxford University Press is a department of the University of Oxford.
It furthers the University's objective of excellence in research, scholarship,
and education by publishing worldwide. Oxford is a registered trade mark of
Oxford University Press in the UK and in certain other countries

Thirteenth edition 1966
Fourteenth edition 1977
Fifteenth edition 1986

Impression: 4

Published in the United States of America by Oxford University Press
198 Madison Avenue, New York, NY 10016, United States of America

British Library Cataloguing in Publication Data

Data available

Library of Congress Control Number: 78301413

ISBN 978-0-19-874937-0

Printed and bound by Replika Press Pvt Ltd, India

I fondly dedicate this book to the late Dr K G Koshi for his encouragement and support when I chose a career in anatomy; and to Dr Mary Jacob, under whose guidance I learned the subject and developed a love for teaching.

Oxford University Press would like to dedicate this book to the memory of the late George John Romanes, Professor of Anatomy at Edinburgh University from 1954–1984, who brought his wisdom to previous editions of *Cunningham's*.

Foreword

It gives me great pleasure to pen down the Foreword to the 16th edition of *Cunningham's Manual of Practical Anatomy*. Just as the curriculum of anatomy is incomplete without dissection, so also learning by dissection is incomplete without a manual.

Cunningham's Manual of Practical Anatomy is one of the oldest dissectors, the first edition of which was published as early as 1893. Since then, the manual has been an inseparable companion to students during dissection.

I remember my days as a first MBBS student, the only dissector known in those days was *Cunningham's* manual. The manual helped me to dissect scientifically, step by step, explore the body, see all structures as mentioned, and admire God's highest creation—the human body—so perfectly. As a postgraduate student I marvelled at the manual and learnt details of structures, in a way as if I had my teacher with me telling me what to do next. The clearly defined steps of dissection, and the comprehensive revision tables at the end, helped me personally to develop a liking for dissection and the subject of anatomy.

Today, as a Professor and Head of Anatomy, teaching anatomy for more than 30 years, I find *Cunningham's* manual extremely useful to all the students dissecting and learning anatomy.

With the explosion of knowledge and ongoing curricular changes, the manual has been revised at frequent intervals.

The 16th edition is more student friendly. The language is simplified, so that the book can be comprehended by one and all. The objectives are well defined. The clinical application notes at the end of each chapter are an academic feast to the learners. The lucidly enumerated steps of dissection make a student explore various structures, the layout, and relations and compare them with the simplified labelled illustrations in the manual. This helps in sequential dissection in a scientific way and for knowledge retention. The text also includes multiple-choice questions for self-assessment and holistic comprehension.

Keeping the concept of 'Adult Learning Principles' in mind, i.e. adults learn when they 'DO', and with a global movement towards 'competency-based curriculum', students learn anatomy when they dissect; *Cunningham's* manual will help students to dissect on their own, at their own speed and time, and become competent doctors, who can cater to the needs of the society in a much better way.

I recommend this invaluable manual to all the learners who want to master the subject of anatomy.

Dr Pritha S Bhuiyan
Professor and Head, Department of Anatomy
Professor and Coordinator, Department of Medical Education
Seth GS Medical College and KEM Hospital, Parel, Mumbai

Preface to the sixteenth edition

Cunningham's Manual of Practical Anatomy has been the most widely used dissection manual in India for many decades. This edition is extensively revised. All anatomical terms are updated using the latest terminology. The language has been modernized and simplified to appeal to the present-day student. Opening remarks have been added at the start of a chapter, or at the beginning of the description of a region where necessary. This volume on the thorax, abdomen, and pelvis and perineum starts with an introduction to the trunk, or torso, defines the boundaries of each constituent part, and provides a general overview of the vertebrae, vertebral column, and autonomic nervous system which are common to all sections of the trunk. The last section in the volume collates and organizes information from the earlier sections to enable further understanding of the body as a whole. Bearing in mind that most examinations test a comprehensive understanding of developmental and microscopic anatomy, the brief sections pertaining to these areas have been removed. Students are requested to read books devoted to these topics. In situations where adult anatomy is better explained based on development, the relevant embryology is briefly described.

Dissection forms an integral part of learning anatomy, and the practice of dissections enables students to retain and recall anatomical details learnt in the first year of medical school during their clinical practice. To make the dissection process easier and more meaningful, in this edition, each dissection is presented with a heading and a list of objectives to be accomplished. The details of dissections have been retained from the earlier edition but are presented as numbered, stepwise easy-to-follow instructions that help students navigate their way through the tissues of the body, and to isolate, define, and study important organs.

This manual contains a number of old and new features that enable students to integrate the anatomy learnt in the dissection hall with clinical practice. Each region has images of living anatomy to help students identify on the skin surface bony or soft tissue landmarks that lie beneath. Numerous X-rays, CTs, and MRIs further enable the student to visualize internal structures in the living. Matters of clinical importance, when mentioned in the text, are highlighted.

A brand new feature of this edition is the presentation of one or more clinical application notes at the end of each chapter. Some of these notes focus attention on the anatomical basis of commonly used physical diagnostic tests such as superficial abdominal reflexes. Others deal with the underlying anatomy of clinical findings in diseases such as flail chest, abdominal hernias, and obstructive jaundice. The clinical anatomy of common procedures, such as vasectomy and thoracotomy, are described. Many clinical application notes are in a Q&A format that challenges the student to brainstorm the material covered in the chapter. Multiple-choice questions on each section are included at the end to help students assess their preparedness for the university examination.

It is hoped that this new edition respects the legacy of *Cunningham's* in producing a text and manual that is accurate, student friendly, comprehensive, and interesting, and that it will serve the community of students who are beginning their career in medicine to gain knowledge and appreciation of the anatomy of the human body.

Dr Rachel Koshi

Contributors

Dr J Suganthy, Professor of Anatomy, Christian Medical College, Vellore, India.
Dr Suganthy wrote the MCQs, reviewed manuscripts, and provided help and advice with the artwork.

Dr Aparna Irodi, Professor of Radiology, Christian Medical College and Hospital, Vellore, India.
Dr Irodi kindly researched, identified, and explained the radiology images.

Dr Ivan James Prithishkumar, Professor of Anatomy, Christian Medical College, Vellore, India.
Dr Prithishkumar wrote some of the clinical applications and reviewed the text as a critical reader.

Dr Tripti Meriel Jacob, Associate Professor of Anatomy, Christian Medical College, Vellore, India.
Dr Jacob wrote some of the clinical applications, reviewed the text as a critical reader, and provided advice and assistance with the artwork.

Acknowledgements

Dr Koshi would like to thank the following:

Dr Benjamin Perakath, Consultant Surgeon and Honorary Senior Lecturer, Dr Gray's Hospital, Elgin, United Kingdom.
Dr Perakath kindly advised on the accuracy and relevance of the clinical anatomy content pertaining to general surgery and critically reviewed the clinical applications in that discipline.

Dr Antony Devasia, Professor of Urology, Christian Medical College and Hospital, Vellore, India.
Dr Devasia kindly advised on the accuracy and relevance of the clinical anatomy content pertaining to urology and critically reviewed the clinical applications in that discipline.

Dr Reuben Thomas Kurien, Associate Professor of Clinical Gastroenterology, Christian Medical College and Hospital, Vellore, India.
Dr Kurien kindly provided the endoscopic images of the stomach and duodenum.

Radiology Department, Christian Medical College, Vellore, India.
The Radiology Department kindly provided the radiology images.

Ms Geraldine Jeffers, Senior Commissioning Editor, and **Karen Moore**, Senior Production Editor, and the wonderful editorial team of Oxford University Press for their assistance, support, and encouragement during the production of this volume.

Reviewers

Oxford University Press would like to thank all those who read draft materials and provided valuable feedback during the writing process and on publication:

Dr TS Roy, MD, PhD, Professor and Head, Department of Anatomy, All India Institute of Medical Sciences, New Delhi 110029, India.

Dr Chittapuram Srinivasan Ramesh Babu (CS Ramesh Babu), Associate Professor of Anatomy, Muzaffarnagar Medical College, India.

Dr Aastha, Associate Professor, Department of Anatomy, Christian Medical College & Hospital, Ludhiana, India.

Dr Aby S Charles, Senior Resident, Department of Anatomy, Christian Medical College, Vellore, India.

Dr Padmavathi G, Professor of Anatomy, Apollo Institute of Medical Sciences and Research, Chittoor, India.

Dr Sunil Jonathan Holla, Professor of Anatomy, Christian Medical College, Vellore, India.

Dr Sabita Mishra, Professor of Anatomy, Maulana Azad Medical College, Delhi, India.

Dr Neerja Rani, Assistant Professor, Department of Anatomy, All India Institute of Medical Sciences (AIIMS), New Delhi-110029, India.

Dr Bertha AD Rathinam, Professor and Head, Department of Anatomy, India Institute of Medical Sciences Bhopal, Madhya Pradesh, India.

Dr Nachiket Shankar, Associate Professor of Anatomy, St John's Medical College, Bangalore, India.

Contents

PART 1

Introduction

1

CHAPTER 1
Introduction to the trunk

The **trunk** or **torso** is an anatomical term for the central part of the human body. It includes the thorax, abdomen, pelvis, and perineum. It does not include the head and neck or upper and lower limbs.

Parts of the trunk

The upper part of the trunk is the thorax. It is separated from the more inferiorly placed abdomen by the diaphragm. The lower part of the abdomen lies in the greater pelvis and is continuous posteriorly and inferiorly with the lesser pelvis or true pelvis. The V-shaped floor of the pelvis is the **pelvic diaphragm**. The part of the trunk inferior to the pelvic diaphragm is the **perineum** [Fig. 1.1].

Superiorly the trunk is continuous with the neck. The upper limbs are attached to the upper part of the torso, and muscles of the upper limb overlie the thoracic cage. The lower limbs articulate with the bony pelvis and posteriorly overlap with the abdominal and pelvic organs.

Most critical organs are placed within the trunk. In the thorax are the heart and lungs, protected by the rib cage. Most of the gastrointestinal tract and the liver, spleen, pancreas, and kidneys are located in the abdomen. The pelvis contains the male and female reproductive organs, the urinary bladder, and the terminal part of the gastrointestinal tract.

The posterior aspect of the trunk is the back, which includes the vertebral column, the deep muscles of the back, and the thoracolumbar fascia.

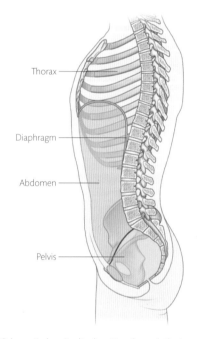

Thorax

Diaphragm

Abdomen

Pelvis

Fig. 1.1 Schematic longitudinal section through the trunk showing the position of the thorax, abdomen, and pelvis.

This figure was published in Gray's Anatomy for Students, 2nd Edition, Drake R et al. Copyright © Elsevier (2009).

Vertebral column

The vertebral column consists of 33 vertebrae arranged one above the other. There are seven cervical, 12 thoracic, five lumbar, five sacral, and four coccygeal vertebrae. The five sacral vertebrae are fused together to form the sacrum, and the coccygeal vertebrae are fused to form the coccyx. The vertebrae articulate with each other at the intervertebral discs and the facet joints [Figs. 1.2A and 1.2B].

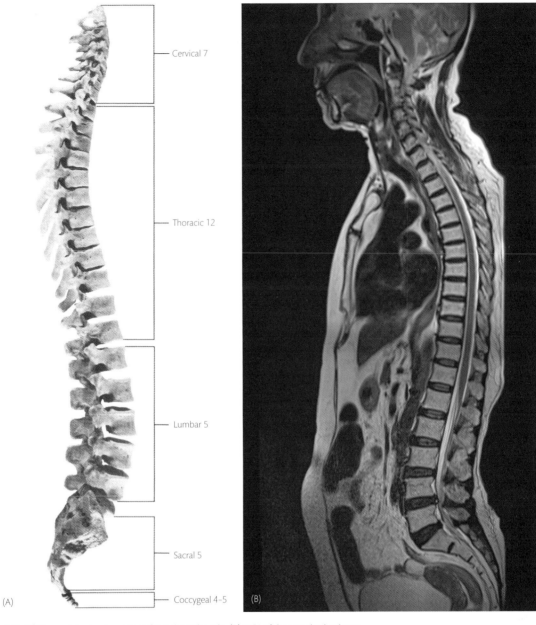

Cervical 7

Thoracic 12

Lumbar 5

Sacral 5

(A)   Coccygeal 4–5   (B)

Fig. 1.2 (A) The vertebral column seen from the right side. (B) MRI of the vertebral column.

Typical vertebra

A typical vertebra has the following elements [Figs. 1.3 and 1.4]—a **vertebral body** which lies anteriorly and the vertebral arch, made up of the **pedicles** and **laminae**, which lies posteriorly. Surrounded by the body and vertebral arch is the **vertebral foramen**. The **vertebral arch** consists of a pedicle and a lamina on each side. The **pedicle** forms the lateral wall of the vertebral foramen. It extends backwards from the posterolateral surface of the body to the base of

the laterally projecting transverse process [Fig. 1.3]. At this point, where the pedicle meets the transverse process, it also meets the **lamina**. The two laminae form the posterior limit of the vertebral foramen. Each lamina passes medially and backwards from the junction of the transverse process and the pedicle to join its fellow at the base of the spine. The **spine** is long and projects downwards and backwards in the midline so that its tip is palpable. Together, the vertebral foramina of all the vertebrae make up the **vertebral**

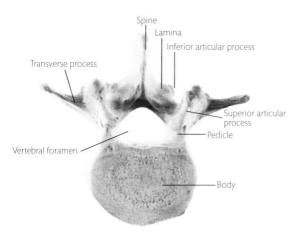

Fig. 1.3 The superior surface of the third lumbar vertebra.

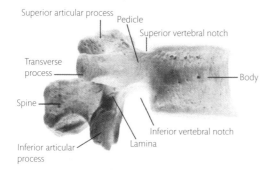

Fig. 1.4 The right surface of the third lumbar vertebra.

canal. The vertebral canal contains the spinal cord, its coverings—the dura, arachnoid, and pia mater—and blood vessels.

The pedicle on each side is deeply notched inferiorly (**inferior vertebral notch**) to form the superior margin of an **intervertebral foramen**. The anterior margin of the foramen is formed by the posterolateral edge of the vertebral body and the intervertebral disc below it. The remainder of the foramen is formed by the vertebra below—inferiorly by the slightly notched margin of the pedicle, and posteriorly by the anterior surface of the wedge-shaped superior articular process. Each intervertebral foramen transmits the spinal nerve, large **intervertebral veins**, and a small spinal artery.

The **superior articular process** projects superiorly from the junction of the pedicle and lamina. It ends in a sharp margin superiorly. The smooth posterior surface of the process is covered with hyaline cartilage and articulates with the anterior surface of the **inferior articular process** of the vertebra above. The **transverse processes** project posterolaterally.

Intervertebral discs

The intervertebral discs lie between adjacent vertebral bodies [Fig. 1.5]. They consist of concentric layers of strong collagenous fibrous tissue known as the **anulus fibrosus**, which lie between the cartilage-covered surfaces of the vertebral bodies. The layers of collagen run at an angle to each other and together surround an inner mass of gelatinous material—the **nucleus pulposus**. The nucleus pulposus is held under pressure by the annulus and lies slightly closer to the posterior surface of the disc. The intervertebral discs confer flexibility on the vertebral column by permitting movement between adjacent vertebrae. This movement takes place around the nucleus pulposus and its range is directly proportional to the thickness of the disc.

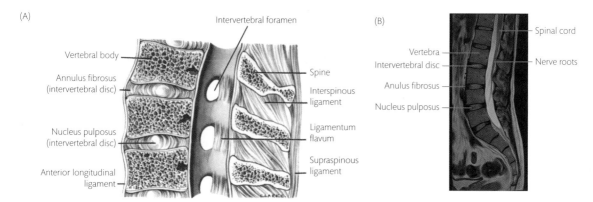

Fig. 1.5 (A) A median section through part of the lumbar vertebral column. (B) A T2-weighted (T2W) sagittal MRI image of lumbosacral spine showing the dark linear nerve roots and the spinal cord in the vertebral canal. The two parts of the intervertebral disc are well demonstrated. Central is the hyperintense nucleus pulposus and around it the hypointense annulus fibrosus.

The discs are thickest in the lumbar region and thinnest in the thoracic region. The direction of the movement is controlled by the position of the articular facets on the vertebral arches.

The intervertebral discs absorb shocks applied to the vertebral column. They also resist the compression forces produced by the contraction of the powerful erector spinae group of muscles. The load on the intervertebral discs is considerable during some activities, for example when an 80-kg man jumps from a height and lands on his feet; or when a person lifts a 50-kg sack.

Herniation of the nucleus pulposus causes loss of pressure within the disc and its consequent narrowing. Progressive narrowing of the discs from this and other causes is seen with increasing age. It leads to a decrease in height of the individual and reduced mobility of the vertebral column.

Articular facets

Paired articular facets lie at the junction of the pedicles, laminae, and transverse processes [Fig. 1.3]. The orientation of the facets determines the type of movements possible between adjacent vertebrae. (This is because the union of the vertebral bodies at the intervertebral discs forces all the axes of movement to pass through the nucleus pulposus [Fig. 1.6].) In the thoracic region, the plane of the articular facets is approximately on the arc of a circle which has the nucleus pulposus at its centre. Hence rotation can take place between the thoracic vertebrae, in addition to flexion and extension. In the lumbar region, the inferior facets of one vertebra fit between the superior facets of the vertebra below. This arrangement effectively prevents rotation but permits free flexion and extension. In the cervical region, the right and left facets are far apart and lie parallel to each other in an oblique coronal plane, sloping upwards and forwards. This orientation also prevents rotation, except in the joints between the first and second cervical vertebrae which permit rotation of the head on the neck.

The range of flexion, extension, and lateral flexion is maximum in the lumbar region because of the thick **lumbar intervertebral** discs. The range is least in the thoracic region and consists principally of rotation. The movements between the typical cervical vertebrae are intermediate in range and in the same directions as in the lumbar region. However, a greater degree of extension is possible in the cervical region because of the small

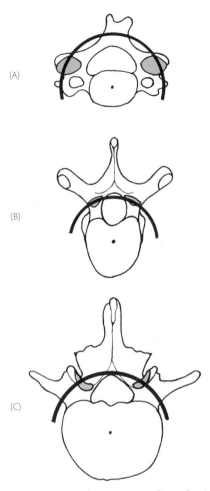

Fig. 1.6 Outline drawings of the superior surfaces of typical cervical (A), thoracic (B), and lumbar (C) vertebrae. In each case, an arc of a circle, with its centre at the nucleus pulposus of the intervertebral disc, has been drawn through the articular facets. In the thoracic region, the arc is parallel to the articular surfaces of the facets, allowing free rotation in this region. Blue = cartilage of the facets.

spines which do not overlap as they do in the thoracic region [Fig. 1.2].

Intervertebral ligaments

Apart from the intervertebral discs, the vertebral bodies are bound together by a number of ligaments.

1. The **anterior longitudinal ligament** lies on the anterior surface of the bodies and stretches from the atlas (C. 1 vertebra) to the sacrum. It is firmly attached to the anterior surfaces of the intervertebral discs and vertebral bodies. Its lateral margin is difficult to define as it fades into the periosteum.

2. The **posterior longitudinal ligament** lies in the vertebral canal. It is attached to the posterior surfaces of the intervertebral discs and the adjacent margins of the vertebral bodies, but not to their posterior surfaces. On the posterior surface of the vertebral body, the ligament is narrowed to permit the passage of veins from the vertebral bodies into the internal vertebral venous plexus—the **basivertebral veins** [Fig. 1.7]. (See Fig. 13.8 for basivertebral veins.)

3. The **ligamenta flava** are strong, yellow, elastic ligaments which unite the posterior surface of the laminae of adjacent vertebrae. They are relatively short and are limited on each side by the articular processes. Together with the laminae, they form a smooth posterior surface of the vertebral canal [Fig. 1.8].

4. A thin **interspinous ligament** unites the adjacent margins of two spines.

5. The strong **supraspinous ligament** is attached to the posterior aspects of the spines throughout the length of the thoracic and lumbar parts of the vertebral column. It is continuous anteriorly with the interspinous ligament [Fig. 1.5].

These ligaments are sufficiently elastic to allow separation of the laminae and spines on flexion of the vertebral column. They also help to return the vertebral column to its resting position when flexion ceases.

Curvatures of the vertebral column

The anteroposterior **curvatures of the vertebral column** (convex anteriorly in the lumbar and cervical regions, concave in the thoracic

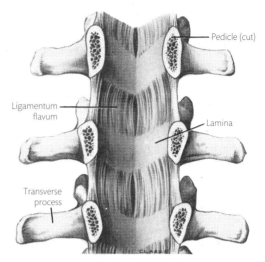

Fig. 1.8 The lumbar vertebral arches and ligamenta flava as seen from in front, after removal of the vertebral bodies.

region) are produced mainly by the intervertebral discs. These curvatures and the discs confer a degree of resilience to the vertebral column.

Muscles and fascia of the back

The deep muscle of the back is the **erector spinae**. The major part of this muscle begins on the sacrum and ascends into the lumbar region. It fills the bony interval between the vertebral spines and transverse processes. The erector spinae splits into three columns which pass upwards into the thorax, deep to the thoracolumbar fascia. Each column is inserted either into the ribs (lateral part) or the vertebrae (medial part), but fresh slips arise from the same situations and continue upwards. From lateral to medial, the three columns are: iliocostalis, longissimus, and spinalis. (The erector spinae is described more fully in Vol. 3.)

The **thoracolumbar fascia** extends from the sacrum to the neck. It binds the **erector spinae** to the posterolateral surfaces of the vertebral bodies and, in the lumbar region, encloses the quadratus lumborum.

Autonomic nervous system

The **autonomic nervous system** is a system of nerves and ganglia that supply cardiac muscle, smooth muscle, glands of the viscera, skin, and

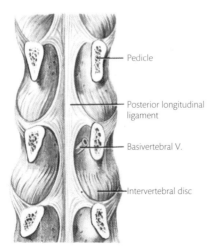

Fig. 1.7 The posterior longitudinal ligament of the vertebral column. The vertebral arches have been removed.

blood vessels. It consists of **sympathetic** and **parasympathetic** parts. The thoracic, abdominal, and pelvic viscera receive dual innervation from the sympathetic and parasympathetic divisions of the autonomic nervous system. The limbs and body wall are supplied by sympathetics alone [Fig. 1.9].

An autonomic nerve pathway involves two nerve cells. The first is the **preganglionic nerve**. It has its cell body in the brainstem or spinal cord. It is connected by the axon to the second nerve cell,

which is located outside the central nervous system in a cluster of nerve cells called the **autonomic ganglion**. Nerve fibres from these peripherally situated autonomic ganglia are distributed to the organs. These are the **post-ganglionic nerves**.

Most of the autonomic ganglia for the sympathetic division are located in the sympathetic trunk, just outside the vertebral column. The autonomic ganglia for the parasympathetic division are located near or in the organs they supply.

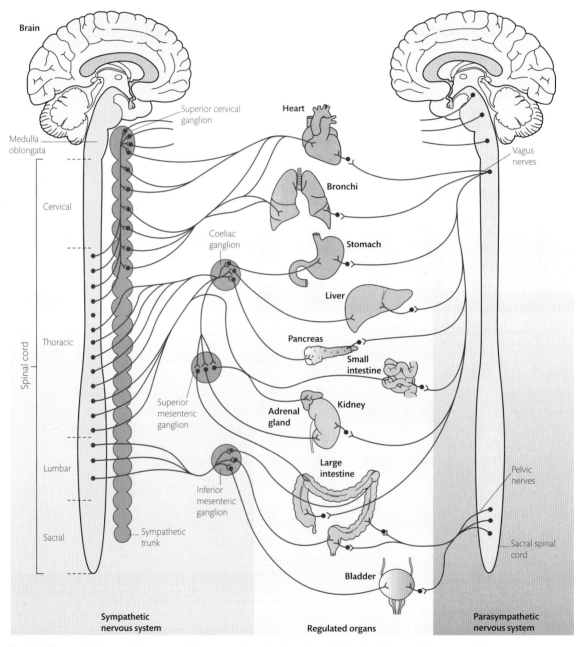

Fig. 1.9 Schematic diagram of the autonomic nerve supply to the thoracic and abdominal viscera. Left = sympathetic nervous system. Right = parasympathetic nervous system.

The autonomic nervous system also transmits **sensory** nerves from the viscera. These have no functional connections with the autonomic ganglia but use the pathways of the preganglionic and post-ganglionic nerve fibres as a route to the central nervous system.

Autonomic nerve plexuses are extensive networks of nerve fibres and cell bodies associated with the autonomic nervous system [see Fig. 4.45]. They are found in the thorax, abdomen, and pelvis and contain sympathetic, parasympathetic, and visceral afferent fibres.

Generally, parasympathetic innervation results in digestion by stimulating peristalsis in the gut and secretion of the gut-associated glands. Sympathetic innervation, on the other hand, decreases blood flow to the abdominal viscera and inhibits digestion. Blood flow is diverted from the viscera to the trunk and limbs to aid the body in the 'fight or flight' response to threat.

Parasympathetic part

The **preganglionic parasympathetic** nerve cells are located in the brain and second to fourth sacral segments of the spinal cord. As such, the parasympathetics are also known as the **craniosacral outflow**. Preganglionic parasympathetic fibres leave the central nervous system through certain cranial nerves and the second and third, or third and fourth, sacral spinal nerves. The **parasympathetic ganglia** containing the **post-ganglionic** neuron lie in or near the structures which they innervate, so the preganglionic fibres end close to these organs. The parasympathetics for the thoracic viscera arise from the vagus. Parasympathetics for the abdominal viscera arise either from the vagus or from the sacral segments of the spinal cord.

Sympathetic part

The **preganglionic sympathetic** nerve cells are located in the spinal cord—thoracic and upper lumbar segments. The **preganglionic sympathetic fibres** arise from all thoracic nerves and the upper two or three lumbar nerves—the thoracolumbar outflow. Sympathetic ganglia are usually confined to ganglia on the sympathetic trunk or in sympathetic plexuses around major arteries. They usually lie at some distance from the organs which they innervate. Their post-ganglionic nerve fibres are often distributed along blood vessels.

Sympathetic trunk

An important part of the sympathetic nervous system are the **sympathetic trunks**. The right and left sympathetic trunks extend from the upper cervical region to the coccyx, one on each side on the front of the vertebral column. The sympathetic trunks consist of a series of ganglia, joined by longitudinal bundles of nerve fibres. The sympathetic ganglia are connected to the ventral rami of the spinal nerve by two fibres. The **white ramus communicans** carries preganglionic nerve fibres from the nerve to the ganglion. The **grey ramus communicans** carries post-ganglionic sympathetic nerve fibres from the ganglion to the nerve for distribution through the branches of the spinal nerve.

The ganglia of the trunks send (1) **post-ganglionic** nerve fibres to most of the cranial and all of the spinal nerves for distribution to the body wall through the grey rami communicantes. The trunks also transmit (2) **preganglionic** fibres to sympathetic ganglia situated more peripherally, (3) some **preganglionic** fibres through visceral branches, e.g. the splanchnic nerves, to the sympathetic plexuses, and (4) **preganglionic** fibres to the adrenal medulla.

Clinical Application 1.1 discusses slipped disc or disc herniation and Clinical Application 1.2 discusses lumbar puncture.

CLINICAL APPLICATION 1.1 Slipped disc or disc herniation

Herniation of the nucleus pulposus or **disc herniation** is a pathological condition when the nucleus pulposus is extruded (pushed out) through the annulus fibrosus. It is one cause of backache and may occur at any age in the cervical or lumbar regions. When herniation occurs posteriorly through the thinnest part of the anulus fibrosus, the nucleus may press on the spinal cord or on one of the spinal nerves where it lies in the intervertebral foramen posterior to the disc. Most commonly, lumbar disc protrusions occur between L. 4–L. 5 and L. 5–S. 1, as seen in Fig. 1.10.

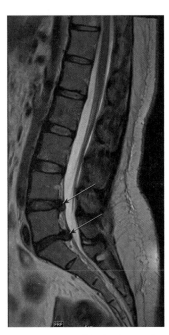

Fig. 1.10 T2W sagittal images of the lumbosacral spine showing disc bulges at L. 4–5 and L. 5–S. 1 levels (arrows).

CLINICAL APPLICATION 1.2 Lumbar puncture

A 15-year-old boy is brought to hospital with a history of fever, severe headache, and stiffness of the neck. In order to exclude the diagnosis of infectious meningitis, a lumbar puncture is done.

Study question 1: what is a lumbar puncture, and how is it done? (Answer 1: lumbar puncture is the tapping of the subarachnoid space (space around the spinal cord) in the lumbar region. It is done for removal of cerebrospinal fluid for testing or for introduction of medication. Lumbar puncture is done by inserting a needle into the vertebral canal from the back. It is done in the lower part of the lumbar spinal column between vertebrae L. 3 and L. 4, or L. 4 and L. 5.)

Study question 2: from your knowledge of the anatomy of this region, list in sequence the structures pierced by the needle before it enters the vertebral canal. (Answer 2: skin, subcutaneous tissue, supraspinous ligament, interspinous ligament, ligamentum flavum.)

PART 2

The thorax

11

CHAPTER 2
Introduction to the thorax

The thorax is that part of the trunk which extends from the root of the neck to the abdomen. The main structures in the thorax are the heart, the lungs, the great vessels which enter and leave the heart, the trachea or windpipe, the oesophagus, and the thoracic duct. (The oesophagus and thoracic duct run all the way through the thorax, between the neck and the abdomen.) A bulky, movable median septum—the **mediastinum**—separates the lungs and their covering from each other and contains the heart and many other thoracic structures.

The **movements of the thorax** are primarily concerned with increasing or decreasing the intrathoracic volume. This volume change alters the pressure in the thorax so that air is drawn into the lungs (inspiration) and expelled from them (expiration) through the respiratory passages. To achieve these movements and to overcome the effects of atmospheric pressure, the walls of the thorax are strengthened by the movable **thoracic cage**. The thoracic cage consists of the 12 **thoracic vertebrae**, the 12 pairs of **ribs** which articulate with these vertebrae, the **sternum** (breastbone), and the flexible **costal cartilages** which unite the ribs to the **sternum** or to each other [Fig. 2.1]. Layers of intercostal muscles fill the spaces between the ribs and their cartilages. When they contract, they move the ribs and cartilages and make the spaces rigid so that the intercostal tissues do not move out and in as the intrathoracic pressure changes.

The thoracic cavity is separated from the abdominal cavity by the musculo-aponeurotic **diaphragm** [Fig. 2.2]. The diaphragm is attached to the lower margin of the thoracic cage (**inferior aperture of the thorax**) and bulges upwards, so that the upper abdominal organs lie under cover of the lower part of the thoracic cage. The diaphragm acts like a piston. When it contracts, it descends and increases the intrathoracic volume (inspiration) [Fig. 2.3A]. When it relaxes, the contracting muscles of the abdominal wall force the abdominal contents and the overlying diaphragm upwards inside the thoracic cage, decreasing the intrathoracic volume (expiration) [Fig. 2.3B]. These are the main movements in quiet respiration.

The changing pressure in the thorax produced by the respiratory movements affects venous return to the heart. The volume of blood received by the heart increases during inspiration and decreases

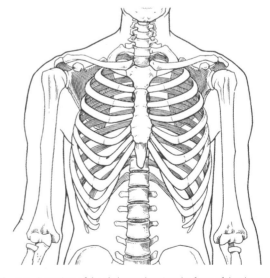

Fig. 2.1 A portion of the skeleton showing the front of the thorax.

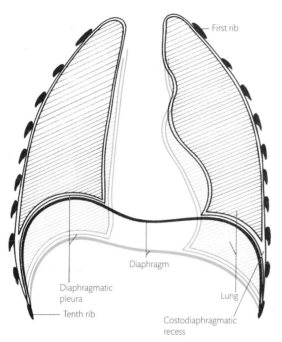

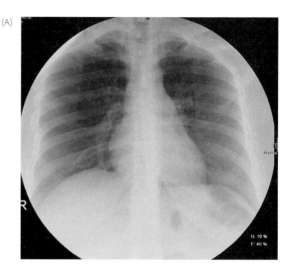

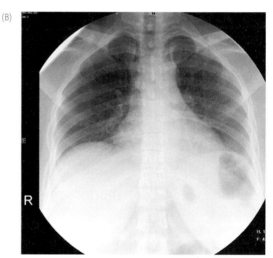

Fig. 2.2 An outline drawing to show the change in shape of the thoracic contents resulting from contraction of the diaphragm alone. The contracted positions are shown in blue. Note that the lungs and mediastinal structures are elongated and that the lungs expand to fill the space vacated by the mediastinal structures and to enter the costodiaphragmatic recesses of the pleura. The movements which the ribs undergo in respiration are not shown.

First rib

Tenth rib

Diaphragmatic
pleura

Diaphragm

Lung

Costodiaphragmatic
recess

during expiration. These changes in venous return cause corresponding changes in the volume of the heart [Figs. 2.3A and B] and in the blood pressure. ➲ During forced expiration against resistance (as in straining or blowing up a balloon), venous return is markedly decreased, and the blood pressure is lowered. This drop in blood pressure may be severe enough to cause fainting.

Shape and framework of the thorax

The thorax has the shape of a truncated cone. It expands inferiorly to surround the upper part of the abdominal cavity. It is flattened anteroposteriorly to fit the scapulae on its posterolateral aspects and to withstand the pull of the powerful upper limb muscles which overlap it anteriorly and posteriorly.

Each **rib** articulates posteriorly with the vertebral column. From there, the rib sweeps backwards and laterally, then obliquely downwards and forwards

Fig. 2.3 (A) An anteroposterior radiograph of the thorax in inspiration. Note that the right dome of the diaphragm is higher than the left, and the outlines of the diaphragm and the costodiaphragmatic recesses are clear owing to the air content in the lungs. (B) An anteroposterior radiograph of the same individual as in Fig. 2.3A, but in expiration. Note that the diaphragm is much higher and that the shadow of the diaphragm and the costodiaphragmatic recesses are poorly defined because of the increased density of the basal parts of the lungs and their withdrawal from the recesses. Note also that the mediastinal shadow is shorter and broader in association with the raised diaphragm.

in the curve of the thoracic wall. It ends anteriorly by articulating with a costal cartilage.

The **costal cartilages** are flexible and extend from the anterior ends of the ribs to the sternum. The cartilages of the upper seven ribs (**true ribs**) articulate with the margins of the sternum. The upper cartilages are in line with their ribs; the lower cartilages become progressively more angulated, the medial part passing upwards to the sternum [Fig. 2.1]. The ribs inferior to the seventh become progressively shorter so that the anterior ends of each successive pair lie further and further apart. The upturned ends of the cartilages of ribs 8–10 (**false ribs**) fail to reach the sternum but articulate with the margin of the cartilage above. Together with the seventh costal cartilage, they form a continuous cartilaginous **costal margin** which diverges from the lower part of the sternum. The **infrasternal angle** lies between the right and left **costal margins**. The costal margins begin at the articulation of the seventh costal cartilage with the xiphisternal joint (the joint between the middle part or body and the lowest part or xiphoid process of the sternum). The costal margins are completed inferiorly by the cartilaginous ends of the eleventh and twelfth ribs and the lower border of the twelfth rib.

The flexibility of the costal cartilages, combined with their synovial joints with the sternum or with each other, permits the ribs to move relative to each other and to the sternum in respiration. The first costal cartilages differ from the others in that they are fused with the upper part of the sternum (manubrium) and are frequently calcified or ossified. This means that the first ribs and the manubrium move together as one piece. The other ribs, especially the floating ribs, have a greater degree of freedom of movement relative to the sternum and to each other.

The progressive shortening of the lower ribs and consequent divergence of the costal margins inferior to the sternum make the anterior wall of the thoracic cage much shorter than the lateral or posterior walls. Thus the thoracic cage overlaps more of the abdominal contents laterally and posteriorly than it does anteriorly. The inferior end of the sternum (xiphoid process) lies approximately at the level of the ninth thoracic vertebra. The lowest part of the costal margin is the tenth costal cartilage in the mid-axillary line. It lies at the level of the third lumbar vertebra, close to the iliac crest [Fig. 2.1].

In transverse section, the thorax is kidney-shaped because the vertebral bodies and posterior parts of the ribs project anteriorly into it [see Fig. 2.5]. This leaves a deep depression—the **paravertebral groove**—on each side of the vertebra formed by the backwards and lateral sweep of the posterior parts of the ribs. The rounded posterior parts of the lungs lie in the paravertebral grooves. The contents of the mediastinum for the most part lie anterior to the vertebral bodies [see Fig. 1.1].

Apertures of the thorax

The small **superior aperture of the thorax** is directed towards the neck. It is formed by the first thoracic vertebra, the inner margin of the first ribs, the first costal cartilages, and the sternum [Fig. 2.4]. This aperture slopes steeply downwards

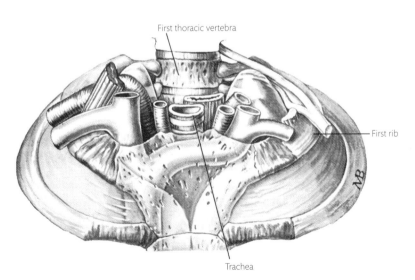

First thoracic vertebra

First rib

Trachea

Fig. 2.4 The superior aperture of the thorax formed by the first thoracic vertebra, the first ribs, and the sternum. Underlying structures are shown through the sternum.

and forwards [Fig. 2.4]. As a result, the apices of the lungs (each surrounded by a dome of parietal pleura) project through the superior aperture up to the level of the neck of the first rib, well above the first costal cartilage. (The two lung apices are separated by the structures which pass between the mediastinum and the upper limbs and neck.) The superior aperture is sealed by a rigid fascia—the **suprapleural membrane**—which extends from the transverse process of the seventh cervical vertebra to the inner margin of the first rib on each side.

The large **inferior aperture of the thorax** slopes downwards and backwards. It is formed by the costal margins, the twelfth ribs, and the twelfth thoracic vertebra. It is closed by the diaphragm which is pierced by structures passing between the thorax and the abdomen.

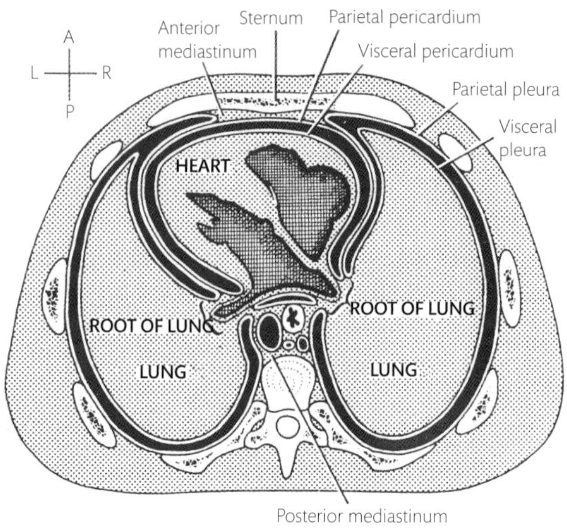

Fig. 2.5 A diagrammatic horizontal section through the thorax to show the positions of the major structures. The pleural and pericardial cavities are shown in black.

Arrangement of main contents

The lungs are a pair of sponge-like, elastic respiratory organs. They fill the greater part of the cavity of the chest and consist of innumerable minute, air-filled cavities called alveoli. The alveoli are connected to the trachea by the branching system of **bronchi** and **bronchioles**. The lungs are covered by pleura.

The **mediastinum** is the broad midline septum which extends from the vertebral column behind to the sternum in front, between the pleura on each side. It contains the heart, trachea, oesophagus, large blood vessels, and other important structures. The medial surface of each lung is united to the mediastinum by a narrow **root of the lung**, through which bronchi, blood vessels, lymph vessels, and nerves enter or leave the lung [Fig. 2.5].

The lungs in the pleural cavities, and the mediastinum between them, are fitted to the convex upper surface of the diaphragm, which separates them from the abdominal contents.

CHAPTER 3
The walls of the thorax

Bones forming the thoracic cage

The thoracic cage consists of the 12 **thoracic vertebrae**, the 12 pairs of **ribs** which articulate with these vertebrae, the **sternum** (breastbone), and the flexible **costal cartilages** which unite the ribs to the sternum or to each other [Figs. 3.1A, 3.1B].

Thoracic vertebrae

The thoracic vertebrae can be differentiated from the other vertebrae by the presence of at least one articular facet on the body for articulation with a rib. The bodies of the thoracic vertebrae enlarge from above downwards, in keeping with the increasing load which each has to carry.

The second to tenth thoracic vertebrae are typical thoracic vertebrae [Figs. 3.2, 3.3]. The **body** is heart-shaped and lies anteriorly. The **vertebral foramen** is circular. The **spine** is long and projects downwards and backwards in the midline so that its tip is palpable. The tip of a typical thoracic spine lies at the level of the upper part of the vertebral body two below in the series. Thus the spines

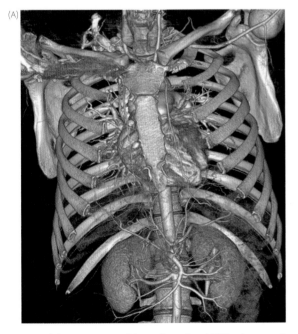 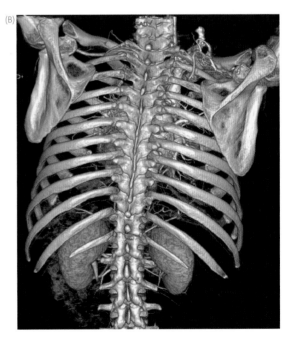

Fig. 3.1 (A) Anterior view of three-dimensional (3D) volume rendered image of the thorax showing the bony thoracic cage. (B) Posterior view of 3D volume rendered image of the thorax showing the bony thoracic cage.

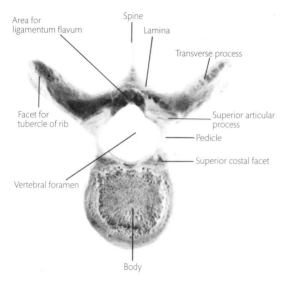

Fig. 3.2 The superior surface of the seventh thoracic vertebra.

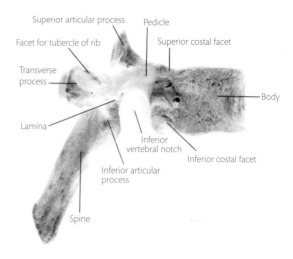

Fig. 3.3 The right surface of the seventh thoracic vertebra.

overlap, effectively hiding the small intervals between the laminae of adjacent vertebrae. The inferior articular process of the thoracic vertebra is at the inferolateral angle of the rectangular lamina. The articulating surfaces on the superior and inferior articular processes lie on an arc of a circle whose centre is in the vertebral body. Thus they permit slight rotatory movements of the vertebrae on each other around a vertical axis passing through the vertebral bodies [see Fig. 1.6]. The stout **transverse processes** project posterolaterally. On the anterolateral surface of the tip of the transverse process is a concave smooth facet for articulation with the tubercle of the corresponding rib. Medial to this, the anterior surface of the process gives attachment to the **costotransverse ligament** from the neck of the rib.

Immediately anterior to the lower part of the intervertebral foramen, the head of a rib articulates with the intervertebral disc and the adjacent parts of the two vertebral bodies. Hence the body of a typical thoracic vertebra has two articular facets on each side [Fig. 3.3]. The upper one to articulate with the corresponding rib, and the lower one for articulation with the head of the rib below.

Thoracic **intervertebral discs** are thin by comparison with the lumbar and cervical discs. This feature, together with the presence of the ribs and the overlapping spinous processes, greatly restricts flexion and extension in the thoracic region.

Atypical thoracic vertebrae

The first and the last four thoracic vertebrae differ from the others in several ways.

- The first and the last three thoracic vertebrae have a single round articulating facet on the body for the head of the corresponding rib.
- In the last three thoracic vertebrae, the costal facet for the head encroaches on to the pedicle.
- The ninth thoracic vertebra has a single demifacet for articulation with the ninth rib.
- The last two thoracic vertebrae have very small transverse processes which do not articulate with the corresponding ribs.
- The lower thoracic spines become progressively shorter and less oblique so that they look more like the rectangular lumbar type of spine.
- The inferior articular processes of the twelfth thoracic vertebra are lumbar in type. Their convex articular surfaces facing laterally and anteriorly to fit within the concave, superior articular facets of the first lumbar vertebra. ➲ This sudden transition from thoracic intervertebral articulations, which permit slight rotation, to lumbar articulations, which effectively prevent rotation [see Fig. 1.6], throws particularly heavy stresses on this region of the vertebral column which is frequently involved in fractures.

Ribs

Ribs are flat, curved bones, slightly twisted on their long axes. Posteriorly, each rib is more cylindrical and ends in an expanded **head**. The head of a typical rib has the shape of a blunt arrowhead with two articular facets—the upper facet for articulation with the body of the vertebra above, and the lower facet for articulation with the body of the numerically corresponding vertebra. The apex of the head articulates with the intervertebral disc between the two [Figs. 3.4, 3.5]. This arrangement places the head of the typical rib at a slightly higher level than the tubercle.

The head is continuous with the slightly narrower **neck** which extends laterally to the tubercle. The **tubercle** is situated on the postero-inferior aspect of the rib and has two parts. The medial, rounded part articulates with the transverse process of the vertebra. The lateral part gives attachment to the **lateral costotransverse ligament**. Lateral to the tubercle is the **body** of the rib [Figs. 3.4, 3.5]. Posteriorly, the external surface of the body is roughened by the attachment of the erector spinae muscles. This area is limited laterally by a vertical ridge which marks the attachment of the **thoracolumbar fascia** covering these muscles. Here the body of the rib is angled slightly forwards in the **angle**

of the rib and continues antero-inferiorly along the curve of the chest wall. The anterior end of the rib has a shallow pit in which the costal cartilage is inserted—the **costochondral joint** [Fig. 3.4].

The **first rib** is short and broad and has a small radius of curvature. It has two flattened surfaces which face anterosuperiorly and postero-inferiorly; and an internal and external margin. The head of the first rib has a single articular facet which articulates with the body of the first thoracic vertebra. The articulations of the heads and tubercles of the first ribs on the two sides lie in the same horizontal plane and move together like a hinge with four bearings [Fig. 3.6]. Inferiorly, the ribs become progressively longer, and have a greater radius of curvature

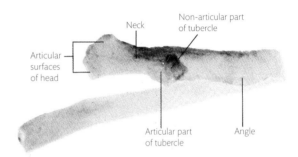

Fig. 3.5 The sixth right rib seen from behind.

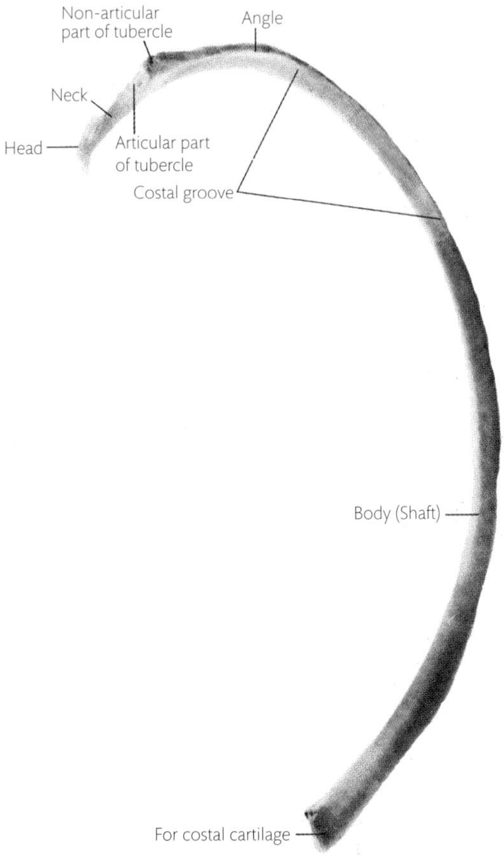

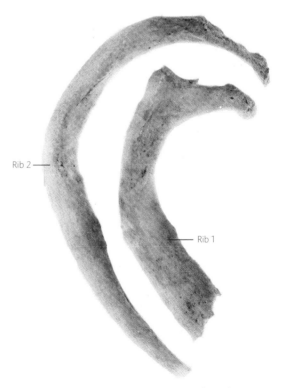

Fig. 3.4 The inferior aspect of a rib from the middle of the series.

Fig. 3.6 The first and second right ribs as seen from above.

until the seventh rib [Fig. 3.1]. Subsequently they decrease in length and the twelfth rib may be just 7–10 cm long. The last two ribs do not articulate with the transverse processes of the corresponding vertebrae. This, and the fact that the costal cartilages of these ribs do not articulate with those of other ribs, makes these ribs highly mobile (**floating ribs**).

The orientation of the ribs also changes gradually from above downwards so that the flattened surfaces lie tangential to the chest wall. Thus the surfaces of the ribs in the middle face internally and externally, with superior and inferior margins. In the lowest ribs, the internal surface faces upwards and inwards, and the external surface faces downwards and outwards. The internal surface of all the ribs are smooth as they lie against the membrane (**pleura**) which lines the chest wall. The external surfaces and margins of the ribs are roughened by the attachment of muscles. The internal surface of the typical ribs has a groove—the **costal groove**—inferiorly in the posterior part, for the posterior intercostal vessels and intercostal nerve. This makes the inferior margin sharp. The superior margin is rounded. Both margins give attachment to intercostal muscles, except in the case of the first and twelfth ribs.

All ribs run downwards and forwards in the chest wall. The articulation of the tubercle of the rib with the transverse process of the vertebra is posterior to the articulation of the head with the body. These two features ensure that the anteroposterior and transverse diameters of the thorax are increased when the ribs are raised [Fig. 3.7]. The increase in transverse diameter is greater in those ribs in which the tubercle articulates at a lower level than the head.

Sternum

The sternum is a flat midline bone on the anterior surface of the thoracic wall. It consists of three parts from above downwards—the manubrium, the body, and the xiphoid process [Fig. 3.8].

The **manubrium** slopes downwards and forwards and is thicker and wider than the other two parts. The superior margin of the manubrium has three notches. In the midline is the **jugular notch**. It can be felt in the front of the root of the neck. On each side is a clavicular notch for articulation with the medial end of the clavicle. Immediately below each clavicular notch, the first costal cartilage (frequently ossified) fuses with the lateral margin of the manubrium. Below this, the manubrium narrows to its articulation with the body of the sternum at the **manubriosternal joint**. The second costal cartilages articulate with the sides of the manubriosternal joint and the adjacent parts of the manubrium and body of the sternum. The **sternal angle** is a bony landmark

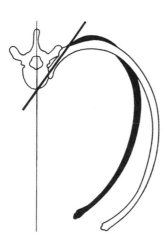

Fig. 3.7 An outline of a thoracic vertebra and one of its ribs as seen from above. The rib is shown in the elevated (white) and depressed (black) positions. The axis of this movement is the solid line passing through the head, neck, and base of the tubercle of the rib. The diagram shows how the anteroposterior and transverse dimensions of the thorax are increased by elevation of the ribs.

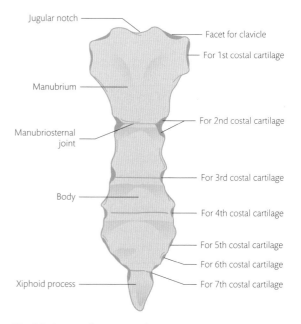

Fig. 3.8 Sternum (anterior view).

at the manubriosternal joint. It is obtuse anteriorly and readily palpable, even in the obese. It forms a landmark for the **second costal cartilage** and rib and permits the identification of the other ribs by counting downwards from the second. (The first rib is not palpable.) The sternal angle also marks the horizontal level between the superior and inferior mediastinum.

The **body of the sternum** is flat and widens from above downwards. It consists of four fused parts, called sternebrae. The **third, fourth, and fifth costal cartilages** articulate with the margins of the body, at the junctions of the sternebrae. The **sixth costal cartilage** articulates with the lowest part of the body, and the **seventh costal cartilage** articulates with the junction of the body and the xiphoid process. All joints between the costal cartilages and sternum (except for the first) are synovial joints.

The **xiphoid process** is a thin cartilaginous plate in young adults that ossifies slowly throughout life. It is fused with the inferior margin of the body of the sternum at the **xiphisternal joint**. A surface depression—the **epigastric fossa**—lies anterior to the xiphoid process in the infrasternal angle.

➲ For the most part, the sternum is covered only by skin, superficial fascia, and the periosteum. It contains red bone marrow which may be obtained for study by a **sternal puncture**. Sternal puncture involves perforating the cortex of the sternum with a wide-bore needle and aspirating the soft bone marrow within it.

Surface landmarks

All **thoracic vertebral spines** are palpable. The first is the lower of two bony prominences at the root of the back of the neck. (The upper one—the **vertebra prominens**—is formed by the spine of the seventh cervical vertebra.)

The lateral surfaces of the upper **ribs** may be palpated by pressing the fingers upwards into the axilla, with the arm by the side to relax the fascia of the axillary floor. The lower ribs are readily palpable, except the twelfth which may not project beyond the lateral margin of the erector spinae muscle. The posterolateral parts of the second to seventh ribs are covered by the scapula and are not palpable.

The **nipple** is very variable in position, especially in the female. It often overlies the fourth inter-

Table 3.1 Vertebral levels of bony landmarks in the thorax

Bony landmark	Vertebral level
Jugular notch	Disc between T. 2 and T. 3
Sternal angle	Disc between T. 4 and T. 5
Xiphisternal joint	Ninth thoracic vertebra
Tip of ninth costal cartilage	First lumbar vertebra
Lowest part of costal margin	Third lumbar vertebra
Root of spine of scapula	Third thoracic spine
Inferior angle of scapula	Seventh thoracic spine

costal space, 10 cm from the median plane in the adult male.

The vertebral levels corresponding to bony landmarks on the thoracic cage are given in Table 3.1. These, and others given elsewhere, are only approximate because of the movements of the thoracic cage and its contents. They also vary with the position of the body, whether standing or lying down, and with the physical type and age of the individual. In the aged, the sternum tends to sag to a lower level and the thoracic vertebral curvature increases. The levels are important because they may be grossly disturbed by pathological curvatures of the vertebral column and diseases of the lungs.

Structures superficial to the thoracic cage

The greater part of the thoracic cage is overlapped by muscles of the upper limb, and the remainder by muscles of the abdomen. The **thoracic spinal nerves** supply the walls of the thorax and send cutaneous branches through or between these muscles to the overlying skin. These nerves innervate the thoracic and abdominal muscles, but not the muscles of the upper limb. Only the first or the first and second thoracic spinal nerves supply muscles of the upper limb through fibres they send to the brachial plexus.

Before going on to study the thoracic cage, identify the remnants of the upper limb muscles still attached to the thorax and the blood vessels and nerves which pierce them [see Fig. 3.11, Vol. 1].

Anteriorly

(1) The **pectoralis major** is attached to the anterior surface of the sternum and the adjacent parts of

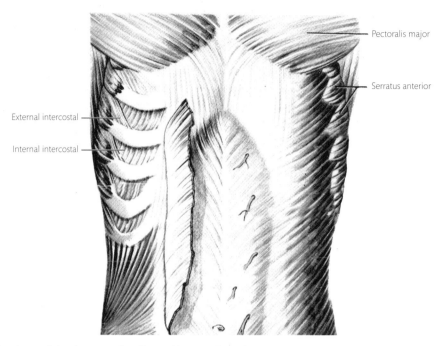

Fig. 3.9 Anterior chest wall showing external and internal intercostal muscles.

the upper six costal cartilages [Fig. 3.9]. Near the sternum, it is pierced by the anterior cutaneous branches of the second to fifth thoracic nerves, the **intercostal nerves**, and branches of the internal thoracic artery [Fig. 3.10]. (The first intercostal nerve has no anterior cutaneous branch.)

(2) The **rectus abdominis** is attached to the xiphoid process and the cartilages of the seventh to fifth ribs.

(3) The **pectoralis minor** is attached to the third to fifth ribs near their costal cartilages.

Laterally

(1) The **serratus anterior** is attached to the upper eight ribs on the side of the thorax. Its lower four attachments interdigitate with the upper four attachments of the external oblique.

(2) The **external oblique** arises from the outer surfaces of the lower eight ribs. The **lateral cutaneous branches** of the intercostal nerves (except the first) emerge between the attachments of these muscles at the mid-axillary line [Fig. 3.9].

Posteriorly

The cutaneous branches of the **dorsal rami** of the thoracic nerves have been removed with the trapezius, rhomboids, and latissimus dorsi which they

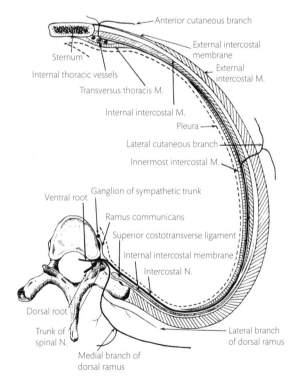

Fig. 3.10 A diagram of the upper thoracic spinal nerve in an intercostal space.

pierce. The cut ends of these nerves may be found where they pierce the thoracolumbar fascia which is deep to these muscles.

Intercostal muscles

Dissection 3.1 explores the intercostal muscles.

Three incomplete layers of muscle lie in each intercostal space—the **external intercostal**, the **internal intercostal**, and the **innermost intercostal** muscles. In addition, there are two small muscles deep to these which may cross more than one intercostal space—the **transversus thoracis**, or **sternocostalis**, and the **subcostales**. (The subcostales will be seen later, when the lungs have been removed.)

The external intercostal muscle originates from the lower margin of the upper rib and is inserted into the rounded superior margin of the rib below. Its fibres run antero-inferiorly [Fig. 3.9]. It extends from the tubercle of the rib posteriorly almost to the costochondral junction anteriorly. Anterior to the costochondral junction, it is replaced in the upper spaces by the **external intercostal membrane**.

The internal intercostal muscle takes origin from the costal groove and is inserted into the upper margin of the rib below. Its fibres run postero-inferiorly [Fig. 3.9]. It extends from the margin of the sternum anteriorly to the angle of the rib, posteriorly. Posterior to this, it is replaced by the **internal intercostal membrane**.

The **innermost intercostal** muscle originates from the internal surface of the rib, just above the costal groove, and is inserted into the upper margin of the rib below. Its extent is variable. Usually it extends further posteriorly than the internal intercostal and not so far anteriorly as the external intercostal. The innermost intercostal is differentiated from the internal intercostal only by the presence of the intercostal nerve and vessels between them.

Nerve supply: the intercostal nerves supply all three muscles. **Actions**: all three muscles prevent the intercostal spaces from being drawn in during inspiration or forced out during forced expiration. The external intercostal is active during inspiration. The internal and innermost intercostals are active during expiration.

Intercostal nerves

The 11 pairs of **intercostal nerves** are the ventral rami of the first to the eleventh thoracic spinal nerves. The twelfth or **subcostal nerve** lies in the

---

DISSECTION 3.1 Intercostal muscles

Objectives

I. To identify and study the external intercostal, internal intercostal, and innermost intercostal muscles. II. To identify and trace the intercostal nerves and their lateral cutaneous branches.

Instructions

1. Remove the remains of the serratus anterior and the pectoral muscles from the upper ribs, but retain the cutaneous branches of the intercostal nerves.

2. In two or more spaces, note the **external intercostal muscle**—its fibres run antero-inferiorly from the upper to the lower rib. Follow it forwards to the external intercostal membrane which replaces it between the costal cartilages.

3. Cut through the external intercostal membrane and muscle along the lower borders of two spaces. Turn them upwards to expose the **internal intercostal muscle**. Its fibres run postero-inferiorly from the upper to the lower rib.

4. Now follow the lateral cutaneous branch of one or more intercostal nerves to the parent trunk, deep to the internal intercostal muscle.

5. Follow the trunk of the **intercostal nerve** forwards and backwards with the accompanying vessels, cutting away as much of the lower margin of the rib and internal intercostal muscle as is necessary to expose them. Note the branches of the nerve to the intercostal muscles and its collateral branch lying along the upper margin of the rib below.

6. The muscle which lies deep to the nerve and vessels is the **innermost intercostal muscle**. This muscle is absent anteriorly and posteriorly. Here the nerve and vessels lie on the parietal pleura, except where the transversus thoracis (sternocostalis) intervenes at the side of the sternum. The innermost intercostal muscles are supplemented internally by the subcostal muscles near the angles of the lower ribs.

abdominal wall below the twelfth rib. The greater part of the first (and sometimes the second) passes to the brachial plexus.

Each intercostal nerve emerges from the intervertebral foramen inferior to the corresponding vertebra. The nerve then runs in the costal groove of the corresponding rib in the intercostal space. More medially it lies between the internal intercostal membrane and the parietal pleura. Further laterally it lies between the internal intercostal muscle, and the innermost intercostal. Where the innermost intercostal muscle is missing, it lies directly on the parietal. Close to the sternum the intercostal nerve lies between the transversus thoracis and the internal intercostal muscle. One centimetre from the sternum, it turns forwards to end as the anterior cutaneous branch [Fig. 3.10].

Branches of the intercostal nerve

1. As the intercostal nerve emerges from the intervertebral foramen, it is connected to a ganglion of the sympathetic trunk by the two rami communicantes.
2. A **collateral branch** arises near the angle of the rib. It runs along the upper margin of the rib below to supply the intercostal muscles. It may rejoin the parent stem or be absent.
3. The **lateral cutaneous branch** arises beyond the angle of the rib. It is thicker than the continuation of the nerve. It pierces the internal and external intercostal muscles obliquely about halfway round the chest and divides into anterior and posterior branches.
4. The **anterior cutaneous branch** pierces the internal intercostal muscle, the external intercostal membrane, and the pectoralis major. It divides into medial and lateral branches.
5. **Muscular branches** supply the intercostal, subcostal, transversus thoracis, and serratus posterior muscles. They do not supply any of the limb muscles which arise from the thorax [Fig. 3.10].

The above description applies only to the third to sixth intercostal nerves. The **first** and **second** run the early part of their course on the pleural surfaces of the corresponding ribs. The first has no lateral or anterior cutaneous branch. It crosses the first rib to join the brachial plexus. The second gives a large lateral cutaneous branch to the floor of the axilla and the medial side of the arm—the **intercostobrachial nerve**. The **seventh** to the **eleventh** intercostal nerves enter the anterior abdominal

wall at the anterior ends of their intercostal spaces either directly (tenth and eleventh) or by passing deep to the upturned end of the next costal cartilage. They run an increasing part of their course in the abdominal wall and supply the skin and muscles of that wall. The anterior cutaneous branches of the fifth to twelfth nerves pierce the rectus abdominis muscle and its sheath to reach the skin. Those of the ninth and tenth nerves supply the skin in the region of the umbilicus.

Intercostal arteries and veins

Each intercostal space receives three arteries. The largest is the single **posterior intercostal artery** which is usually a branch of the thoracic aorta. It accompanies the intercostal nerve and gives a **collateral branch** along the superior margin of the lower rib. There are two anterior intercostal arteries in each space. In the upper six spaces, these arteries are branches of the internal thoracic artery. In the seventh to ninth spaces, they are branches of the musculophrenic branch of the internal thoracic artery [Fig. 3.11]. In the last two spaces, there are no anterior intercostal arteries. The posterior intercostal artery and its collateral branch end by anastomosing with the two smaller **anterior intercostal arteries**. In the last two spaces, the posterior intercostal artery and its collateral branch continue into the anterior abdominal wall. The corresponding **anterior intercostal veins** drain into the musculophrenic and internal thoracic veins. The arteries and veins which lie subjacent to the **mammary gland** play a part in supplying it and become greatly enlarged during pregnancy and lactation.

The remaining parts of the posterior intercostal arteries and the posterior intercostal veins will be seen later.

Transversus thoracis (sternocostalis)

This muscle consists of four or five slips which arise from the inner surface of the xiphoid process and the lower part of the body of the sternum. They pass superolaterally to the second to sixth costal cartilages, close to their junctions with the ribs [Fig. 3.11]. This muscle is continuous with the deepest muscle

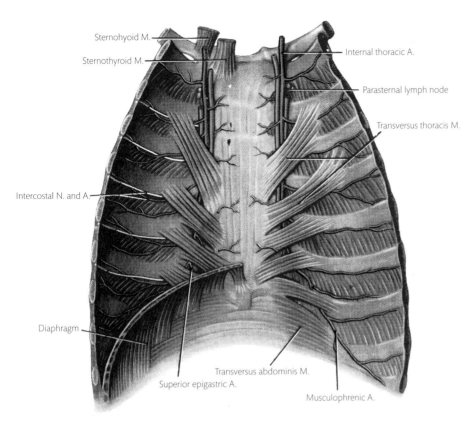

Fig. 3.11 Posterior surface of the anterior thoracic wall.

Labels in figure:
Sternohyoid M.
Sternothyroid M.
Internal thoracic A.
Parasternal lymph node
Transversus thoracis M.
Intercostal N. and A.
Diaphragm
Transversus abdominis M.
Superior epigastric A.
Musculophrenic A.

of the anterior abdominal wall—the **transversus abdominis**. **Nerve supply**: the corresponding intercostal nerves. **Action**: a weak expiratory muscle.

Subcostales muscle

These irregular muscle slips lie internally near the angles of the lower ribs. When present, they cross the internal surface of two or three intercostal spaces, parallel to the internal intercostal muscle. They are part of an incomplete muscle layer formed by the transversus thoracis and the innermost intercostal muscles. These muscles will be identified after the lungs have been removed.

Internal intercostal membrane

These fascial sheets extend from the internal intercostal muscles to the superior costotransverse ligament on the neck of each rib. They separate the intercostal vessels and nerve from the external intercostal muscle in the posterior part of the intercostal space. This membrane will be identified after the lungs have been removed.

Internal thoracic artery

The internal thoracic artery is a branch of the first part of the subclavian artery. It descends posterior to the medial end of the clavicle and the costal cartilages. This first part of the artery gives the small pericardiacophrenic branch to the phrenic nerve. The internal thoracic artery descends about 1 cm from the margin of the sternum, anterior to the pleura and the transversus thoracis, and posterior to the upper six costal cartilages, the spaces between them, and the terminal parts of the intercostal nerves. It ends by dividing into the superior epigastric and musculophrenic arteries at the sixth intercostal space [Fig. 3.11].

In Dissection 3.2 the anterior wall of the thorax is cut and reflected down to open the thoracic cavity.

The walls of the thorax

26

Objective

I. To cut through the manubrium sternum and lateral parts of the ribs and reflect the anterior thoracic wall downwards.

Instructions

1. Remove the intercostal muscles and membrane from the anterior parts of the first and second intercostal spaces. This exposes a part of the **internal thoracic artery** and veins, about 1 cm from the side of the sternum.

2. Cut through the internal thoracic vessels in the first intercostal space.

3. Cut transversely through the manubrium sternum, immediately inferior to its junction with the first costal cartilage. Take care not to cut into the underlying soft tissue.

4. Cut through the parietal pleura in the first intercostal space on both sides. Carry this cut as far back as possible.

5. In the mid-axillary line, make a vertical cut through the second and subsequent ribs and the intercostal spaces. Extend this cut to the level of the xiphisternal joint.

6. Gently elevate the inferior part of the cut sternum with the costal cartilages and anterior parts of the ribs.

7. Close to the midline, the parietal pleura passes from the back of the sternum on to the mediastinum on both sides. Cut through this pleura where it leaves the sternum. As the anterior part of the sternum is lifted away and turned back on the superior part of the abdominal wall, continue to cut through the pleura along the line of its reflection from the sternum on to the mediastinum, up to the level of the lower border of the heart. Note the position of this reflection and the differences on the two sides [see Fig. 4.5A].

8. When the anterior thoracic wall has been turned down, trace the cut edges of the **parietal pleura** and note its smooth internal surface where it lines the thoracic wall and covers the lateral aspects of the mediastinum.

9. Strip the pleura and the endothoracic fascia external to it from the back of the sternum and costal cartilages. This exposes the transversus thoracis (sternocostalis) muscle and the internal thoracic vessels [Fig. 3.11].

10. If the line on which the thoracic wall is turned down is lower than the inferior border of the heart, the attachment of the diaphragm to the xiphoid process and costal cartilages will be stretched and torn. Note these attachments and divide them as necessary.

11. This exposes the upper part of the transversus abdominis muscle and the posterior wall of the fibrous sheath of the rectus abdominis muscle.

Branches of the internal thoracic artery

(1) The **pericardiacophrenic artery** which accompanies the phrenic nerve.
(2) Many small branches to the sternum, thymus, and pericardium.
(3) Anterior intercostal arteries of the upper six spaces.
(4) **Perforating branches** which accompany the anterior cutaneous branches of the intercostal nerves. These are large in the second, third, and fourth spaces in the female as they supply the **mammary gland**.
(5) **Superior epigastric artery**. This terminal branch passes between the sternal and costal origins of the diaphragm into the rectus sheath in the anterior abdominal wall. Here it anastomoses with the inferior epigastric branch of the external iliac artery.

(6) **Musculophrenic artery**. This terminal branch runs inferolaterally along the superior surface of the costal origin of the diaphragm, deep to the costal cartilages. Near the eighth costal cartilage, it pierces the diaphragm and runs on its abdominal surface to supply it.

Internal thoracic veins

Two venae comitantes of each internal thoracic artery drain the territory supplied by it. They usually unite opposite the third costal cartilage and enter the corresponding brachiocephalic vein [Fig. 3.11].

DISSECTION 3.3 Intercostal nerve

Objective

I. To identify and trace the anterior part of the intercostal nerve on the deep surface of the anterior thoracic wall.

Instructions

1. Find the anterior part of the intercostal nerve in one or more spaces. Trace it laterally and medially. Laterally it disappears superficial to the innermost intercostal muscle. Medially it passes superficial to the internal thoracic vessels.

Parasternal lymph nodes

Small **parasternal lymph nodes** lie along the internal thoracic artery. They drain lymph from the anterior thoracic wall and the medial part of the mammary gland.

Dissection 3.3 explores the anterior part of the intercostal nerve.

Respiratory movements

These have already been dealt with but are now summarized [Figs. 3.7, 3.12; see also Table 20.2].

Inspiration

Raising the ribs increases the anteroposterior and transverse diameters of the thorax. The contracting diaphragm [see Fig. 2.2] lowers the dome of the diaphragm. This action increases the vertical extent of the thorax, opens the costodiaphragmatic recesses, and elongates and narrows the mediastinum. Muscles of the posterior abdominal wall hold down the lower ribs to make the diaphragmatic contraction effective.

Expiration

This is the reverse movement. In quiet respiration, expiration is achieved by the elastic recoil of the lungs. In forced expiration, the ribs are pulled down mainly by contraction of the abdominal muscles, which also increases the intra-abdominal pressure and forces the relaxed diaphragm upwards.

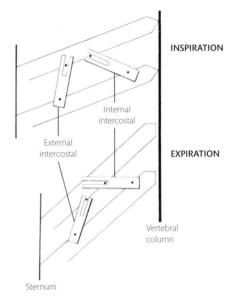

Fig. 3.12 A diagram to demonstrate that depression of the ribs decreases the anteroposterior diameter of the thorax. Note also that the internal intercostal muscle fibres are elongated in elevation of the ribs, while the external intercostal muscle fibres are shortened. The opposite occurs in depression of the ribs, i.e. on expiration.

➔ If the elasticity of the lungs is lost, the thorax tends to remain permanently in a position of inspiration. There is also considerable expiratory difficulty and the tidal volume of air in each respiratory cycle is greatly reduced.

See Clinical Applications 3.1, 3.2, and 3.3 for the practical implications of the anatomy in this chapter.

CLINICAL APPLICATION 3.1 Rib fractures

Rib fractures are extremely painful, as splinting of the disrupted segments is difficult and the ribs move with every breath.

Study question 1: which nerves should be anaesthetized to relieve pain due to a fractured rib? (Answer: an intercostal nerve block is an effective way of relieving the pain of fractured ribs. However, due to overlap of segmental nerve supply, the nerves of the spaces above and below the fractured rib should also be blocked. The needle is inserted into the chest wall proximal to the fracture site, until the resistance of the inferior margin of the rib is felt. The needle is then withdrawn slightly and slid

further below the inferior margin. After checking that the needle tip is not in a vessel, the local anaesthetic agent is injected.) Intercostal nerve blocks could also be used as an anaesthetic technique for repairing lacerations of the anterior chest or abdominal wall.

Study question 2: what is the distribution of the intercostal nerve? (Answer: the intercostal nerve supplies areas of overlying skin, the intercostal muscles of that space, the rib with its costal cartilage, and the parietal pleura lining that space. The lower intercostal nerves also supply corresponding segments of the skin, the muscle of the anterior abdominal wall, and the parietal peritoneum.)

CLINICAL APPLICATION 3.2 Flail chest

Severe trauma can result in fracture of multiple ribs in several places. In such cases, a loose or 'flail' segment of the chest wall is produced. During respiration, the flail segment moves in a direction that is opposite to that of the

rest of the chest wall, i.e. it moves in on inspiration and out in expiration. This is known as paradoxical movement. Paradoxical movement impedes lung expansion, and it is necessary to fix the loose segment with hooks or wires.

CLINICAL APPLICATION 3.3 Surgical approaches to the thoracic cavity

A **median sternotomy**, followed by gradual retraction of the cut halves of the sternum, offers exposure to the thymus and other mediastinal structures like the heart, the pericardium, the great vessels, and the lower trachea. Sternal wires are used at the end of surgery to secure the cut bone. This procedure often results in periosteal oozing.

Study question 1: which artery supplies the sternum and where does this artery lie? (Answer: the internal thoracic arteries which run on the posterolateral aspect of the sternum (anterior to the slips of the transversus thoracis) supply the sternum.)

Thoracotomy incisions, combined with partial rib excision, allow surgical access to thoracic structures and the diaphragm. A **posterior** or **posterolateral thoracotomy** is performed with the patient lying on his side with the arm completely abducted so the scapula is laterally rotated. The incision traditionally begins in front of the anterior axillary line and curves posterosuperiorly

below the inferior angle of the scapula.

Study question 2: which large extrinsic muscles of the chest wall would be encountered by this incision? (Answer: (1) the latissimus dorsi. It is divided from medial to lateral. Alternatively, a vertical axillary incision can be made anterior to the latissimus dorsi. (2) The serratus anterior is detached from its costal origins.)

An **anterior** or **anterolateral thoracotomy** is done with the patient supine and with the operative side elevated about 45° with a sandbag. An incision is made along the inframammary fold to access the fourth or fifth intercostal space.

A **transverse thoracosternotomy** or **clam shell incision** (so named because of the appearance of the retracted chest wall) provides access to both sides of the thoracic cavity. It combines two anterior thoracotomy incisions with a transverse division of the sternum at the fourth intercostal space.

CHAPTER 4
The cavity of the thorax

Introduction

In this chapter, the thoracic organs, blood vessels, nerves, and lymphatics supplying them, and the pleural and pericardial cavities are described. The mediastinum in the midline and the right and left pleural cavities on either side have already been identified.

Mediastinum

The mediastinum is the bulky midline septum between the pleural cavities and their contents—the lungs. It is thick and extends from the root of the neck to the diaphragm and from the sternum to the vertebral column [see Figs. 2.2, 2.5]. The mediastinum is elongated in inspiration and may be displaced to one side or the other if the pressures in the two pleural cavities are unequal. For descriptive purposes, the mediastinum is subdivided by an imaginary horizontal plane, drawn from the sternal angle in front to the intervertebral disc between the fourth and fifth thoracic vertebrae behind. The **superior mediastinum** lies above this plane. Below the plane, the **inferior mediastinum** is further subdivided into: (1) the **middle mediastinum** which contains the heart in the pericardial sac, and a phrenic nerve on each side; (2) the **anterior mediastinum** between the pericardium and the sternum; and (3) the **posterior mediastinum** between the pericardium and the diaphragm anteriorly and the vertebral column posteriorly [Fig. 4.1].

The superior mediastinum has a smaller anteroposterior depth than the inferior mediastinum. The posterior mediastinum extends furthest inferiorly because it passes into the angle between the diaphragm and the vertebral column to reach down to the level of the twelfth thoracic vertebra [Fig. 4.1].

Pleura

On each side of the mediastinum is a lung covered with a double layer of pleura. The inner layer of the pleura is the **pulmonary** or **visceral pleura**, and the outer layer is the **parietal pleura** [see Fig. 2.5]. The narrow space between the two layers is the **pleural cavity**. The smooth, glistening layer of visceral pleura invests the lung closely, except on a small part of its medial surface [see Figs. 4.11, 4.12]. The parietal pleura lies in close contact with the structures adjacent to the lungs. These include the inner aspect of the thoracic cage, the upper surface of the diaphragm, the mediastinum, and structures in the root of the lung. Different parts of the parietal pleura are given different names, depending on the structure on which they lie [Fig. 4.2]. The part of the parietal pleura that lines the inner surfaces of the thoracic wall is known as the **costal pleura**. Inferiorly, the part which covers the superior surface of the diaphragm is the **diaphragmatic pleura**. Superiorly, the **dome of the pleura** extends through the superior aperture of the thorax into the root of the neck. The **mediastinal pleura** covers the mediastinum laterally. Anteriorly and posteriorly, the mediastinal pleura is continuous with the costal pleura at the anterior and posterior margins. The mediastinal and costal pleura continue with the **dome of the pleura** at the margin of the first rib. The costal pleura continues with the diaphragmatic pleura at the margins of the diaphragm. The parietal pleura

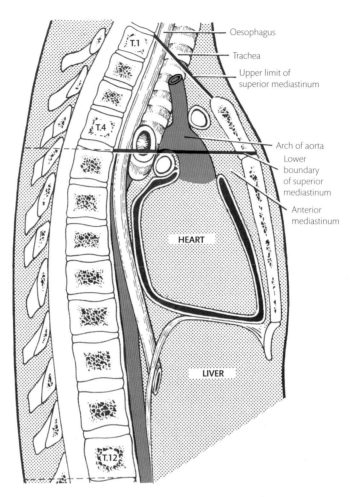

Oesophagus

Trachea

Upper limit of
superior mediastinum

Arch of aorta

Lower
boundary
of superior
mediastinum

Anterior
mediastinum

HEART

LIVER

Fig. 4.1 A diagram of a median section through the thorax to show the general disposition of the structures in the mediastinum. The heart in the pericardium forms the middle mediastinum. The anterior and posterior mediastina lie between it and the sternum and vertebral column, respectively. The posterior mediastinum also extends downwards behind the diaphragm.

has a thick, fibrous layer (endothoracic fascia) external to it.

The visceral pleura invests the lung closely, except on a small part of its medial surface where the structures in the **root of the lung**—the bronchi and the pulmonary vessels and nerves—enter or leave the lung. In this region, the pulmonary pleura which surrounds the root of the lung is continuous with the parietal pleura which covers the surface of the mediastinum (mediastinal pleura). The pleura which surrounds the root of the lung extends inferiorly as a narrow fold—the **pulmonary ligament**. This fold attaches the pleura on the medial surface of the lung to the adjacent mediastinal pleura below the root of the lung [see Figs. 4.11, 4.12].

The arrangement of the parietal and visceral pleura to the lungs and to each other is the result of the embryonic lung growing laterally into the hollow pleural cavity [Fig. 4.3]. The invaginated medial wall of the primitive pleural cavity now invests the lung closely and forms the pulmonary pleura covering the lung. As the lung expands outwards, the pleural cavity is reduced to a mere slit between the outer wall of the cavity (parietal pleura) and the pleura covering the lung (pulmonary pleura). The original point of outgrowth from the mediastinum remains as the relatively narrow root of the lung around which the pulmonary and parietal parts of the pleura are continuous with each other. The lung moves freely within the pleural cavity during respiration. (A similar arrangement permits free movement of the heart within the pericardial cavity and parts of the gut tube within the peritoneal cavity.) The pleural cavity contains a small quantity of thin serous pleural fluid which

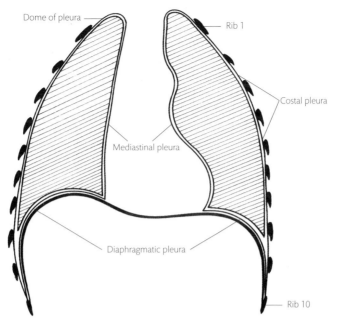

Fig. 4.2 Schematic diagram showing parts of the parietal pleura.

lubricates the pleural surfaces and allows them to slide freely on each other.

If the pleural cavity is opened in the body of an individual who has healthy lungs, the lung is free to be lifted away from the parietal pleura, except at the root and pulmonary ligament. In the aged, it is common to find the pulmonary and parietal pleura adherent at various points because of the spread of inflammatory or cancerous processes from the lung. Such adhesion makes it difficult to confirm the extent of the pleural cavity by dissection. Nev-

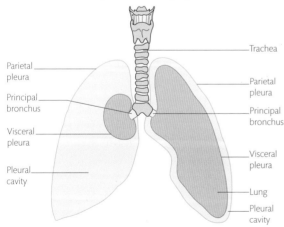

Fig. 4.3 Schematic diagram to show how the lungs expand into the pleural cavity, carrying part of the pleura in front of it as a covering. By expanding within the cavity, the lungs reduce the cavity to a mere slit between the outer (parietal) and the inner (visceral) layers of the pleura. Right side: during development. Left side: adult.

ertheless, the cavity should be carefully explored and the root of the lung and pulmonary ligament identified.

Dissection 4.1 describes the identification of lung root, removal of lungs, and exploration of the pleural cavity.

Dome of the pleura

The dome of the pleura is that part of the parietal pleura which bulges into the root of the neck above the inner margin of the first rib [Fig. 4.4]. The apex of the dome lies at the level of the neck of the first rib. Because of the obliquity of the first rib, the apex is 4.5 cm above the anterior end of the first rib and 2.5 cm above the medial third of the clavicle. The right and left domes are separated by the midline structures of the neck.

The **subclavian vessels** arch across the anterior surface of the dome, the artery near its highest point, with the vein antero-inferior to the artery. The internal thoracic artery descends on the front of the dome from the subclavian artery to the back of the first costal cartilage. Between these vessels and the dome is a layer of dense fascia called the **suprapleural membrane**. The suprapleural membrane extends from the transverse process of the seventh cervical vertebra to the inner margin of the first rib. The membrane may contain some muscle fibres—the **scalenus minimus**—which

DISSECTION 4.1 Identification of the pleura and removal of the lungs

Objectives

I. To identify the layers of the pleura, the root of the lung, and the pulmonary ligament.   II. To remove the lungs.

Instructions

1. Pull the lung laterally from the mediastinum and find the root of the lung and the pulmonary ligament extending laterally from it.

2. Cut through the root and pulmonary ligament from above downwards close to the lung.

3. Remove the lung on each side and store in a plastic bag to prevent from drying.

4. Examine the extent of the pleural cavity.

---

tighten it and help to maintain the pleural dome despite changes in intrapleural pressure.

Margins of the parietal pleura

The anterior margins of the right and left parietal pleura start at a point posterior to the sternoclavicular joint, and converge towards the midline as they descend from the domes. They come close to each other at the sternal angle and below this remain in apposition till the level of the fourth costal cartilage [Fig. 4.5A]. At the fourth costal cartilage, the left pleural margin deviates to the left and descends posterior to the fifth and sixth costal cartilages, close to the sternum. (The heart and pericardium project to the left here.) The right pleural margin continues its vertical descent, close to the midline. Each anterior margin becomes contin-

uous with the corresponding inferior margin of the pleura at the level of the xiphisternal joint.

Trace the inferior margin of each pleural cavity with a finger in the costodiaphragmatic recess. This margin passes postero-inferiorly deep to the seventh costal cartilage and crosses the tenth rib in the mid-axillary line, about 5 cm superior to the costal margin [Fig. 4.5B]. It then passes anterior to the eleventh and twelfth ribs to reach the side of the vertebral column inferior to the medial part of the twelfth rib, at the level of the twelfth thoracic spine. It is important to remember how far inferiorly the pleural cavity extends, so as to avoid entering it during clinical procedures of the upper abdomen.

The rounded posterior margin of the pleura extends along the vertebral column, from the dome to the inferior margin [Fig. 4.5C].

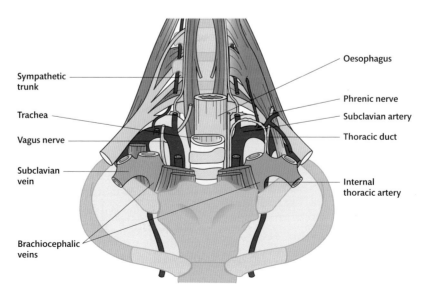

Fig. 4.4 The root of the neck to show the structures adjacent to the dome of the pleura (green).

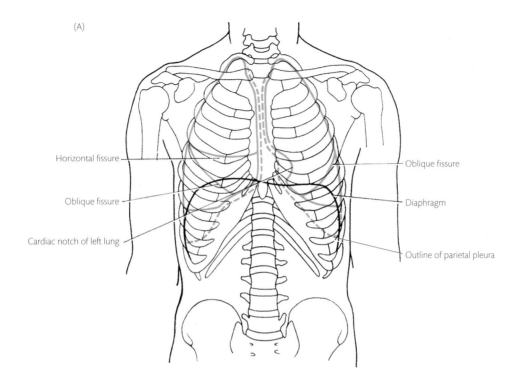

- Horizontal fissure
- Oblique fissure
- Cardiac notch of left lung
- Oblique fissure
- Diaphragm
- Outline of parietal pleura

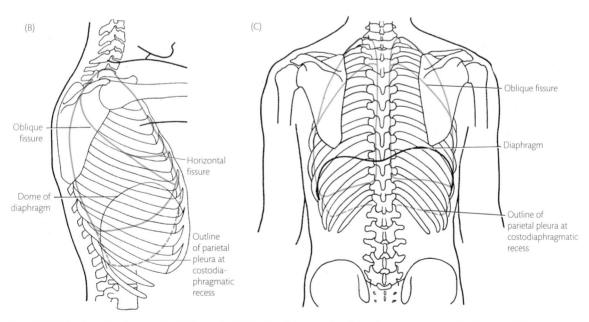

- Oblique fissure
- Dome of diaphragm
- Horizontal fissure
- Outline of parietal pleura at costodia-phragmatic recess
- Oblique fissure
- Diaphragm
- Outline of parietal pleura at costodiaphragmatic recess

Fig. 4.5 (A) Position of the lungs and their fissures (solid blue lines), the margins of the pleural sacs (broken blue lines), and the diaphragm, as seen from the anterior aspect of the trunk. The same structures seen (B) from the right lateral aspect and (C) from the posterior aspect.

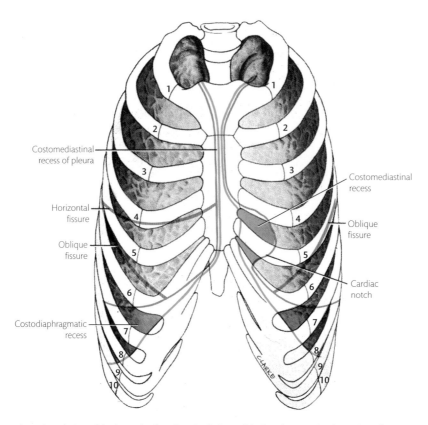

Fig. 4.6 Diagram to show the relation of the lungs (red) and parietal pleura (blue) to the anterior thoracic wall.

Pleural recesses

Pleural recesses are empty parts of the pleural cavity, which are occupied by the lung only in full inspiration. They lie where different parts of the parietal pleura meet at an acute angle and are in apposition to each other [Fig. 4.6]. (1) The **costomediastinal recess** lies where the anterior margin of the costal pleura meets the mediastinal pleura. (2) The **costodiaphragmatic recess** lies inferiorly where the lower margin of the costal pleura meets the diaphragmatic pleura along the lateral and posterior parts of the diaphragm. The costodiaphragmatic recess extends inferiorly between the thoracic wall and the diaphragm. The sharp inferior margins of the lungs pass into the costodiaphragmatic recesses in full inspiration so that the pleural cavities and lungs overlap the contents of the upper abdomen. ➲ Thus penetrating wounds of the lower thorax frequently involve the abdomen. Where the costal and diaphragmatic parts of the pleura meet, they are bound down to the costal cartilages and diaphragm by a narrow thickening of the endothoracic fascia—the **phrenicopleural fascia**.

General structure and position of the heart

Before studying the lungs, it is useful to have an idea of the general arrangement of the heart. The heart and the great arteries which arise from it form a U-shaped tube which lies obliquely across the thorax. The bend of the U lies antero-inferiorly (close to the sternum), and the ends of the two limbs of the U are posterosuperior (close to the vertebral column), one end anterosuperior to the other [Fig. 4.7]. The tube is divided longitudinally into right and left channels by a continuous septum. Each channel is further subdivided by two transversely placed valves. The valves in the postero-inferior limb are the **atrioventricular valves**, and they lie between the atria and ventricles. The valves in the anterosuperior limb are the **aortic** and **pulmonary valves**, and they lie between the ventricles and the great arteries (aorta and pulmonary trunk). The valves ensure that the blood which enters the atria from the veins passes into the

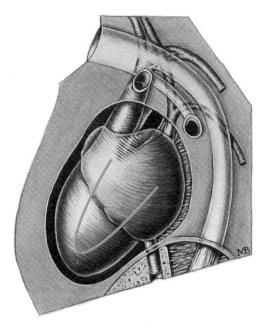

Fig. 4.7 Diagram of the embryonic heart in the pericardial cavity to show the folding of the heart tube.

ventricles and emerges from them through the great arteries. The atria and ventricles are distended muscular chambers, each of which shares one wall with the corresponding chamber of the other channel (the **interatrial septum** and the **interventricular septum**). The great arteries are parallel-sided elastic tubes which are completely separate from each other (no shared wall). (The right channel is made up of: (1) the veins entering the right atrium; (2) the right atrium; (3) the right ventricle; and (4) the pulmonary trunk. The two valves in this stream are the right atrioventricular valve and the pulmonary valve. In the same way, the left channel is made up of: (1) the veins entering the left atrium; (2) the left atrium; (3) the left ventricle; and (4) the aorta. The two valves in this stream are the left atrioventricular valve and the aortic valve.)

The U-shaped heart lies in the pericardial cavity in the same manner as the lungs lie in the pleural cavities. The two ends of the U (veins entering the atria and the great arteries leaving the ventricles) correspond to the root of the lung and are relatively fixed. It is here that the **parietal pericardium**—the outer wall of the pericardial cavity—becomes continuous with the **visceral pericardium** which immediately covers the heart. The ventricles

are fully surrounded by the pericardial cavity and have the greatest freedom of movement.

The **left atrium** receives oxygenated blood from the lungs through two pairs of pulmonary veins. The **right atrium** receives deoxygenated blood from the rest of the body through the superior and inferior venae cavae and the main vein of the heart (the coronary sinus). The thin-walled atria discharge blood into the corresponding thick-walled ventricles through the atrioventricular valves. The ventricles pump the blood either through the pulmonary trunk to the lungs (**right ventricle**) or through the aorta to the rest of the body (**left ventricle**).

As the thorax is flattened anteroposteriorly, the heart is rotated to the left, with the bend of the U (**apex of the heart**) displaced to that side. As a result, the relative positions of the chambers of the heart are altered [Figs. 4.8, 4.9].

1. The longitudinal septum (which forms the interatrial and interventricular septa) lies obliquely, with the right atria and ventricle lying anterior to, and to the right of, the left atria and ventricles.
2. The left atrium lies posteriorly towards the vertebral column. (It forms the **base of the heart**.)
3. The left ventricle forms the greater part of the left surface.
4. The displacement of the **apex** causes it to lie in the fifth left intercostal space, just medial to the midclavicular line.
5. The displacement also moves the right ventricle from the **right margin** of the heart so that the right margin is formed entirely by the right atrium.
6. The heart in its pericardial cavity bulges the left wall of the mediastinum far to the left, thus deeply indenting the left pleural cavity and lung.
7. On the right, the gently convex surface of the right atrium indents the right pleural cavity and lung to a lesser extent.

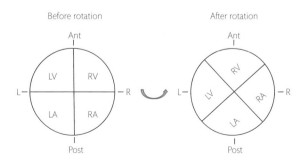

Fig. 4.8 Diagram to show the change in position of the four cavities of the heart as a result of its rotation. LV, RV = left and right ventricles; LA, RA = left and right atria.

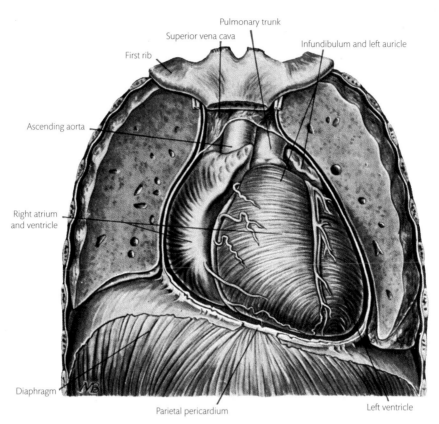

First rib

Superior vena cava

Pulmonary trunk

Infundibulum and left auricle

Ascending aorta

Right atrium
and ventricle

Diaphragm

Parietal pericardium

Left ventricle

Fig. 4.9 The sternocostal surface of the heart *in situ*. The front of the pericardium has been removed, together with the anterior parts of both lungs.

The lungs

The lungs are a pair of sponge-like, elastic respiratory organs. They fill the greater part of the pleural cavity and consist of innumerable (approximately 300 million) minute air-filled cavities—the **alveoli**. The alveoli are connected to the trachea by a branching system of **bronchi** and **bronchioles**. Each lung is shaped like half a cone [Fig. 4.10]. Lungs are comparatively light because they contain air (right, approximately 600 g and left, 550 g in a healthy adult) and they float freely in water, unless filled with fluid or consolidated by disease.

In children, the lungs are yellowish pink. In the adult, deposition of carbon particles which are ingested by phagocytes makes the surface mottled with dark patches and lines. The lines indicate the position of lymph channels in the interlobular fibrous septa.

Each lung lies free in its own pleural cavity, attached only to the mediastinum by the root. When the lungs are fixed *in situ*, their elasticity is destroyed and they retain the shape of the structures against which they lie in the thorax.

Apex

The apex of the lung extends into the root of the neck, 3–5 cm above the anterior part of the first rib and 1–2 cm above the medial third of the clavicle. The subclavian artery and vein cross the anterior surface of this part and may groove it [Fig. 4.4]. These vessels are separated from the lung by the pleura and the suprapleural membrane.

Base

The base of the lung is semilunar in shape. It is fitted to the dome of the diaphragm and is deep-

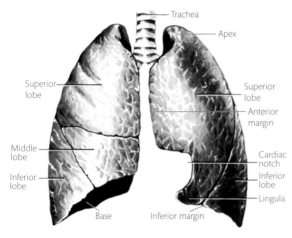

Labels on figure:
Trachea
Apex
Superior lobe
Superior lobe
Anterior margin
Middle lobe
Cardiac notch
Inferior lobe
Inferior lobe
Lingula
Base
Inferior margin

Fig. 4.10 The trachea, bronchi, and lungs.

ly concave, especially on the right side where the dome is higher [Fig. 4.2].

Inferior margin

The concave base meets the costal surface of the lung at the sharp inferior margin. The inferior margin extends into the costodiaphragmatic recess of the pleura but does not reach the lower limit of the recess, except in deep inspiration. The inferior margin is blunt medially where it abuts on the pericardium. The inferior margin follows a course from a point lateral to the xiphisternal joint to the eighth rib in the mid-axillary line and the level of the tenth thoracic vertebral spine at the vertebral column [Fig. 4.10].

Anterior margin

The thin anterior margin of the lung extends into the narrow costomediastinal recess of the pleura. It passes posterior to the sternoclavicular joint as it descends from the apex of the lung to the middle of the sternal angle. From there on the right side, the anterior margin descends vertically to meet the inferior margin at the xiphisternal joint. On the left side, the anterior margin is deeply notched posterior to the fifth left costal cartilage by the bulging pericardium. This notch is the **cardiac notch**. A part of the lung extends medially below the cardiac notch. This is the **lingula** [Fig. 4.10]. The cardiac notch leaves a part of the pericardium uncovered by the lung. ↪ Percussion in this area gives a dull note (known as the area of superficial cardiac dull-

ness), in comparison with the resonant note obtained over the lung [see Fig. 4.20].

Posterior border

The thick, rounded posterior border of each lung fits into the deep paravertebral gutter.

Medial surface

The medial surface of the lung consists of a more posterior part in contact with the vertebral column—the **vertebral part**—and the anterior **mediastinal part** that is indented by the heart and other mediastinal structures. The **hilus** of the lung is a depressed area near the centre of the mediastinal surface, through which structures enter and leave the lung [Figs. 4.11, 4.12].

Mediastinal surface of the lung

The mediastinal surface of the lung is indented by the larger structures projecting laterally from the mediastinum. With the help of Figs. 4.11, 4.12, 4.13, and 4.14, identify these structures on the mediastinum and the impressions they leave on the lung. On the right lung, the impressions of the heart, right brachiocephalic vein, superior vena cava, inferior vena cava, azygos vein, trachea, and oesophagus are seen. On the mediastinal surface of the left lung are seen the impressions of the heart, arch of the aorta, descending aorta, left common carotid and left subclavian arteries, and oesophagus.

Smaller structures on the surface of the mediastinum leave no mark on the lungs. These are: (1) the **phrenic nerve** and associated vessels on both sides; (2) the **right vagus** on the trachea and the **left vagus** on the aortic arch; (3) the **left superior intercostal vein** on the aortic arch; and (4) the **thoracic duct** on the left side of the oesophagus [Figs. 4.13A, 4.13B, 4.14A, 4.14B].

Roots of the lungs

All the structures which enter or leave the lung do so through the root of the lung. The root is enclosed in a short tubular sheath of pleura which joins the pulmonary and parietal pleura and extends inferiorly as a narrow fold—the pulmonary ligament [Figs. 4.11, 4.12].

In the root of the lung, one principal **bronchus** passes inferolaterally from the termination of the trachea to the hilus of each lung. A pulmonary artery passes transversely into each lung, anterior to

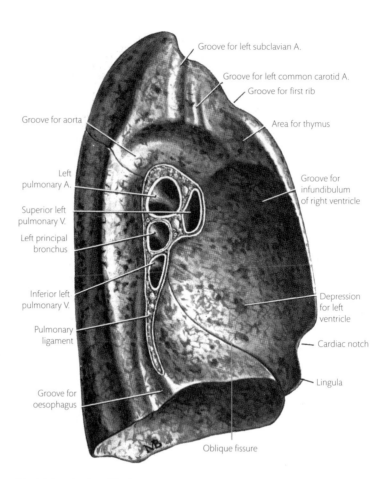

Groove for left subclavian A.

Groove for left common carotid A.

Groove for first rib

Groove for aorta

Area for thymus

Left pulmonary A.

Groove for infundibulum of right ventricle

Superior left pulmonary V.

Left principal bronchus

Inferior left pulmonary V.

Depression for left ventricle

Pulmonary ligament

Cardiac notch

Lingula

Groove for oesophagus

Oblique fissure

Fig. 4.11 The medial surface of the left lung hardened *in situ*.

the bronchus. Two pulmonary veins pass from the anterior and inferior part of each hilus into the left atrium [Figs. 4.11, 4.12]. This relationship of pulmonary veins most anterior, then pulmonary artery, and posteriorly the bronchus should be confirmed on the hilus of the lungs.

Contents of each lung root

(1) The right and left **principal bronchi** which transmit air to and from the lungs. The right principal bronchus gives off the superior lobar bronchus in the root of the heart.
(2) A **pulmonary artery** which carries deoxygenated blood to the lungs.
(3) Superior and inferior **pulmonary veins** which transmit oxygenated blood from the heart.
(4) **Lymph vessels** and **nodes** which drain the lung and pulmonary pleura.

(5) **Bronchial arteries** which carry oxygenated blood to the bronchi and lymph nodes. (They anastomose with the branches of the pulmonary arteries in the lungs.)
(6) **Bronchial veins**.
(7) Branches of the vagus nerve and sympathetic trunk which form the **pulmonary plexus** and innervate all the structures in the lungs.

The relative positions of the larger structures in the lung roots can be seen in Figs. 4.11 and 4.12. The bronchi can be recognized by the firm hyaline **cartilages** in their wall. These cartilages maintain the patency of the lumen despite changes in external pressure and are found in all but the smallest branches of the bronchial tree. The single pulmonary artery in each root may be differentiated from the two veins by its position and by the greater thickness of its wall.

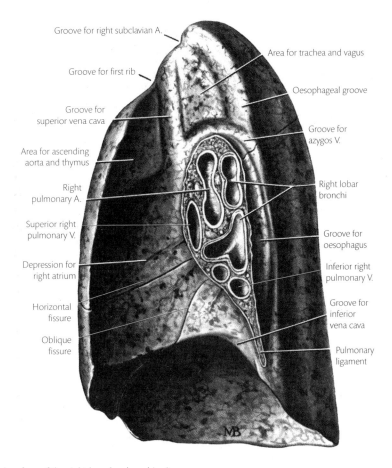

Groove for right subclavian A.

Groove for first rib

Groove for
superior vena cava

Area for ascending
aorta and thymus

Right
pulmonary A.

Superior right
pulmonary V.

Depression for
right atrium

Horizontal
fissure

Oblique
fissure

Area for trachea and vagus

Oesophageal groove

Groove for
azygos V.

Right lobar
bronchi

Groove for
oesophagus

Inferior right
pulmonary V.

Groove for
inferior
vena cava

Pulmonary
ligament

MB

Fig. 4.12 The medial surface of the right lung hardened *in situ*.

Lobes of the lungs

The **left lung** is divided into two lobes—a superior and inferior lobe—by a deep **oblique fissure**. This fissure begins posteriorly at the level of the fifth thoracic vertebra. It passes antero-inferiorly in a spiral course to meet the inferior margin of the lung, close to the sixth costochondral junction. It extends into the lung almost to the hilus [Figs. 4.6, 4.10, 4.11, 4.15A]. The **superior lobe** forms the apex, the anterior margin, and much of the anterior surface of the lung. The **inferior lobe** makes up the diaphragmatic and the greater part of the posterior surfaces.

The **right lung** is divided by a similar **oblique fissure**. A second, **horizontal fissure** extends horizontally backwards from the anterior margin at the fourth right costal cartilage to meet the oblique fissure in the mid-axillary line [Figs. 4.5B, 4.6, 4.10,

4.12, 4.15B]. The oblique fissure separates the **superior** and **middle lobes** from the **inferior lobe**. The horizontal fissure separates the wedge-shaped **middle lobe** from the superior lobe.

The pulmonary (visceral) pleura extends into the fissures of the lungs so that the lobes of the lungs can move on each other during respiration. ➲ The fissures may be obliterated by inflammation of the pleura (pleurisy). Infection may become localized in the fissure to form an abscess between the lobes of the lung. In both cases, the pleura in the fissure is thickened and may be visible in radiographs.

Not all the fissures are constantly present. The horizontal fissure is commonly absent in whole or in part.

The right lung may be differentiated from the left by the three lobes. It is shorter, broader, and has no cardiac notch.

Bronchi

Each principal bronchus arises as a terminal branch of the trachea and enters the lung [Figs. 4.16, 4.17]. The bronchi divide in a tree-like fashion within the lung and each branch supplies a clearly defined sector of the lung [Fig. 4.18]. Each **principal bronchus** divides into secondary or **lobar bronchi**, one to each lobe of the lung. Thus, the principal bronchus on the right gives rise to three lobar bronchi—the **right superior lobar bronchus**, the **right middle lobar bronchus**, and the **right inferior lobar bronchus**. The left principal bronchus gives rise to two lobar bronchi—the **left superior lobar bronchus** and the **left inferior lobar bronchus**. Each lobar bronchus divides into tertiary bronchi. These tertiary or **segmental**

bronchi supply sectors known as **bronchopulmonary segments** within the lobe. Each bronchopulmonary segment is pyramidal in shape, with its apex directed towards the root of the lung and its base at the pleural surface [Fig. 4.16].

Bronchopulmonary segments

➲ Bronchopulmonary segments are of considerable clinical significance as disease in the lung may be limited to one or more bronchopulmonary segments. The arrangement of lung tissue into segments also permits the surgeon to remove diseased parts of the lung, with minimal disturbance to the surrounding healthy lung tissue.

The general arrangement of the segments can best be understood by reference to Fig. 4.16 and

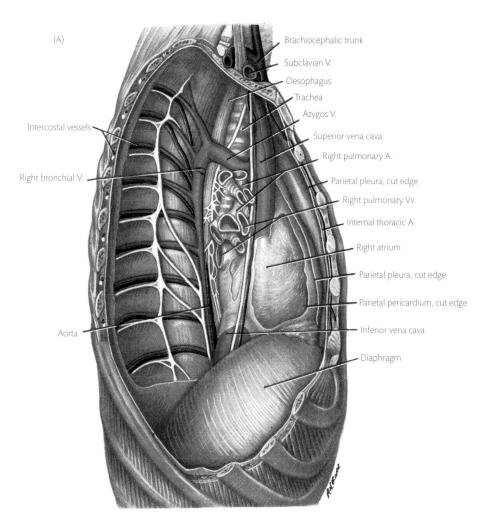

(A)

Brachiocephalic trunk

Subclavian V.

Oesophagus

Trachea

Azygos V.

Superior vena cava

Right pulmonary A.

Parietal pleura, cut edge

Right pulmonary Vv.

Internal thoracic A.

Right atrium

Parietal pleura, cut edge

Parietal pericardium, cut edge

Inferior vena cava

Diaphragm

Intercostal vessels

Right bronchial V.

Aorta

Fig. 4.13 (A, B) The right side of the mediastinum and thoracic vertebral column. The pleura has been removed, together with part of the pericardium.

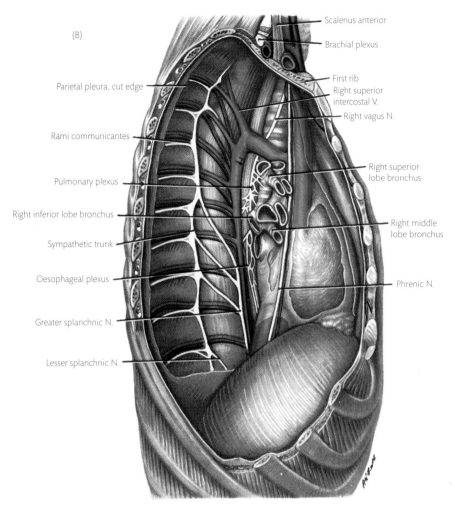

(B)

Scalenus anterior

Brachial plexus

First rib

Right superior intercostal V.

Right vagus N.

Parietal pleura, cut edge

Rami communicantes

Pulmonary plexus

Right superior lobe bronchus

Right inferior lobe bronchus

Sympathetic trunk

Right middle lobe bronchus

Oesophageal plexus

Phrenic N.

Greater splanchnic N.

Lesser splanchnic N.

Fig. 4.13 (*Continued*)

by dissecting out the main branches of the bronchi and vessels close to the hilus of the lung. The pattern in the superior lobes of the two lungs differs because of the presence of a middle lobe in the right lung and the resulting earlier division of the right principal bronchus. The right superior lobar bronchus (also known as the eparterial bronchus as it lies superior to the pulmonary artery) divides into three to supply the **apical, posterior**, and **anterior** bronchopulmonary segments. The right middle lobar bronchus divides to supply the **lateral** and **medial segments** of the middle lobe. The left superior lobar bronchus is larger than the right one because the superior lobe of the left lung corresponds to the superior and middle lobes of the right. The **upper branch of the left superior lobar bronchus** supplies three segments—**apical, posterior**, and **anterior**. These correspond to the same three segments

of the right upper lobe. The **lower branch of the left superior lobar bronchus** supplies the **superior lingular** and **inferior lingular segments**. The lingular segments make up a section which corresponds to, but is smaller than, the middle lobe of the right. The arrangement of the tertiary bronchi to the inferior lobe is similar in both lungs. The inferior lobar bronchus supplies five bronchopulmonary segments—**apical, medial basal, anterior basal, lateral basal**, and **posterior basal**. (A separate **medial basal bronchus** is not normally recognized in the left lung because it is usually a small branch of the anterior basal bronchus.)

Smaller units of lung tissue are bound by connective tissue and are known as **pulmonary lobules**. They are not discernable in gross specimens.

Dissection 4.2 instructs how the structures in the root of the lung should be identified.

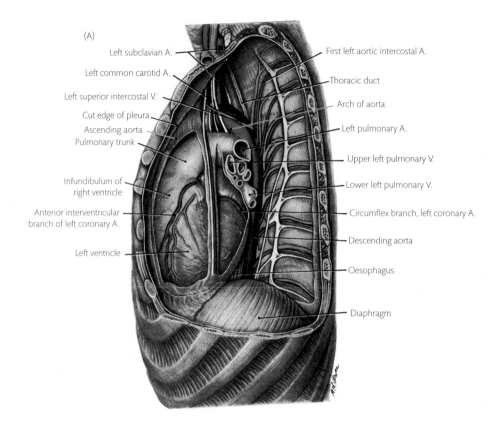

(A)

Left subclavian A.

Left common carotid A.

Left superior intercostal V.

Cut edge of pleura

Ascending aorta

Pulmonary trunk

Infundibulum of right ventricle

Anterior interventricular branch of left coronary A.

Left ventricle

First left aortic intercostal A.

Thoracic duct

Arch of aorta

Left pulmonary A.

Upper left pulmonary V.

Lower left pulmonary V.

Circumflex branch, left coronary A.

Descending aorta

Oesophagus

Diaphragm

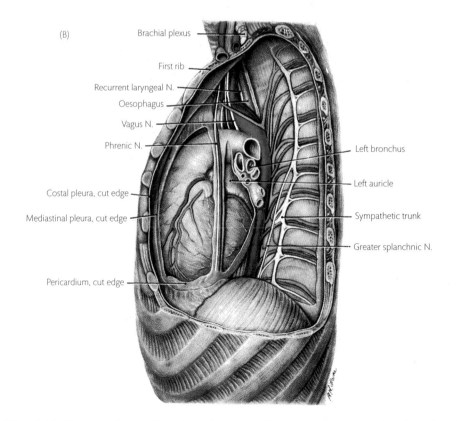

(B)

Brachial plexus

First rib

Recurrent laryngeal N.

Oesophagus

Vagus N.

Phrenic N.

Costal pleura, cut edge

Mediastinal pleura, cut edge

Pericardium, cut edge

Left bronchus

Left auricle

Sympathetic trunk

Greater splanchnic N.

Fig. 4.14 (A, B) The left side of the mediastinum and thoracic vertebral column. The pleura has been removed, together with part of the pericardium.

DISSECTION 4.2 Root of the lungs

Objective

I. To study the structures in the roots of the lungs.

Instructions

1. With the help of Figs. 4.11, 4.12, 4.13, and 4.14, check the positions of the structures in the sectioned **roots of the lungs**. These are the bronchi, pulmonary artery, and pulmonary veins. Note the difference in the arrangement of the bronchi in the two lung roots due to the earlier division of the right principal bronchus. In addition to these structures, there are a number of lymph nodes which are easily distinguished by the black carbon deposits in them. It may be possible to see the branches of the bronchial arteries on the posterior surfaces of the main bronchi.

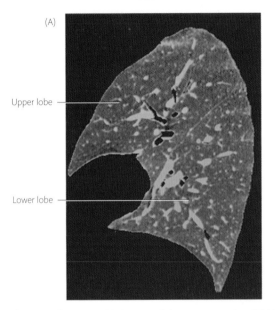
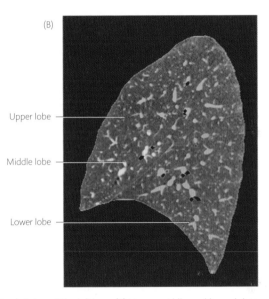

Fig. 4.15 Computer-aided automatic lung segmentation. (A) Upper and lower lobes of the left lung. (B) Upper, middle, and lower lobes of the right lung.

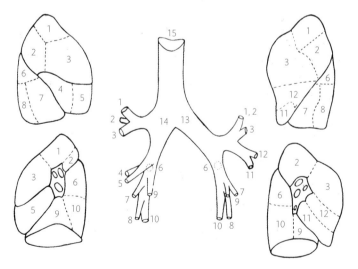

Fig. 4.16 The bronchi and bronchopulmonary segments. Each segmental bronchus has the same name as the subdivision of the lung supplied by it. The anterior and medial basal bronchi arise from a common stem in the left lung. This is often called the anteromedial basal bronchus. 1 = apical; 2 = posterior; 3 = anterior; 4 = lateral–middle lobe; 5 = medial–middle lobe; 6 = apical (inferior lobe); 7 = anterior basal; 8 = lateral basal; 9 = medial basal; 10 = posterior basal; 11 = inferior lingular; 12 = superior lingular; 13 = left principal bronchus; 14 = right principal bronchus; 15 = trachea.

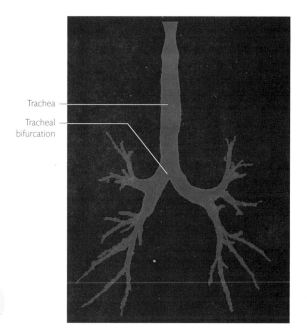

Trachea

Tracheal
bifurcation

Fig. 4.17 Volume-rendered image of the central tracheobronchial
tree.

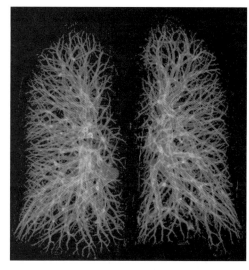

Fig. 4.18 Volume-rendered image of the intraparenchymal
tracheobronchial tree.

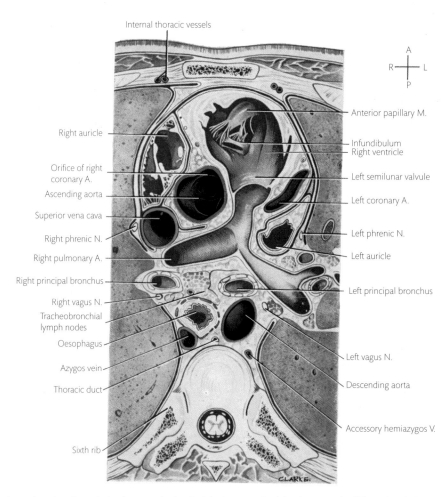

Internal thoracic vessels

Right auricle

Orifice of right
coronary A.

Ascending aorta

Superior vena cava

Right phrenic N.

Right pulmonary A.

Right principal bronchus

Right vagus N.

Tracheobronchial
lymph nodes

Oesophagus

Azygos vein

Thoracic duct

Sixth rib

Anterior papillary M.

Infundibulum
Right ventricle

Left semilunar valvule

Left coronary A.

Left phrenic N.

Left auricle

Left principal bronchus

Left vagus N.

Descending aorta

Accessory hemiazygos V.

Fig. 4.19 A horizontal section through the thorax at the level of the intervertebral disc between the fifth and sixth thoracic vertebrae.

Blood vessels

Branches of the **pulmonary artery** distribute venous blood to the lungs. They follow the bronchi and lie mainly on their posterior surfaces. (Note that, at the root of the lung, the artery lies anterior to the bronchus [Figs. 4.11, 4.12, 4.19].) There is a branch of the pulmonary artery to each lobe, each bronchopulmonary segment, and each lobule of the lung. The artery and bronchi are centrally placed within the bronchopulmonary segment. The terminal capillaries lie in the walls of the alveoli and respiratory bronchioles where gaseous exchange takes place between blood and air.

The **pulmonary veins** drain oxygenated blood from the lungs to the left atrium of the heart. One main vein drains each bronchopulmonary segment and usually lies on the anterior surface of the corresponding tertiary bronchus. Veins also run between the segments and on the mediastinal and fissural surfaces of the lungs. Some may even cross the line of a fissure when the fissure is incomplete. The **right superior pulmonary vein** drains the right superior and middle lobes and corresponds to the **left superior pulmonary vein** which drains the left superior lobe. The **right and left inferior pulmonary veins** drain the corresponding inferior lobes.

There are usually two **bronchial arteries** to the left lung and one to the right. The left bronchial arteries arise from the descending aorta. The right arises either from the first right posterior intercostal artery or from the superior left bronchial artery. The bronchial arteries are the nutrient arteries of the lung. The blood they carry is returned either through the pulmonary veins or through the **bronchial veins**. The bronchial veins drain into the azygos vein on the right and into the accessory hemiazygos vein on the left. ↪ In some congenital abnormalities of the heart or of the great vessels, the blood going to the lungs through the pulmonary arteries is inadequate. In these cases, the bronchial arteries may enlarge to take over this function.

Dissection 4.3 describes the dissection of the intrapulmonary structures.

Lymph vessels and nodes of the lung

The lymph nodes of the lungs are very obvious because of their black colour and the dense connective tissue which binds them to the bronchi. The lymph vessels of the lung cannot be demonstrated in dissecting room specimens. A **superficial plexus** of lymph vessels lies deep to the pulmonary pleura. It drains either over the surface of the lung to the **bronchopulmonary lymph nodes** in the hilus or along the interlobular septa into deep lymph

---

DISSECTION 4.3 Intrapulmonary structures

Objectives

I. To identify and trace the bronchi, pulmonary arteries, and veins within the lungs.   II. To identify the bronchial vessels.

Instructions

1. Begin by washing out the bronchi in the lungs as far as possible. Then shine a light into the main bronchus and attempt to see the apertures of its various branches.

2. When the surface of the lung has been broken at the hilus, it is simple to scrape away the alveolar tissue from the main veins, bronchi, and arteries. In both lungs, begin by cleaning the superior pulmonary vein and its tributaries. Then clean the corresponding bronchi posterior to the veins. Repeat this procedure with the inferior pulmonary vein and corresponding

bronchi. Note the small grey or black **pulmonary lymph nodes** at the angles formed by the bifurcation of the bronchi.

3. In the left lung, identify the superior and inferior lobar bronchi.

4. In the right lung, identify the superior, middle, and inferior lobar bronchi. Note that the right superior lobar bronchus passes superior to the pulmonary artery. It is also known as the **eparterial bronchus**.

5. Follow the branches of the pulmonary arteries. They follow the bronchi and lie mainly on their posterior surface.

6. As the principal bronchi are lifted forwards to expose the arterial branches, look for the **bronchial arteries** on their posterior surfaces. There are usually two bronchial arteries to the left lung and one to the right.

vessels. The deep lymph vessels drain along the bronchi, pass through the **pulmonary nodes** within the lungs, and reach the bronchopulmonary nodes in the hilus. The bronchopulmonary nodes form the most lateral part of a collection of nodes stretching from the tracheal bifurcation, along the principal bronchus, to the hilus of the lungs. Lymph from the bronchopulmonary nodes drains into the superior and inferior **tracheobronchial nodes** which lie along the trachea and principal bronchi. The nodes below the tracheal bifurcation are the **inferior tracheobronchial nodes**. The tracheobronchial nodes drain through the **bronchomediastinal lymph trunk** on each side to the corresponding brachiocephalic vein or to the thoracic duct on the left. Each bronchomediastinal trunk ascends lateral to the trachea and receives efferent vessels from the **parasternal nodes**. Some of the lymph from the lungs may drain to posterior mediastinal nodes or even to the lower deep cervical nodes. (See Clinical Application 4.3.)

➲ When the bronchopulmonary nodes are enlarged by disease in the lung, they may be visible in radiographs as shadows of increased density at the lung root.

The mediastinum

Mediastinal structures visible through the pleura

Before proceeding to the study of the mediastinum, the structures visible through the mediastinal pleura should be identified. The following mediastinal structures are usually visible through the pleura, unless it is thickened by disease or by excessive fat deposition.

On the right side [Figs. 4.13A, 4.13B], identify (1) the bulge of the heart and the pericardium antero-inferior to the lung root. A vertical ridge descending to the superior extremity of the cardiac bulge is formed by (2) the **right brachiocephalic vein** down to the first costal cartilage and (3) the **superior vena cava** inferior to this. (4) The **inferior vena cava** forms a similar, but shorter, ridge between the diaphragm and the postero-inferior end of the cardiac bulge. (5) The **phrenic nerve** and its accompanying vessels form a vertical ridge on the superior vena cava,

pericardium and inferior vena cava, anterior to the lung root. (6) The **azygos vein** arches over the lung root to enter the superior vena cava. Above the arch of the azygos vein, (7) the **trachea** and (8) **oesophagus** may be seen or felt posterior to the phrenic nerve and superior vena cava. (9) The **right vagus nerve** descends postero-inferiorly across the trachea to pass behind the lung root with the oesophagus. Posterior to the oesophagus are (10) the thoracic vertebral bodies with (11) the posterior intercostal vessels and the azygos vein lying on them. (12) The **sympathetic trunk** may be seen or felt on the heads of the upper ribs and the sides of the lower vertebral bodies. (13) The posterior intercostal vessels and the initial parts of the intercostal nerves can be seen on the vertebral body. (14) The roots of the **greater splanchnic nerve** may be seen passing antero-inferiorly from the lower part of the sympathetic trunk.

On the left side [Figs. 4.14A, 4.14B], identify (1) the large bulge of the **heart** in the pericardium antero-inferior to the lung root and (2) the **descending aorta** behind the heart and root of the lung. (3) The **arch of the aorta** curves over the superior surface of the lung root. (4) The **left common carotid artery** and (5) the **left subclavian artery** pass superiorly from the convex side of the arch, anterior to the oesophagus. (6) The **oesophagus** is hidden by the aorta, except superior to the arch and inferiorly where it lies between the pericardium and the aorta. (7) The **phrenic** and (8) **vagus nerves** descend between the left common carotid and left subclavian arteries on to the lateral surface of the aortic arch. The vagus passes posterior to the lung root. The phrenic nerve runs vertically in front of the lung root, over the pericardium to the diaphragm. (9) The thoracic duct may be seen on the oesophagus superior to the aortic arch. (10) The parts of the sympathetic system are arranged as on the right, though they may be partly hidden by the aorta.

Use the instructions given in Dissection 4.4 to identify structures lying medial to the mediastinal pleura.

Before proceeding to the study of the mediastinum, complete the dissection and study of the phrenic nerves. These nerves lie in the superior and middle mediastinum.

Dissection 4.5 describes the dissection of the phrenic nerve.

DISSECTION 4.4 Right and left sides of the mediastinum

Objectives

I. To strip the mediastinal pleura covering the pericardium, phrenic nerves, vagus, superior and inferior venae cavae, sympathetic trunks, trachea, oesophagus, and posterior intercostal vessels. II. To identify the trace of the left superior intercostal vein, the left cervical cardiac branches, the left recurrent laryngeal nerve, and the left subclavian artery.

Instructions

1. Make a longitudinal incision through the pleura parallel to, and on each side of, the phrenic nerve.

2. Strip the pleura posterior to the phrenic nerve backwards to the intercostal spaces. Avoid injury to the underlying structures.

3. Strip the pleura anterior to the cut forwards to uncover the remainder of the pericardium and superior vena cava on the right and the arch of the aorta on the left.

4. Remove the fat and connective tissue from the sympathetic trunk and its anterior branches. Superiorly, these anterior branches pass to the pulmonary plexus and inferiorly to the splanchnic nerves. In two or three ganglia, identify the **rami communicantes** which pass backwards to the corresponding intercostal nerve. Usually there are two to each nerve, but they may be combined into one [Figs. 4.13, 4.14].

5. Follow the **posterior intercostal vessels** on the vertebral column and in the posterior parts of the intercostal spaces. Trace those in the first two spaces of each side to the neck of the first rib.

6. On the right, the remaining posterior intercostal veins drain into the **azygos vein**. On the left, they drain into the left superior intercostal or hemiazygos vein. (The azygos and hemiazygos veins will be seen later.) Trace the **left superior intercostal vein** obliquely across the arch of the aorta to the left brachiocephalic vein, posterior to the manubrium of the sternum.

7. Find the vagus nerve on each side [Figs. 4.13, 4.14]. Trace it to the posterior surface of the corresponding lung root and find its branches to the pulmonary plexus.

8. On the right, identify the trachea and follow the bronchi to the lung root.

9. Trace the superior and inferior venae cavae to the pericardium. Leave the phrenic nerve *in situ*.

10. On the left side, on the arch of the aorta, find the superior cervical cardiac branch of the left sympathetic trunk and the inferior cervical cardiac branch of the left vagus between the vagus and phrenic nerves. Trace them superiorly. Inferiorly, they pass medially under the concavity of the aortic arch.

11. Trace the left subclavian artery and the oesophagus, superior to the aortic arch. Avoid injury to the thoracic duct on the left surface of the oesophagus and to the recurrent laryngeal nerve on its anterolateral surface.

DISSECTION 4.5 Phrenic nerves

Objective

I. To identify and trace the phrenic nerves.

Instructions

1. Remove the pleura covering the phrenic nerves.

2. Trace the phrenic nerves and the pericardiacophrenic vessels which accompany them as far as possible.

Phrenic nerves

Phrenic nerves are the sole motor supply to the diaphragm. They also transmit sensory nerve fibres from the diaphragm, pericardium, mediastinal and diaphragmatic pleura, inferior vena cava, liver, and biliary apparatus (that is, structures developed in or from the septum transversum).

The phrenic nerve arises from the ventral rami of the third, fourth, and fifth cervical nerves. It descends into the thorax, posterolateral to the corresponding internal jugular vein. At the root of the neck, it is joined by the **pericardiacophrenic branch** of the internal thoracic artery. Each nerve descends on the side of the mediastinum, a short distance anterior to the root of the lung, immediately medial to the mediastinal pleura.

The **right phrenic nerve** lies posterolateral to the right brachiocephalic vein and superior vena cava. It then lies on the fibrous pericardium covering the right atrium of the heart and passes to the diaphragm on the right surface of the inferior vena cava [Fig. 4.13A].

The **left phrenic nerve** descends on to the left surface of the arch of the aorta between the left common carotid and subclavian arteries. It then lies on, and supplies, the pericardium covering the left auricle and left ventricle of the heart [Fig. 4.14A].

Both nerves pierce the diaphragm and are distributed to its inferior surface.

➲ The common origin of the phrenic and supraclavicular nerves from the **third and fourth cervical** ventral rami accounts for the pain felt in the right shoulder in biliary disease.

The anterior mediastinum

The anterior mediastinum is a narrow space posterior to the body of the sternum. It contains the remains of the lower part of the thymus, down to the level of the third or fourth costal cartilages, and some loose fatty tissue [Fig. 4.20]. Two condensations of fibrous tissue—the **sternopericardial ligaments**—lie in the anterior mediastinum and connect the pericardium to the superior and inferior parts of the body of the sternum.

Thymus

In the child, the thymus is a bilobed mass of lymph tissue. In dissecting room subjects, it is usually reduced to two strips of lymph tissue infiltrated with fat and fibrous tissue [Fig. 4.20]. The thymus develops from the third pharyngeal pouch of the embryo, in common with the inferior parathyroid glands. Subsequently, it descends with the pericardium into the thorax. (It may retain a fibrous connection with one or both inferior parathyroid glands in the neck.) In the fetus and newborn [Fig. 4.21], the thymus is nearly as large as the heart. It continues to grow until puberty but is progressively reduced in size thereafter.

Dissection 4.6 provides instructions for dissecting the thymus.

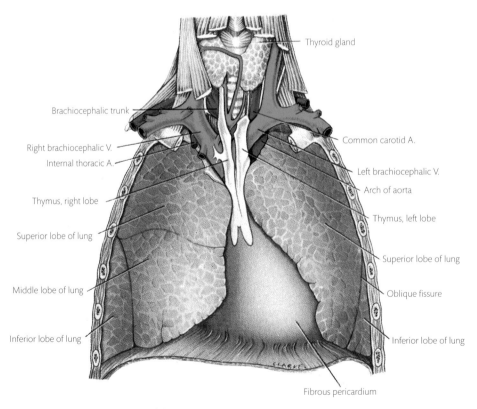

Fig. 4.20 The thyroid gland and thymus in the adult.

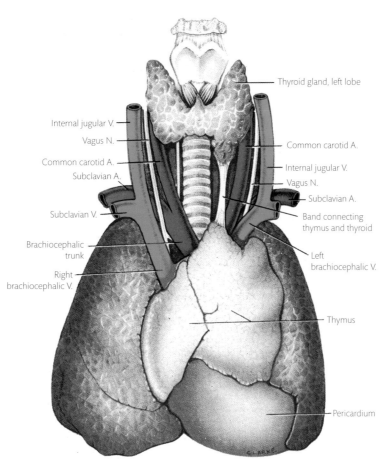

Fig. 4.21 The thymus in a full-term fetus.

Thyroid gland, left lobe

Internal jugular V.

Vagus N.

Common carotid A.

Subclavian A.

Subclavian V.

Brachiocephalic trunk

Right brachiocephalic V.

Common carotid A.

Internal jugular V.

Vagus N.

Subclavian A.

Band connecting thymus and thyroid

Left brachiocephalic V.

Thymus

Pericardium

DISSECTION 4.6 Thymus

Objective

I. To identify and study the thymus.

Instructions

1. Remove the fat and fibrous tissue from the thymus as far as possible. Separate it from the pericardium and turn it superiorly. Note any blood vessels entering it.

The middle mediastinum

Pericardium

The pericardium is the covering of the heart. It consists of an outer **fibrous** [Fig. 4.20] and an inner **serous** part. The fibrous pericardium also extends to cover the great vessels (the aorta, pulmonary trunk, superior and inferior venae cavae, and pulmonary veins) as they enter or leave the heart. The serous pericardium has two layers—an **outer parietal layer** which adheres to, and lines, the fibrous pericardium, and **an inner visceral layer** which adheres to the heart. The narrow space between the two layers of the serous pericardium is the **pericardial cavity** [see Fig. 2.5]. It contains the pericardial fluid. The two layers slide freely on each other as the heart beats within the pericardium. (The cut edges of the fibrous and serous pericardium are seen in Fig. 4.22.)

Fibrous pericardium

The fibrous pericardium is the outer covering of the heart. Superiorly, it fuses with the walls of the aorta and pulmonary trunk. Inferiorly, the fibrous pericardium is attached to the central tendon of the diaphragm [Fig. 4.20]. The pericardium and

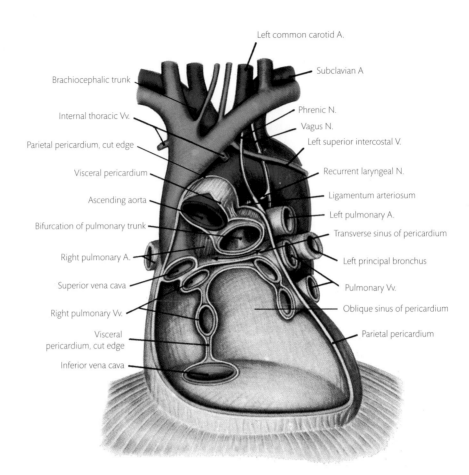

Left common carotid A.

Subclavian A

Brachiocephalic trunk

Phrenic N.

Vagus N.

Internal thoracic Vv.

Left superior intercostal V.

Parietal pericardium, cut edge

Recurrent laryngeal N.

Visceral pericardium

Ligamentum arteriosum

Ascending aorta

Left pulmonary A.

Bifurcation of pulmonary trunk

Transverse sinus of pericardium

Right pulmonary A.

Left principal bronchus

Superior vena cava

Pulmonary Vv.

Right pulmonary Vv.

Oblique sinus of pericardium

Visceral pericardium, cut edge

Parietal pericardium

Inferior vena cava

Fig. 4.22 The pericardium and great vessels after removal of the heart. The arrow lies in the transverse sinus of the pericardium, and the posterior wall of the oblique sinus lies between the right and left pulmonary veins.

diaphragm are both pierced by the inferior vena cava posteriorly and to the right [Fig. 4.22]. The central tendon of the diaphragm separates the pericardium from the liver and the fundus of the stomach in the abdomen. The fibrous pericardium lies posterior to the body of the sternum and the costal cartilages of the second to sixth ribs. The anterior surface of the pericardium is covered by the tissues of the anterior mediastinum and the lungs and pleura, except where the left pleura deviates to the left and leaves the pericardium directly in contact with the thoracic wall. To the left of this, the pericardium is covered by the anterior extremity of the left pleural sac which is filled by the cardiac notch of the left lung in deep inspiration [Figs. 4.21, 4.23].

The lateral surfaces of the fibrous pericardium are in contact with the phrenic nerves and mediastinal pleura. The posterior surface is in contact with the oesophagus and descending aorta which separate it from the vertebral column. The pulmonary veins pierce the pericardium where the lateral and posterior surfaces meet [Fig. 4.22].

Using the instructions given in Dissection 4.7, cut open the pericardium and examine the pericardial cavity.

Serous pericardium and pericardial sinuses

The outer parietal layer of the serous pericardium lines the fibrous pericardium, and the inner visceral layer covers the heart and adjacent parts of the great vessels. At points where the blood vessels enter or leave the heart, the serous pericardium forms a sheath over them, and the parietal and visceral layers become continuous with each other. The arteries (pulmonary trunk and aorta) are surrounded together in one sheath, and the veins (superior and inferior vena cavae and pulmonary veins) in another [Fig. 4.22].

The aorta and pulmonary trunk are enclosed in a common sheath of serous pericardium—the arterial sheath. On the right, the venous sheath surrounds the superior and inferior venae cavae, with the right pulmonary veins between them. On the left, it encloses the two left pulmonary veins. Between

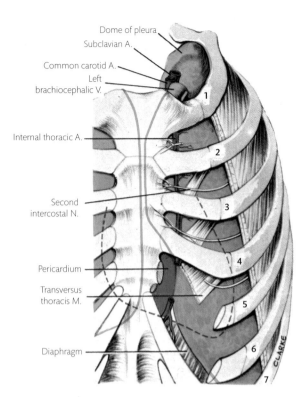

Dome of pleura
Subclavian A.
Common carotid A.
Left brachiocephalic V.
Internal thoracic A.
Second intercostal N.
Pericardium
Transversus thoracis M.
Diaphragm

1
2
3
4
5
6
7

CLARKE

Fig. 4.23 A diagram to show the structures anterior to the pericardium and the heart. Broken red line = outline of the pericardium and heart; blue = parietal pleura; 1–7 = ribs and costal cartilages.

the right and left venous sheaths is the **oblique sinus of the pericardium**. Between the arterial and venous sheaths of the serous pericardium is the **transverse sinus of the pericardium**. This

sinus permits some movement between the arterial and venous ends of the heart [Fig. 4.22].

The **transverse sinus** of the pericardium lies between the pericardial sheath enclosing the great arteries and that enclosing the veins. During development, the transverse sinus is an aperture in the dorsal mesentery of the heart between its venous and arterial ends. As the straight heart tube folds, the two ends of the heart tube come together and the sinus is caught between the ends [Fig. 4.7].

The **oblique sinus** of the pericardium is a blind pocket of the pericardial cavity which lies posterior to the heart. It lies between the right and left pulmonary veins as they enter the left atrium [Fig. 4.22].

Dissection 4.8 describes the examination of the pericardial cavity, the external features of the heart, and pericardial sinuses.

Surface anatomy of the heart

An understanding of the surface anatomy of the heart is essential for clinical examination of the heart. The **superior border** of the heart is formed by the upper margins of the atria. It is largely hidden by the ascending aorta and the pulmonary trunk. The border extends from the upper part of the left second intercostal space, 1–2 cm from the margin of the sternum, to the lower part of the same space on the right, close to the margin of the sternum. A line joining these points also marks the position of the pulmonary arteries which lie along the upper border [Fig. 4.25].

DISSECTION 4.7 Pericardium

Objective

I. To open the fibrous pericardium and examine the pericardial cavity and sinuses.

Instructions

1. Make a vertical cut on each side of the pericardium, immediately anterior to the phrenic nerve.

2. Join the lower ends of these two cuts by a transverse incision, approximately 1 cm above the diaphragm. (Note that these cuts will include the parietal layer of the serous pericardium which is fused to the deep surface of the fibrous pericardium.)

3. Turn the flap of the pericardium upwards and examine the pericardial cavity. Note the smooth, shiny

parietal layer of the serous pericardium on the inner surface of the upturned fibrous pericardium and the visceral layer of the serous pericardium adherent to the heart.

4. Determine the attachment of the flap of the pericardium to the superior vena cava, aorta, and pulmonary trunk.

5. Cut through these attachments, leaving a narrow strip of the pericardium on the vessels so that its position may be determined later [Fig. 4.22].

6. Identify the superior vena cava, ascending aorta, and pulmonary trunk [Fig. 4.22].

DISSECTION 4.8 External features of the heart and pericardial sinuses

Objectives

I. To identify the right atrium, right and left ventricles, and apex of the heart.   II. To explore the transverse and oblique pericardial sinuses.

Instructions

1. Using Fig. 4.24, examine the heart and identify the right atrium, right ventricle, and left ventricle.

2. Identify the apex of the heart.

3. Identify the coronary sulcus and the anterior interventricular sulcus. On the right side the coronary sulcus lies between the right atrium and the right ventricle. On the left it lies between the left auricle and the left ventricle. The anterior interventricular sulcus lies on the interventricular septum between the two ventricles.

4. Identify the borders of the heart—the right border formed by the right atrium. The inferior border formed mostly by the right ventricle and a small part by the left ventricle. The left border formed by the left ventricle. (The superior border is formed by the right and left atria but is not seen in this view as it is overlapped by the pulmonary trunk and ascending aorta.)

5. To explore the **transverse sinus of the pericardium** place one finger anterior to the lowest part of the superior vena cava and push it to the left, posterior to the ascending aorta. The finger passes behind the aorta and pulmonary trunk and appears on the left between the pulmonary trunk and the left auricle.

6. Lift the apex of the heart and slip your fingers behind the heart. The space entered is the **oblique sinus of the pericardium**.

7. Place a probe in one of the pulmonary veins and note that it is felt by the fingers in the oblique sinus. The left atrium lies immediately anterior to the fingers in the oblique sinus, but is separated from them by its covering of visceral pericardium.

8. Note also that the finger tips in the oblique sinus lie close to the finger in the transverse sinus.

9. Replace the anterior thoracic wall in position. Note the relation of the various parts of the sternocostal surface of the heart to the sternum and costal cartilages.

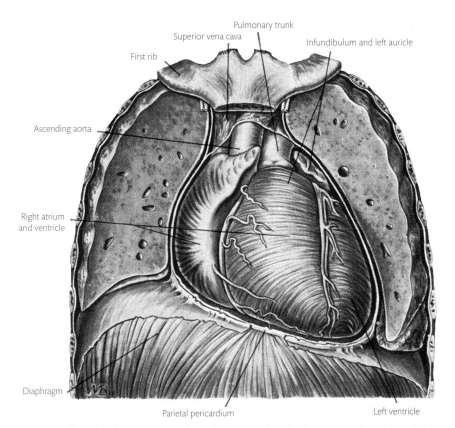

Fig. 4.24 The sternocostal surface of the heart *in situ*. The front of the pericardium has been removed, together with the anterior parts of both lungs.

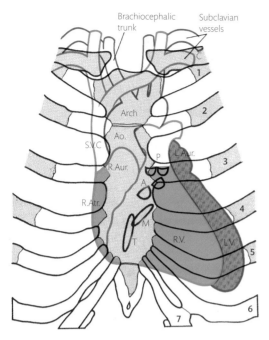

Brachiocephalic trunk   Subclavian vessels

Arch
Ao.
S.V.C
R.Aur.
P L.Aur.
A
R.Atr.
M
T   R.V.   L.V.

1 2 3 4 5 6 7
C

Fig. 4.25 The relation of the heart and the great vessels to the anterior wall of the thorax. 1–7 = ribs and costal cartilages; A = aortic valve; Ao. = ascending aorta; C = clavicle; L.Aur. = left auricle; L.V. = left ventricle; M = left atrioventricular (mitral) orifice; P = pulmonary valve; R.Atr. = right atrium; R.Aur. = right auricle; R.V. = right ventricle; S.V.C. = superior vena cava; T = right atrioventricular (tricuspid) orifice.

The **right border** of the heart extends from the right end of the superior border to a point on the right sixth costal cartilage, 1–2 cm from the margin of the sternum. This border is convex and is formed by the **right atrium** [Figs. 4.24, 4.25].

The **inferior border** extends from the lower end of the right border to the **apex of the heart**. The apex lies in the fifth left intercostal space, immediately medial to the mid-clavicular line. It is formed mainly by the right ventricle, except for a small part on the left which is formed by the left ventricle. This border is normally slightly concave [Fig. 4.25].
➲ Any condition leading to hypertrophy of the right ventricle, e.g. increased pulmonary arterial pressure, makes the lower border convex and gives the heart a globular shape.

The **left border** is marked by a convex line joining the left ends of the superior and inferior borders. It is formed by the **left ventricle**, except for a small part superiorly which is formed by the left auricle [Figs. 4.24, 4.25].

The **coronary sulcus** lies deep to a line joining the sternal ends of the third left and sixth right costal cartilages [Fig. 4.25].

The great **orifices** of the heart and the four cardiac **valves**—the right and left atrioventricular

valves, aortic valve, and pulmonary valve—lie on a line parallel and slightly inferior to the coronary sulcus. They will be seen when the heart is opened. The **pulmonary orifice** and **valve** lie posterior to the sternal end of the third left costal cartilage. The **aortic orifice** and **valve** are posterior to the left margin of the sternum at the level of the third intercostal space. The **left atrioventricular** (mitral) **orifice** and **valve** are posterior to the left half of the sternum at the level of the fourth costal cartilage. The **right atrioventricular** (tricuspid) **orifice** and **valve** are posterior to the middle of the sternum at the level of the fourth intercostal space [Fig. 4.25].

The positions given above are only approximate because the heart is a mobile organ whose shape and position vary with diaphragmatic movements and with venous return.

Surfaces of the heart

Sternocostal surface

The heart is rotated so that the **right ventricle** and **atrium** form the greater part of the sternocostal (anterior) surface, with the left ventricle forming a small strip which includes the apex. The apex points to the left and anteriorly.

The **atria** lie posterosuperior to the ventricles. The upper parts of the atria lie behind and partially surround the ascending aorta and pulmonary trunk. The **right** and **left auricles** project anteriorly from the atria and overlap the anterior aspect of the pulmonary trunk (left auricle) and aorta (right auricle) [Fig. 4.24].

The right border of the heart is formed by the right atrium. On the sternocostal surface, the right atrium is separated from the right ventricle by the deep **coronary sulcus**. This sulcus passes obliquely from the root of the ascending aorta to the junction of the right border of the heart with the diaphragmatic surface. The ventricular part of the sternocostal surface lies to the left of this sulcus. It is divided by the **anterior interventricular sulcus** into a right two-thirds formed by the right ventricle and a left one-third formed by the left ventricle. The anterior interventricular sulcus marks the line along which the **interventricular septum** meets the sternocostal surface. It contains the anterior interventricular branch of the left coronary artery and the great cardiac vein, usually buried in fat. The sternocostal surface of the right ventricle narrows superiorly to become continuous with the pulmonary trunk. This narrow part is the **infundibulum** of the right ventricle. The continuity of the left ventricle with the aorta is not visible on this surface because it lies posterior to the infundibulum [Fig. 4.24].

The **left border** of the sternocostal surface is formed largely by the convex, bulging wall of the left ventricle and superiorly by the **left auricle** [Fig. 4.24].

Diaphragmatic surface

This slightly concave surface is formed entirely by the ventricles which are separated from each other by the **posterior interventricular sulcus**. The sulcus is often visible as a line of fat. It contains the posterior interventricular branch of the right coronary artery and the middle cardiac vein. The left ventricle forms the left two-thirds of this surface [Fig. 4.26].

Base

The base is the posterior or vertebral surface of the heart. It is formed entirely by the **atria**, principally the left atrium [Figs. 4.26, 4.27]. The base is separated from the diaphragmatic surface by the pos-

terior part of the **coronary sulcus**. This part of the coronary sulcus contains parts of the right coronary artery, a branch of the left coronary artery, and a large vein—the **coronary sinus**—which drains the heart [Figs. 4.26, 4.27].

Arteries of the heart

The heart is supplied by the **right** and **left coronary arteries**. They are large vasa vasorum which arise from the **aortic sinuses** or dilatations, found at the root of the ascending aorta [Figs. 4.28, 4.29].

The right coronary artery arises from the **anterior** or **right aortic sinus** of the ascending aorta. It passes forwards between the right auricle and the upper part of the infundibulum and runs in the coronary sulcus to the inferior border of the heart. Here it gives off the **marginal branch** [Figs. 4.24, 4.30] and then turns to the left in the posterior part of the coronary sulcus. On the diaphragmatic surface of the heart, it gives a large **posterior interventricular artery**, which runs along the posterior interventricular sulcus towards the apex [Fig. 4.26]. The right coronary artery continues in the coronary sulcus supplying a variable amount

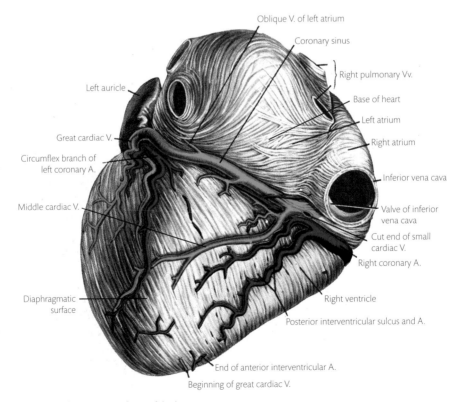

Fig. 4.26 Diaphragmatic and posterior surfaces of the heart.

Labels (clockwise):
Oblique V. of left atrium
Coronary sinus
Right pulmonary Vv.
Base of heart
Left atrium
Right atrium
Inferior vena cava
Valve of inferior vena cava
Cut end of small cardiac V.
Right coronary A.
Right ventricle
Posterior interventricular sulcus and A.
End of anterior interventricular A.
Beginning of great cardiac V.
Diaphragmatic surface
Middle cardiac V.
Circumflex branch of left coronary A.
Great cardiac V.
Left auricle

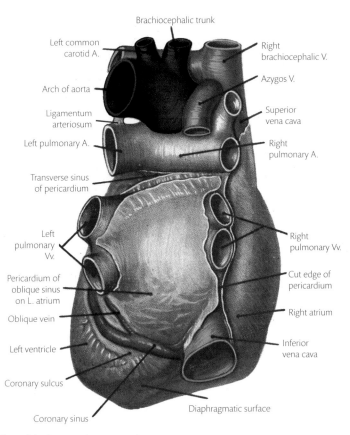

Brachiocephalic trunk

Left common
carotid A.

Arch of aorta

Ligamentum
arteriosum

Left pulmonary A.

Transverse sinus
of pericardium

Left
pulmonary
Vv.

Pericardium of
oblique sinus
on L. atrium

Oblique vein

Left ventricle

Coronary sulcus

Coronary sinus

Right
brachiocephalic V.

Azygos V.

Superior
vena cava

Right
pulmonary A.

Right
pulmonary Vv.

Cut edge of
pericardium

Right atrium

Inferior
vena cava

Diaphragmatic surface

Fig. 4.27 The posterior surface of the heart and great vessels.

of the left ventricle and atrium. On the sternocostal surface, the right coronary artery supplies the right atrium, the sino-atrial node, and a large part of the right ventricle. In the posterior part of the coronary sulcus, it supplies the remainder of the right atrium, all of the diaphragmatic part of the right ventricle, and a variable amount of the left atrium and ventricle. The posterior interventricular artery supplies the postero-inferior part of the interventricular septum, including the atrioventricular node and bundle (part of the conducting system of the heart). It anastomoses with the anterior interventricular branch of the left coronary artery in the interventricular septum.

The left coronary artery arises from the **left posterior** or **left aortic sinus** of the ascending aorta [Figs. 4.28, 4.29]. It runs to the left between the pulmonary trunk and the left auricle. Emerging on the surface from between them, it divides into the **anterior interventricular artery** and the **circumflex artery** [Fig. 4.29]. The anterior interventricular branch descends in the anterior interventricular sulcus and runs towards the apex

[Figs. 4.24, 4.29]. It supplies both ventricles and the anterosuperior part of the interventricular septum. The **circumflex branch** curves postero-inferiorly with the great cardiac vein in the left part of the coronary sulcus [Figs. 4.26, 4.29]. It ends to the left of the posterior interventricular sulcus and gives branches to the left atrium and ventricle, including a **left marginal branch**.

➲ The coronary arteries are the only arterial supply to the heart. The two arteries anastomose so inadequately that blockage (coronary thrombosis) of any one artery usually leads to death of the muscle which it supplies. The damaged muscle is replaced by fibrous tissue, if the individual survives the blockage. If the node or other parts of the conducting tissue of the heart are affected by the blockage, the ventricles may continue to contract at their own slow rate, independent of the atrial contractions (heart block).

Veins of the heart

The coronary sinus will be seen later, but the main tributaries of this principal vein of the heart are seen

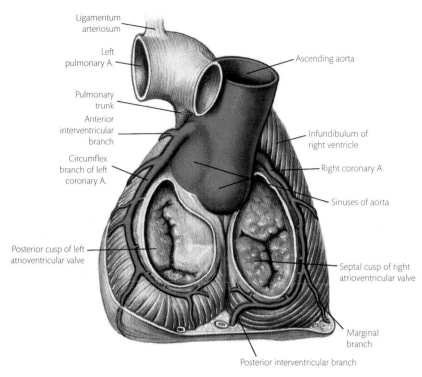

Ligamentum arteriosum

Left pulmonary A.

Pulmonary trunk

Anterior interventricular branch

Circumflex branch of left coronary A.

Posterior cusp of left atrioventricular valve

Ascending aorta

Infundibulum of right ventricle

Right coronary A.

Sinuses of aorta

Septal cusp of right atrioventricular valve

Marginal branch

Posterior interventricular branch

Fig. 4.28 The ventricular part of the heart as seen after removal of the atria. The right coronary artery usually extends further to the left than in this specimen. The sternocostal surface is to the right.

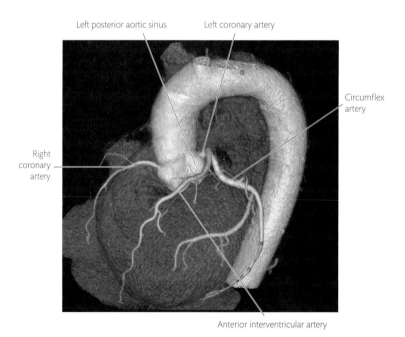

Left posterior aortic sinus

Left coronary artery

Circumflex artery

Right coronary artery

Anterior interventricular artery

Fig. 4.29 3D volume-rendered image of the left coronary artery.

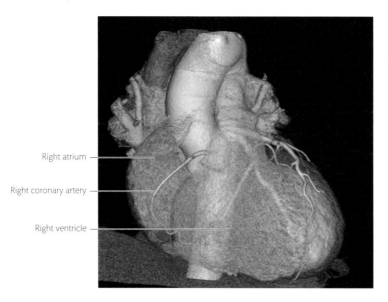

Fig. 4.30 3D volume-rendered image of the right coronary artery.

now [Figs. 4.26, 4.31]. The **great cardiac vein** runs with the anterior interventricular and circumflex branches of the left coronary artery. The **small cardiac vein** runs with the marginal branch of the right coronary artery. It accompanies the right coronary artery in the posterior part of the coronary sulcus to the right extremity of the coronary sinus. The **middle cardiac vein** accompanies the posterior interventricular artery. Most of the veins of the heart enter the coronary sinus. However, the **anterior cardiac veins** and some small venous channels—**venae cordis minimae**—which lie in the walls of the heart open directly into the right atrium.

Dissection 4.9 describes the procedure for removal of the heart.

Dissection 4.10 provides instructions to trace the blood vessels of the heart.

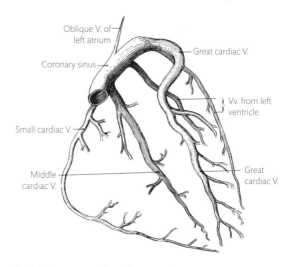

Fig. 4.31 Diagram of the tributaries of the coronary sinus viewed from in front.

DISSECTION 4.9 Removal of the heart

Objective

I. To remove the heart from the pericardial cavity by cutting through the large vessels opening into it.

Instructions

1. Place a probe in the transverse sinus and cut the ascending aorta and pulmonary trunk in front of the probe.

2. Cut the superior vena cava about 1 cm superior to its entry into the right atrium.

3. Lift the apex of the heart, and cut the inferior vena cava close to the diaphragm.

4. Cut the four pulmonary veins and the serous pericardium between.

5. Lift the heart out of the pericardial sac.

6. Examine the posterior aspect of the pericardium [Fig. 4.22] and identify the cut ends of the inferior and superior venae cavae and the pulmonary veins.

DISSECTION 4.10 Blood vessels of the heart

Objectives

I. To identify and trace the right and left coronary arteries and their branches.   II. To identify and study the coronary sinus and its tributaries.

Instructions

1. Strip the visceral pericardium from the sternocostal surface of the heart.

2. Expose the **anterior interventricular branch** of the **left coronary artery** and the **great cardiac vein** by scraping the fat from the anterior interventricular sulcus [Fig. 4.24].

3. Note the branches of the artery to both ventricles and to the interventricular septum which lies deep to it. Trace the artery inferiorly to the diaphragmatic surface.

4. Carefully remove the fat from the coronary sulcus. Avoid damage to the small **anterior cardiac veins**, which cross the sulcus from the right ventricle to enter the right atrium directly.

5. Trace the **anterior interventricular artery** superiorly to the left of the pulmonary trunk [Fig. 4.24] to its origin from the left coronary artery.

6. Trace the left coronary artery to the left posterior aortic sinus (a swelling at the root of the ascending aorta).

7. Trace the **circumflex branch** of the **left coronary artery** in the left part of the coronary sulcus to the diaphragmatic surface of the heart [Fig. 4.29].

8. Find the **right coronary artery** in the depths of the sulcus between the right atrium and ventricle [Fig. 4.24]. Follow the artery superiorly to its origin from the **right aortic sinus** (a swelling at the root of the ascending aorta, deep to the right auricle). Trace the artery inferiorly till it turns on to the posterior surface of the heart. Note the branches to the right ventricle and atrium. One of these—the **nodal artery**—passes to the left of the auricle towards the superior vena cava. It supplies part of the atrium and the sino-atrial node.

9. Trace the **coronary sinus** to its opening into the right atrium.

10. Note that the right coronary artery supplies a considerable part of the diaphragmatic surface of the left ventricle and that large branches of the two coronary arteries do not anastomose in the coronary sulcus. Attempt to find the **oblique vein of the left atrium** [Fig. 4.26].

11. Define the vessels on the diaphragmatic surface [Fig. 4.26]. In particular, follow the **posterior interventricular artery** posteriorly and to the right to its origin from the right coronary artery. The **middle cardiac vein** runs a similar course to the right end of the coronary sinus.

Chambers of the heart and the great vessels

The chambers of the heart and the valves between them are best displayed by opening into each chamber.

Right atrium

Dissection 4.11 gives instructions on how to study the interior of the right atrium.

The right atrium consists of smooth-walled and rough-walled parts. The smooth-walled part is more posterior and receives the superior and inferior venae cavae and the coronary sinus. The rough-walled part is anterior and is ridged by parallel muscle bundles called **musculi pectinati**. The two parts are separated on the right by an external groove—the **sulcus terminalis**—and a corresponding internal vertical ridge—the **crista terminalis** [Fig. 4.33]. The crista terminalis begins superiorly, anterior to the opening of the superior vena cava. It curves to the right, extends downwards, and becomes continuous with a sharper ridge in front of the opening of the inferior vena cava—the **valve of the inferior vena cava**. A small flap—the **valve of the coronary sinus**—lies in front of the opening of the coronary sinus.

The posteromedial wall of the right atrium is the **inter-atrial septum** [Fig. 4.34]. A shallow, oval, thumb-print sized depression on the right atrial side of the inter-atrial septum is the **fossa ovalis** [Figs. 4.33, 4.34]. The upper margin of the fossa ovalis is limited by a thickened rim, the limbus fossa ovalis.

The crista terminalis, the valve of the inferior vena cava, and the valve of the coronary sinus to-

DISSECTION 4.11 Right atrium

Objective

I. To study the internal surface of the right atrium.

Instructions

1. Identify the right auricle.

2. Identify the groove—the **sulcus terminalis**—on the right side. This separates the right atrium from the right auricle.

3. Follow the incisions shown in Fig. 4.32 to open into the right atrium.

4. Turn the flap to the left and remove the clotted blood.

5. Identify the **crista terminalis** separating the smooth-walled and rough-walled parts [Fig. 4.33].

6. Identify the smooth-walled part of the right atrium and the openings of the superior vena cava, inferior vena cava, and coronary sinus in it. Identify the **valve of the coronary sinus** and the **valve of the inferior vena cava** [Fig. 4.33].

7. On the posterior wall of the right atrium, identify the **fossa ovalis** and the thickened superior margin—the **limbus fossa ovalis**.

8. Note the continuity of the crista terminalis, the valve of the inferior vena cava, the valve of the coronary sinus, and the limbus fossa ovalis [Fig. 4.34].

9. Identify the right atrioventricular orifice.

gether represent the remains of the embryological right venous valve. In the embryo, the right venous valve guards the opening of the **sinus venosus** into the right atrium.

(In the fetus, the foramen ovale is an oblique valvular opening in the interatrial septum. It allows blood reaching the right atrium through the inferior vena cava to enter the left atrium. The interatrial septum consists of two incomplete septae—to the right, the rigid septum secundum

and to the left the thin, flexible septum primum.) The foramen ovale remains open in the fetus as the pressure in the left atrium is lower than that in the right atrium. After birth, the pressure in the left atrium rises; the septum primum is forced against the septum secundum, and the foramen ovale is closed. Subsequently, the two septae fuse, the septum primum forms the floor of the fossa ovalis and becomes adherent to the limbus fossa ovalis. If the foramen ovale persists, it lies

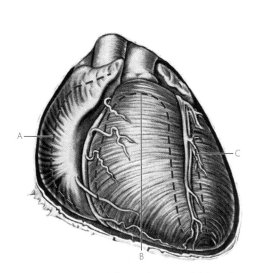

Fig. 4.32 Incision to open (A) the right atrium, (B) the right ventricle, and (C) the left ventricle.

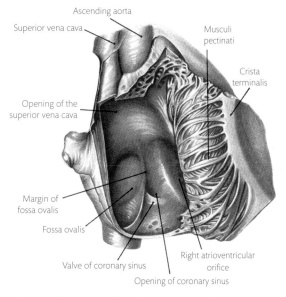

Fig. 4.33 The interior of the right atrium exposed by turning its right and anterior walls towards the left.

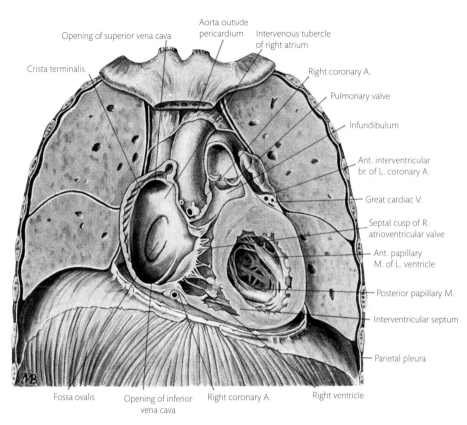

Aorta outside pericardium

Opening of superior vena cava

Intervenous tubercle of right atrium

Crista terminalis

Right coronary A.

Pulmonary valve

Infundibulum

Ant. interventricular br. of L. coronary A.

Great cardiac V.

Septal cusp of R. atrioventricular valve

Ant. papillary M. of L. ventricle

Posterior papillary M.

Interventricular septum

Parietal pleura

Fossa ovalis

Opening of inferior vena cava

Right coronary A.

Right ventricle

Fig. 4.34 The heart *in situ*. A coronal section through the right atrium, right ventricle, infundibulum of the right ventricle, pulmonary valve, and left ventricle.

between the fossa ovalis and the upper margin of the limbus.

The opening of the inferior vena cava into the right atrium is directed towards the fossa ovalis on the interatrial septum. The valve of the inferior vena cava directs blood towards the fossa. The opening of the superior vena cava into the right atrium lies on a more anterior plane, and faces the right atrioventricular orifice. This arrangement produces an almost complete separation of the two venous streams before birth.

Veins entering the right atrium

Superior vena cava

The superior vena cava lies on the right side and drains blood from the head and neck, upper limbs, walls of the thorax, and the upper abdomen. The upper part lies in the superior mediastinum and will be described later. The lower part of the superior vena cava lies in the middle mediastinum

and is covered by the pericardium. It opens into the superior part of the right atrium [Fig. 4.34]. The azygos vein arches over the superior surface of the right lung root [Fig. 4.13A] and enters the posterior surface of the superior vena cava at its midpoint, just before it enters the pericardium.

The superior vena cava is anterolateral to the trachea, anterior to the lung root, and lateral to the ascending aorta. ⊃ The phrenic nerve and the right mediastinal pleura lie on its right surface. The close association of the superior vena cava with the right lung root and its contained pulmonary veins [Fig. 4.13A] makes it possible for an abnormal pulmonary vein to drain into the superior vena cava.

Inferior vena cava

The intrathoracic part of the inferior vena cava is short [Fig. 4.13A]. It pierces the central tendon of the diaphragm and pericardium approximately at the level of the eighth thoracic vertebra. It immediately enters the inferior part of the right atrium at the level of the sixth right chondrosternal joint. The right pleura and lung are wrapped round the right and posterior surfaces of the inferior vena cava and separate it from the vertebral column posteriorly. The right phrenic nerve descends on its right surface.

Coronary sinus

The coronary sinus is the main vein of the heart. It is formed by the union of the great cardiac vein and the oblique vein of the left atrium [Fig. 4.26]. It runs from left to right in the posterior part of the coronary sulcus and empties into the right atrium. The main tributaries of the coronary sinus are the **great cardiac vein** at its left extremity, and the **middle** and **small cardiac veins** at its right extremity [Fig. 4.31]. It also drains the veins of the left ventricle and the oblique vein of the left atrium. It enters the right atrium immediately to the left of the valve of the inferior vena cava.

The **oblique vein of the left atrium** corresponds developmentally to the inferior half of the superior vena cava. Thus a persistent left superior vena cava may replace the oblique vein and enter the coronary sinus. Both the oblique vein and the coronary sinus are partly covered by cardiac muscle on their posterior aspects.

The right atrium also receives (1) the **anterior cardiac veins** which pierce the anterior wall of the right atrium and (2) small **venae cordis minimae** which enter the right atrium through irregularly scattered openings which are difficult to identify.

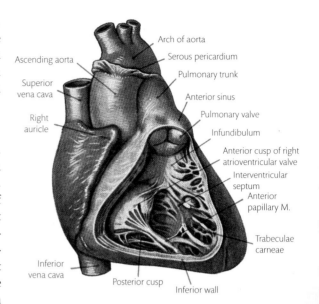

Fig. 4.35 The interior of the right ventricle exposed from in front.

Right atrioventricular orifice and valve

The right atrioventricular orifice lies between the antero-inferior part of the right atrium and the postero-inferior part of the right ventricle [Fig. 4.35]. It is approximately 2.5 cm in diameter and is guarded by the right atrioventricular, or tricuspid valve. The atrioventricular orifice is surrounded by a **fibrous ring** which gives attachment to the cusps of the atrioventricular valve, the atrial and ventricular muscle. This fibrous ring is part of the fibrous skeleton of the heart [Fig. 4.36]. The three cusps of the tricuspid

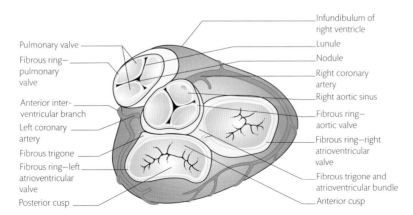

Fig. 4.36 A diagram of the ventricular part of the heart with the atria and great vessels removed.

valve are the anterior, posterior, and septal cusps. Further details of the valve are described after the right ventricle is studied.

Right ventricle

Dissection 4.12 gives instructions on the dissection of the right ventricle.

The cavity of the right ventricle is approximately triangular in shape when seen from in front [Fig. 4.35]. Blood enters the right ventricle through the right **atrioventricular orifice** at the right inferior angle and leaves through the **pulmonary orifice** at the superior angle. The smooth-walled anterosuperior part of the right ventricle is the **infundibulum** (= a funnel). It leads to the pulmonary orifice. The remainder of the wall of the right ventricle has irregular muscle ridges called **trabeculae carneae**. Three conical **papillary muscles** arise from the wall of the ventricle and project into the cavity of the ventricle [Fig. 4.35]. They are inserted by tendinous strands called **chordae tendineae** into the margins and ventricular surfaces of the cusps of the right atrioventricular valve. The large **posterior papillary muscle** arises from the inferior wall

DISSECTION 4.12 Right ventricle

Objective

I. To study the interior of the right ventricle.

Instructions

1. Follow the incisions shown in Fig. 4.32 to open into the right ventricle.

2. Turn the flap inferiorly and remove the clotted blood.

3. Examine the cavity of the right ventricle and note the trabeculae carneae.

4. Identify the interventricular septum and the anterior and inferior walls of the right ventricle.

5. Identify the anterior, posterior, and septal papillary muscles, and the chordae tendinae arising from them. Identify the septomarginal trabecula which extends from the septum to the anterior papillary muscle.

6. Examine the infundibulum, pulmonary valve, and trunk.

and sends chordae tendineae to the posterior and septal cusps of the valve. A larger anterior papillary muscle is attached to the anterior wall and sends chordae tendinae into the anterior and posterior cusps. Several small septal papillary muscles arise from the septum and send chordae tendineae into the anterior and septal cusps. The anterior and posterior muscles are occasionally divided into a number of smaller projections.

When the papillary muscles contract, they draw the margins of adjacent cusps together and close the atrioventricular valve. They also prevent the valve from being forced back into the atrium as the intraventricular pressure rises. This mechanism increases the efficiency of the ventricular contraction and permits the atrium to fill completely while the ventricle is contracting.

The **septomarginal trabecula** is one of the trabeculae carneae which passes from the septum to the anterior papillary muscle. It carries part of the right crus of the **atrioventricular bundle** (a part of the conducting system of the heart) [Fig. 4.35]. This and similar parts of the conducting system pass to the other papillary muscles and ensure early contraction of these muscles. Thus the chordae tendineae are already taut when ventricular contraction begins.

In a transverse section, the right ventricle is crescentic in shape because the interventricular septum bulges to the right. The wall of the right ventricle is thinner than that of the left. The difference in thickness of the muscle of the two ventricles is directly related to the work done by each in overcoming the vascular resistance against which it pumps. (The pulmonary systolic arterial pressure is low at 25–35 mmHg, compared with the much higher systolic pressure of 120 mmHg in the systemic circulation.) ➲ Any condition which increases the pulmonary arterial resistance raises the right ventricular pressure and produces a compensatory hypertrophy of the right ventricular wall.

Right atrioventricular (tricuspid) valve

The three cusps of the right atrioventricular valve are named from their position. The anterior cusp separates the atrioventricular orifice from the infundibulum. The posterior cusp lies on the inferior wall of the right ventricle. The septal cusp lies on the interventricular septum. The anterior and posterior cusps are more nearly horizontal. The chordae tendineae are attached to the margins and ventricular surfaces of the cusps. The atrial surfaces of the cusps are smooth as blood flows over them during ventricular filling [Fig. 4.35].

Pulmonary orifice and pulmonary valve

The pulmonary orifice lies at the apex of the infundibulum [Fig. 4.35]. It is surrounded by a slender fibrous ring which gives attachment to the cusps of the pulmonary valve. This fibrous ring is part of the fibrous skeleton of the heart which is described later.

The pulmonary valve is a **semilunar valve** with three **semilunar cusps** [Fig. 4.36]. Each cusp is deeply concave on its arterial surface and is composed of a thin endothelial-covered layer of fibrous tissue. The free margin of the cusp is thickened near the middle to form a small, rounded structure—the **nodule**. The crescentic edges on each side of the nodule are thinner and are called the **lunules**. The semilunar cusps are forced apart as blood is ejected from the contracting ventricle [Fig. 4.36]. At the end of ventricular contraction, the elastic recoil of the pulmonary trunk forces blood back towards the ventricle. This back thrust distends the semilunar cusps, forces the margins of the valve together, and closes the valve. The valve margins come together in the form of a 'Y' with the nodules pressed together at the centre. The pulmonary cusps are named **anterior**, **right**, and **left**. The wall of the pulmonary trunk is slightly dilated opposite each cusp to form a **sinus**.

Pulmonary trunk

This great artery begins at the level of the pulmonary valve [Fig. 4.35]. It is anterior to, and to the left of, the ascending aorta and posterior to the sternal end of the third left costal cartilage. The trunk is approximately 5 cm long and 2 cm wide. It winds round the left side of the ascending aorta to end in the concavity of the aortic arch by dividing into the **right** and **left pulmonary arteries** [Fig. 4.19]. This division occurs posterior to the sternal end of the second left costal cartilage. The transverse sinus of the pericardium separates the pulmonary trunk from the superior margin of the left atrium. The trunk and ascending aorta are enclosed in a common sheath of serous pericardium.

Left ventricle

Dissection 4.13 gives instructions on the dissection of the left ventricle.

The cavity of the left ventricle is longer than that of the right ventricle. It is circular in transverse section, and its walls are much thicker [Figs. 4.37, 4.38]. The trabeculae carneae are finer and more numerous than in the right ventricle. They are particularly marked at the apex, but the surfaces of the septum and the upper part of the anterior wall are relatively smooth.

There are two large papillary muscles in the left ventricle—the **anterior** and **posterior papillary** muscles [Fig. 4.39]. The anterior papillary

---

DISSECTION 4.13 Left ventricle

Objective

I. To study the interior of the left ventricle.

Instructions

1. Identify the three cusps of the aortic valve—anterior, left posterior, and right posterior cusps—by examining the valve from above [Fig. 4.36].

2. Make the incisions shown in Fig. 4.32. The cut should pass through the aorta, aortic vestibule, and left ventricle.

3. Turn the flap to the left and remove the clotted blood.

4. Identify the anterior and posterior cusps of the left atrioventricular valve.

5. Identify the anterior and posterior papillary muscles. Follow the chordae tendineae arising from them to both cusps of the left atrioventricular valve.

6. Examine the trabeculae carneae on the inner surface of the left ventricle.

7. Examine the interventricular septum by holding it between your finger and thumb.

8. Note the position of the muscular part of the interventricular septum, its relation to the membranous part, and the septal cusp of the right atrioventricular valve.

9. Examine the anterior cusp of the left atrioventricular valve by placing a finger in the mitral valve and another in the aortic orifice. Appreciate how this cusp separates the inflow and outflow tracts of the left ventricle.

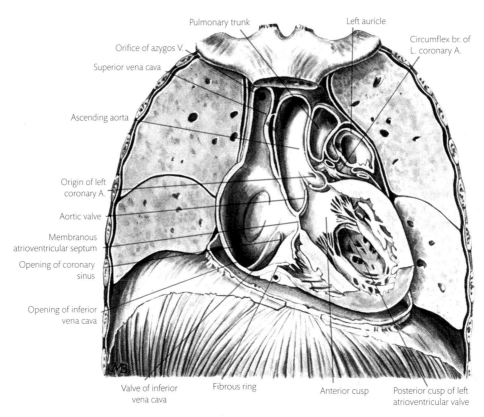

Pulmonary trunk
Left auricle
Orifice of azygos V.
Circumflex br. of
L. coronary A.
Superior vena cava
Ascending aorta
Origin of left
coronary A.
Aortic valve
Membranous
atrioventricular septum
Opening of coronary
sinus
Opening of inferior
vena cava
Valve of inferior
vena cava
Fibrous ring
Anterior cusp
Posterior cusp of left
atrioventricular valve

Fig. 4.37 The heart *in situ*. A coronal section through the right atrium, right ventricle, left auricle, left ventricle, aortic vestibule, aortic valve, and aorta. The arrow lies in the transverse sinus of the pericardium.

muscle is attached to the anterior part of the left wall. The posterior papillary muscle arises from the inferior wall further posteriorly. Each papillary muscle sends chordae tendineae to both cusps of the left atrioventricular (mitral) valve [Figs. 4.38, 4.39].

The **aortic vestibule** is the outflow tract of the left ventricle. Its smooth walls are mainly fibrous and not muscular [Fig. 4.39].

Aortic orifice and aortic valve

The aortic orifice lies in the right posterosuperior part of the left ventricle. It is surrounded by a fibrous ring to which the cusps of the aortic valve are attached [Fig. 4.36]. It is separated from the left atrioventricular orifice only by the anterior cusp of the mitral valve [Figs. 4.36, 4.37, 4.39]. The anterior cusp of the mitral valve separates two blood streams. Blood entering the ventricle from the atrium, and that leaving the ventricle through the aorta. As a result, the cusp is smooth on both

surfaces. Note also that the aortic orifice is superior to the interventricular septum.

Aortic valve

The aortic valve is similar to the pulmonary valve in having three cusps. The cusps of the aortic valve are thicker and differently placed (anterior, left posterior, and right posterior), and the **aortic sinuses** are larger [Fig. 4.36].

Interventricular septum

The interventricular septum is mostly thick and muscular. Posterosuperiorly, it is thin and membranous [Figs. 4.37, 4.38] and connected to the fibrous skeleton. The **muscular interventricular septum** is placed obliquely between the anterior and posterior interventricular sulci. The right surface of the septum faces forwards and to the right and bulges into the right ventricle [Fig. 4.37]. Towards the aortic orifice, the septum becomes thin and collagenous to form the **membranous part of**

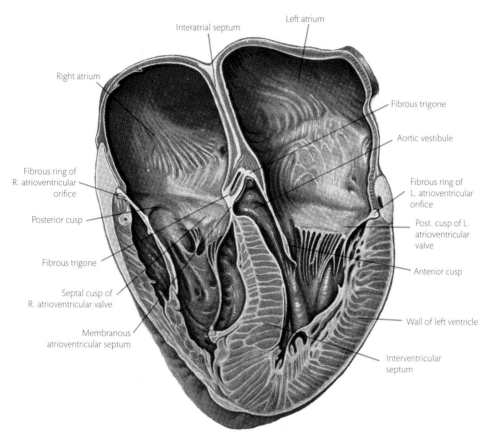

Interatrial septum

Left atrium

Right atrium

Fibrous trigone

Aortic vestibule

Fibrous ring of
R. atrioventricular
orifice

Fibrous ring of
L. atrioventricular
orifice

Posterior cusp

Post. cusp of L.
atrioventricular
valve

Fibrous trigone

Anterior cusp

Septal cusp of
R. atrioventricular valve

Wall of left ventricle

Membranous
atrioventricular septum

Interventricular
septum

Fig. 4.38 A section through the heart to show the interatrial, atrioventricular, and interventricular septae, and the fibrous rings that surround the atrioventricular orifices.

the interventricular septum. Superiorly, the posterior part of the membranous interventricular septum narrows and continues with a septum between the right atrium and the left ventricle. This is the **membranous atrioventricular septum**. The membranous interventricular septum is developed from the same tissue that forms the valves of the heart. ➲ Since the membranous interventricular septum develops separately from the muscular part of the septum, it may be deficient, leaving an interventricular foramen immediately inferior to the aortic orifice. The presence of such an **interventricular foramen** inevitably means that the pressures in both ventricles are the same—a situation which leads to hypertrophy of the right ventricular wall.

The aorta

The aorta arises from the aortic orifice behind the third left intercostal space at the margin of the sternum [Fig. 4.25]. It runs through the thorax and abdomen and ends on the anterior surface of the fourth lumbar vertebra by dividing into the right and left common iliac arteries. For descriptive purposes, the thoracic part of the aorta is divided into the ascending aorta, the arch of the aorta, and the descending aorta. The ascending aorta lies in the middle mediastinum, the arch in the superior mediastinum, and the descending aorta in the posterior mediastinum [Fig. 4.14B].

Ascending aorta

The ascending aorta lies in the middle mediastinum. It is the first part of the aorta. It runs upwards, forwards, and to the right [Fig. 4.39]. Behind the right half of the sternal angle, it continues as the arch of the aorta. It is enclosed with the pulmonary trunk in a sheath of serous pericardium. The ascending aorta has four dilatations of its wall, three **aortic sinuses** at its root corresponding to the cusps of the aortic valve [Figs. 4.29, 4.39]. These are the right, left anterior, and left posterior aortic

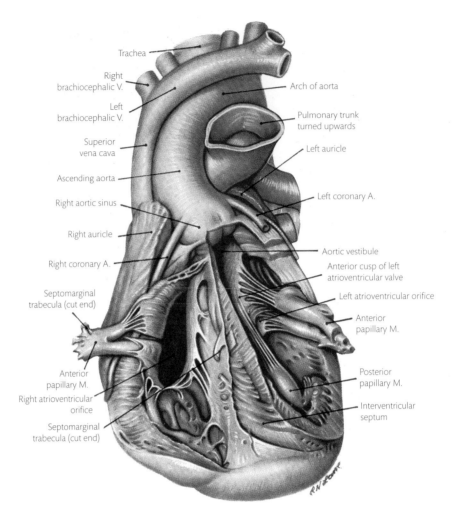

Fig. 4.39 A diagrammatic representation of the dissected ventricles of the heart. The root of the aorta has been exposed by separating the pulmonary trunk from the right ventricle and turning the trunk upwards.

sinuses. The right and left coronary arteries arise from the right and left posterior aortic sinuses. At the right border of the aorta is a fourth swelling where the full thrust of the blood discharged from the left ventricle is felt. This is the **bulb of the aorta**. ➲ The bulb is a common site for the formation of an abnormal dilatation or aneurysm.

Initially, the ascending aorta lies between the left atrium and the infundibulum of the right ventricle. The right atrium is on its right side. It then ascends anterior to the right pulmonary artery and right bronchus, with the superior vena cava on the right and the pulmonary trunk running posteriorly on its left [Figs. 4.19, 4.33, 4.35]. The ascending aorta is separated from the sternum by the pericardium, pleura, lung, and the remains of

the thymus. The **vasa vasorum** of the ascending aorta arises principally from a branch of the left coronary artery.

Left atrium

Dissection 4.14 provides instructions on the dissection of the left atrium.

The left atrium lies posteriorly and forms the base of the heart [Fig. 4.27]. The long, narrow left auricle projects forwards on the left side and partly overlaps the beginning of the pulmonary trunk [Fig. 4.24]. The **right** and **left superior** and **inferior pulmonary veins** enter the upper half of the left atrium, close to the lateral margins of the posterior surface. The superior veins are on a plane anterior to that of the inferior veins [Fig. 4.41].

DISSECTION 4.14 Left atrium

Objective

I. To study the interior of the left atrium.

Instructions

1. Examine the posterior surface of the heart and identify the four pulmonary veins.

2. Make the incision shown in Fig. 4.40.

3. Turn the flap inferiorly and remove the clotted blood.

4. Note the smooth wall of the left atrium and the rough wall of the small left auricle.

5. Examine the left atrioventricular opening and valve.

The upper part of the anterior surface of the left atrium is covered by the ascending aorta and the pulmonary trunk. The pulmonary arteries course along its superior margin. The coronary sinus in the coronary sulcus runs along the inferior margin [Fig. 4.27].

The interior of the left atrium is almost entirely smooth. Musculi pectinati are seen only in the auricle. A prominent muscular ridge projects into the left atrium anterior to the left pulmonary veins so that the orifices of these veins are not visible from in front. The **interatrial septum** [Fig. 4.41] slopes posteriorly and to the right so that a considerable part of the left atrium lies posterior to the right atrium.

Veins entering the left atrium

The four pulmonary veins enter the left atrium [Figs. 4.41, 4.42, 4.43]. Their openings are not guarded by valves.

Left atrioventricular valve

The **left atrioventricular orifice** lies at the antero-inferior part of the left atrium [Figs. 4.38, 4.41, 4.43]. The orifice is smaller (2 cm) than the right atrioventricular orifice and is guarded by the **left atrioventricular** (mitral) **valve**. The left atrioventricular valve has two cusps. The larger anterior cusp lies anterior to, and to the right of, the poste-

67

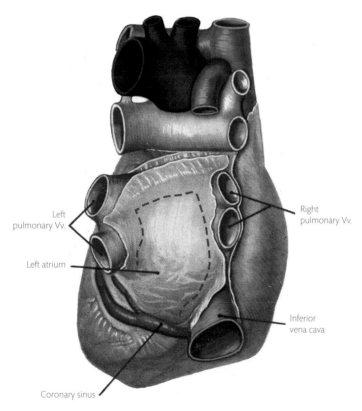

Left
pulmonary Vv.

Right
pulmonary Vv.

Left atrium

Inferior
vena cava

Coronary sinus

Fig. 4.40 Position of incision to open the left atrium.

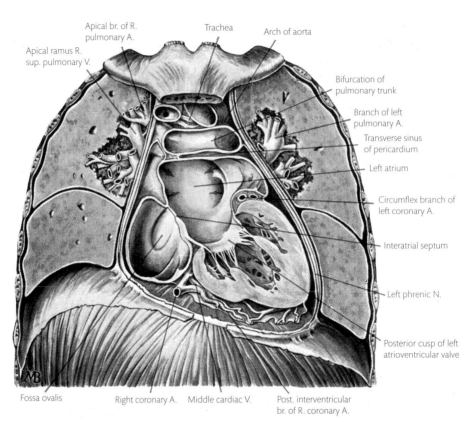

Apical br. of R.
pulmonary A.

Apical ramus R.
sup. pulmonary V.

Trachea

Arch of aorta

Bifurcation of
pulmonary trunk

Branch of left
pulmonary A.

Transverse sinus
of pericardium

Left atrium

Circumflex branch of
left coronary A.

Interatrial septum

Left phrenic N.

Posterior cusp of left
atrioventricular valve

Fossa ovalis

Right coronary A.

Middle cardiac V.

Post. interventricular
br. of R. coronary A.

Fig. 4.41 The heart *in situ*. A section through the heart to show the left atrium, interatrial septum, right atrium, left atrioventricular valve, and left ventricle. The arrows emerge from the pulmonary veins.

rior cusp. The cusps are attached to the fibrous ring of the left atrioventricular orifice [Figs. 4.36, 4.41] and project into the ventricle. The anterior papillary muscle sends chordae tendineae to the left or anterior halves of both cusps. The posterior papillary muscle is similarly attached to the posterior or right halves of both cusps. The anterior cusp forms the anterior wall of the atrioventricular orifice and the posterior wall of the aortic vestibule. It has blood flowing over both surfaces and, as a result,

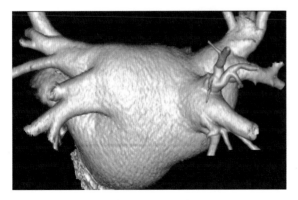

Fig. 4.42 Posterior view of 3D volume-rendered image of the left atrium and pulmonary veins.

both surfaces are smooth, with only a few chordae tendineae attached to its ventricular surface.

Fibrous skeleton of heart

The **fibrous skeleton** of the heart is made up of dense fibrous tissue. It surrounds the atrioventricular, pulmonary, and aortic orifices. The cusps of all four cardiac valves are attached to the fibrous skeleton. At the junction of the atrioventricular valves and the aortic valve are fibrous tissue triangles called fibrous trigones [Fig. 4.36]. The atrioventricular part of the skeleton prevents conduction of impulses from atrial to ventricular muscle in all areas, except through the atrioventricular bundle. The atrioventricular bundle pierces the fibrous tissue at the postero-inferior part of the interventricular septum. This arrangement ensures a time delay between atrial and ventricular contractions.

Conducting system of the heart

The conducting system of the heart is made up of muscle fibres specialized for generating and con-

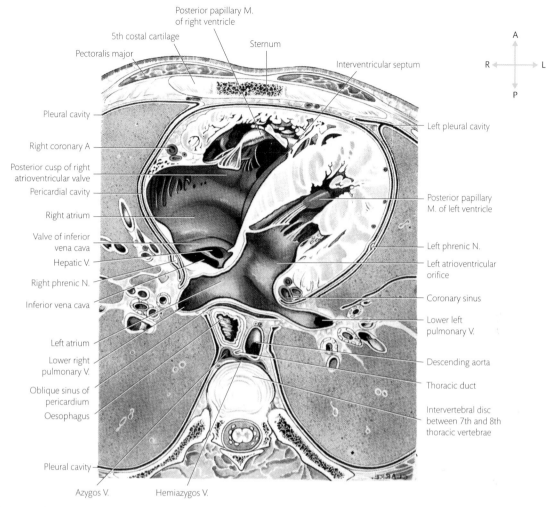

Posterior papillary M.
of right ventricle

5th costal cartilage

Sternum

Pectoralis major

Interventricular septum

A

R ←——→ L

P

Pleural cavity

Left pleural cavity

Right coronary A

Posterior cusp of right
atrioventricular valve

Pericardial cavity

Posterior papillary
M. of left ventricle

Right atrium

Valve of inferior
vena cava

Left phrenic N.

Hepatic V.

Left atrioventricular
orifice

Right phrenic N.

Inferior vena cava

Coronary sinus

Left atrium

Lower left
pulmonary V.

Lower right
pulmonary V.

Descending aorta

Oblique sinus of
pericardium

Thoracic duct

Oesophagus

Intervertebral disc
between 7th and 8th
thoracic vertebrae

Pleural cavity

Azygos V.

Hemiazygos V.

Fig. 4.43 A horizontal section through the thorax at the level of the intervertebral disc between the seventh and eighth thoracic vertebrae.

ducting electrical impulses in the heart. It cannot be demonstrated in fixed human hearts but is shown in the sheep's heart [Fig. 4.44]. The normal heartbeat is initiated in the **sino-atrial node** and spreads through the atrial muscles to the **atrioventricular node**. The impulses then run in the **trunk of the atrioventricular bundle** (a direct continuation of the atrioventricular node) and are disseminated rapidly through the ventricles through the **crura of the atrioventricular bundle** and their branches.

The sino-atrial node lies in the superior end of the crista terminalis in the right atrium, anterior to, and to the right of, the opening of the superior vena cava [Fig. 4.44]. The cells of the sino-atrial node generate the most rapid rhythm of all heart cells and hence function as the **pacemaker** of the heart. The impulse initiated in the sino-atrial node spreads through the atrial muscle and causes

it to contract. The rate at which the node generates impulses can be altered by nervous stimulation. It is accelerated by sympathetic stimulation and slowed, or even stopped, by vagal stimulation. If the sino-atrial node is destroyed, a slower heart rate initiated by the atrioventricular node is established.

The atrioventricular node consists of the same kind of tissue as the sino-atrial node. It lies in the postero-inferior part of the interatrial septum, immediately above the opening of the coronary sinus. It receives impulses from the atrial muscle and transmits them to the atrioventricular bundle.

The atrioventricular bundle or trunk passes antero-inferiorly from the atrioventricular node. It pierces the fibrous atrioventricular tissue and passes along the upper edge of the muscular interventricular septum. Here it lies inferior to the line of attachment of the septal cusp of the right atrioventricular

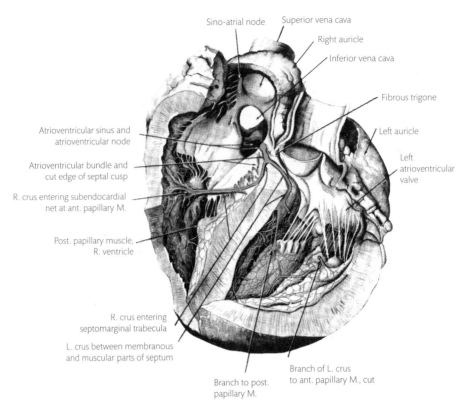

Fig. 4.44 The conducting system of the sheep's heart as seen in an injected specimen.

valve. The atrioventricular trunk divides into the right and left **crura** which straddle the muscular interventricular septum [Fig. 4.44] and lie beneath the endocardium—the inner lining of the heart.

The right crus passes towards the septal end of the septomarginal trabecula. It gives branches to the septum and posterior papillary muscle and runs in the septomarginal trabecula to the anterior papillary muscle. It supplies this muscle and spreads out on the wall of the right ventricle.

The left crus pierces the interventricular septum between its membranous and muscular parts. It descends on the left of the septum to the posterior papillary muscle of the left ventricle and gives fine strands around the cavity of the ventricle to the anterior papillary muscle. Branches of this crus also spread out to form a subendocardial network [Fig. 4.44]. The sino-atrial node, atrioventricular node, and atrioventricular bundle are supplied by the right coronary artery.

Nerves of the heart

The nerves which supply the heart are from the cardiac plexuses which lie on the bifurcation of the trachea. They consist of sympathetic, parasympathetic, and sensory fibres. **Sympathetic fibres** come from the cervical and upper thoracic ganglia of the sympathetic trunk. Sensory fibres transmitting pain run with the sympathetics. **Parasympathetic fibres** arise in the cells of the cardiac plexuses and in ganglion cells scattered along the vessels of the heart. The preganglionic fibres come from the vagus. The vagus also transmits sensory fibres. Stimulation of the sympathetic fibres dilates the coronary arteries and causes an increase in the rate and strength of cardiac contraction. Vagal stimulation slows or even stops the heart. The nerve fibres reach the heart along the great arteries (forming coronary plexuses on the coronary vessels) and veins. Many nerves accompany the conducting tissue of the heart [Fig. 4.45].

Superficial cardiac plexus

The superficial cardiac plexus is the left extremity of a complicated plexus of nerve cells and fibres which extends from the bifurcation of the trachea to the concavity of the arch of the aorta.

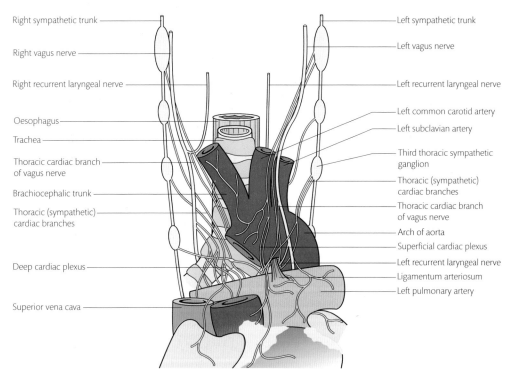

Right sympathetic trunk

Right vagus nerve

Right recurrent laryngeal nerve

Oesophagus

Trachea

Thoracic cardiac branch
of vagus nerve

Brachiocephalic trunk

Thoracic (sympathetic)
cardiac branches

Deep cardiac plexus

Superior vena cava

Left sympathetic trunk

Left vagus nerve

Left recurrent laryngeal nerve

Left common carotid artery

Left subclavian artery

Third thoracic sympathetic
ganglion

Thoracic (sympathetic)
cardiac branches

Thoracic cardiac branch
of vagus nerve

Arch of aorta

Superficial cardiac plexus

Left recurrent laryngeal nerve

Ligamentum arteriosum

Left pulmonary artery

Fig. 4.45 The cardiac plexus.

This figure was published in Gray's Anatomy: The Anatomical Basis of Clinical Practice, 40th Edition, Standring S. Copyright © Elsevier (2008).

It is continuous on the surface of the principal bronchi with the **pulmonary plexuses**. Together these plexuses send nerve fibres to the heart and lungs. The superficial cardiac plexus receives nerve fibres from the **superior cervical cardiac branch** of the left sympathetic trunk and the **inferior cervical cardiac branch** of the left vagus. (The deeper part receives the remaining cardiac branches from the sympathetic trunk and the vagus on both sides.) The **cardiac branch-es** of the vagus and sympathetic trunks descend obliquely from the neck as a result of the caudal displacement of the heart during development. Branches from the superficial part of the cardiac plexus pass to the heart predominantly on the pulmonary trunk, but it is virtually impossible to demonstrate the cardiac plexus satisfactorily by dissection.

Using instructions given in Dissection 4.15 trace the branches of the left vagus to the heart.

DISSECTION 4.15 Branches of the left vagus

Objective

I. To identify the ligamentum arteriosum, left recurrent laryngeal nerve, and cardiac nerves arising from the left vagus.

Instructions

1. Find the left vagus on the aortic arch. Follow its **re-current laryngeal** branch beneath the concavity of the arch. The nerve lies postero-inferior to the **liga-mentum arteriosum** which unites the root of the left pulmonary artery to the aortic arch.

2. Identify the cardiac nerves on the aortic arch. They turn medially under the arch to join a plexus of nerve cells and fibres—the superficial cardiac plexus. This is the left extremity of the extensive **cardiac plexus** which sends branches to the heart and great vessels.

Deep cardiac plexus

This interlacing plexus of parasympathetic (vagus) and sympathetic nerve fibres lies on the lowest part of the trachea, posterior to the arch of the aorta. It contains scattered groups of ganglion cells which are mainly parasympathetic.

The deep cardiac plexus receives numerous **cardiac nerves** from the sympathetic trunks and the vagus. (1) **Cervical sympathetic** branches from the right superior cardiac nerve, right and left middle cardiac nerves, and right and left inferior cardiac nerves (the left superior cervical cardiac nerve goes to the superficial cardiac plexus). (2) **Thoracic sympathetic** cardiac branches from the second to fourth thoracic sympathetic ganglia. (3) Cervical cardiac branches of the **vagi** through their superior cervical, middle cervical, and right inferior cervical cardiac branches (the inferior cervical cardiac branch of the left vagus goes to the superficial cardiac plexus). (4) Thoracic cardiac branch of the right vagus. (5) Cardiac branches of both recurrent laryngeal nerves.

The deep and **superficial** cardiac plexuses form a single mass. Together they send **efferent (motor) fibres**: (1) directly to the atria and great vessels, and to the rest of the heart through the **coronary plexuses**; (2) to the lungs through the anterior parts of the lung roots (**anterior part of the pulmonary plexus**).

The cardiac plexuses are pathways through which the central nervous system controls the action of the heart and monitors blood pressure and respiration. In addition to efferent fibres, the plexuses transmit afferent (sensory) fibres from the great arteries, veins, and lungs through the vagus and upper thoracic ganglia of the sympathetic trunk. These fibres are responsible for carrying the pain of ischaemic disease of the heart (angina pectoris).

Bronchi

The right and left principal bronchi are branches of the trachea [Figs. 4.16, 4.46, 4.47]. Each bronchus passes inferolaterally into the hilus of the corresponding lung, in line with the inferior lobar bronchus. The extrapulmonary parts of the principal bronchi contain U-shaped cartilaginous bars similar to those in the trachea. As such, they are flattened posteriorly. The intrapulmonary parts of the bronchial tree are supported by irregular cartilage plates and tend to be cylindrical in shape.

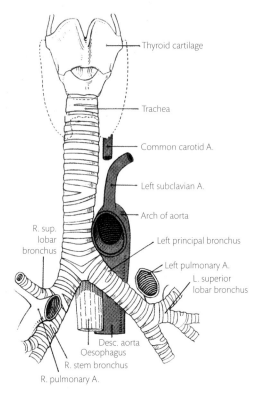

Fig. 4.46 The larynx, trachea, and bronchi. The thyroid gland is shown by the broken line.

Right principal bronchus

The right principal bronchus is approximately 2.5 cm long. This bronchus is wider and more vertical than the left. ⊃ As such foreign bodies which enter the trachea tend to fall into the right bronchus, and lodge in one or other of its branches, most usually in the right inferior lobar bronchus [Figs. 4.46, 4.48]. When this happens, the air distal to the block is rapidly absorbed and that part of the lung collapses and becomes solid.

The right principal bronchus begins anterior to the right margin of the oesophagus and has the azygos vein posterior and superior to it. More laterally, it is posterior to the ascending aorta, superior

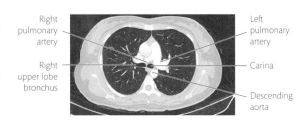

Fig. 4.47 Axial CT image through the upper thorax, in the lung window, showing the carina and the right upper lobe bronchus.

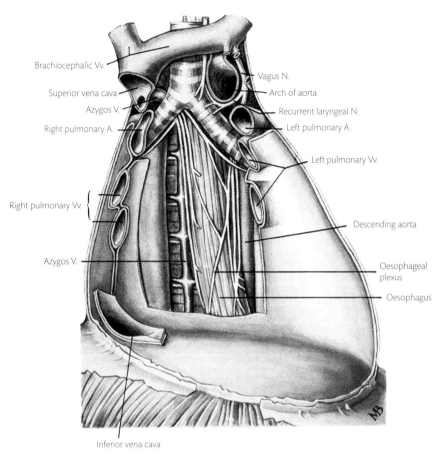

Brachiocephalic Vv.
Superior vena cava
Azygos V.
Right pulmonary A.

Right pulmonary Vv.

Azygos V.

Vagus N.
Arch of aorta
Recurrent laryngeal N.
Left pulmonary A.
Left pulmonary Vv.

Descending aorta

Oesophageal plexus
Oesophagus

Inferior vena cava

Fig. 4.48 Upper part of the posterior mediastinum as seen after removal of the heart and the posterior wall of the pericardium.

vena cava, and right pulmonary artery. The **right superior lobar bronchus** is the first branch of the right principal bronchus. It is also known as the **eparterial bronchus**. It arises immediately medial to the hilus of the lung, posterior to the right pulmonary artery [Fig. 4.13A].

Left principal bronchus

The left principal bronchus is more horizontal and longer (approximately 5 cm) than the right bronchus. This is because the distance from the tracheal bifurcation to the hilus of the left lung is greater, and because its first branch (the **left superior lobar bronchus**) arises within the lung substance [Figs. 4.46, 4.48].

Anterior to the left principal bronchus are the left pulmonary artery (which separates it from the left atrium) and the left superior pulmonary vein at the hilus [Fig. 4.14A]. The arch of the aorta is superior, and the descending aorta and oesophagus are posterior, to it.

Both bronchi have the corresponding bronchial vessels and pulmonary plexus on their posterior surface.

The superior mediastinum

Begin by reviewing the boundaries of the superior mediastinum. It extends from the inlet of the thorax to an imaginary horizontal plane drawn from the sternal angle to the intervertebral disc between the fourth and fifth thoracic vertebrae [Fig. 4.1].

Dissection 4.16 describes the dissection of the anterior structures of the superior mediastinum.

Brachiocephalic veins

The right and left brachiocephalic veins are formed by the union of the corresponding internal jugular and subclavian veins, posterior to the medial end of the clavicle. The two brachiocephalic veins

DISSECTION 4.16 Superior mediastinum-1

Objectives

I. To identify and trace the brachiocephalic veins, superior vena cava, and tributaries of the brachiocephalic veins.   II. To identify the arch of the aorta and its branches.   III. To identify and trace the left vagus and left phrenic nerves.   IV. To identify the ligamentum arteriosum and left recurrent laryngeal nerve.

Instructions

1a. If the upper limbs have been dissected and the clavicles divided, cut through the first ribs immediately anterior to the subclavian veins. Turn the manubrium of the sternum upwards to expose the superior mediastinum.

1b. If the upper limbs have not been dissected, make two drill holes through the middle of each clavicle approximately 1 cm apart. Cut through the clavicles between these holes with a fine saw; divide the first ribs as above, and turn the manubrium sterni upwards, together with

the medial parts of the clavicles and first costal cartilages. (Later, the cut ends of the clavicles may be drawn together by a wire passed through the drill holes.)

2. Identify the right and left brachiocephalic veins and the upper part of the superior vena cava [Fig. 4.22].

3. Find the inferior thyroid, internal thoracic, and left superior intercostal veins, and follow them into the brachiocephalic veins [Fig. 4.22].

4. Displace the veins and expose the remainder of the aortic arch and the branches arising from its convex surface. These are the brachiocephalic trunk, left subclavian artery, and left common carotid artery.

5. Find the left vagus and left phrenic nerves on the left surface of the aortic arch. Trace them superiorly between the left common carotid and subclavian arteries.

6. Find the left recurrent laryngeal nerve and the ligamentum arteriosum in the concavity of the aortic arch.

unite to form the superior vena cava posterior to the lower border of the first right costal cartilage at the margin of the sternum [Figs. 4.22, 4.25, 4.49, 4.50, 4.51].

The **right brachiocephalic vein** has a short, vertical course. It is lateral to the brachiocephalic

trunk and has the right phrenic nerve posterolateral to it. The **left brachiocephalic vein** passes downwards from left to right, posterior to the upper part of the manubrium sterni. It lies anterior to the origin of the left common carotid artery and the brachiocephalic trunk [Figs. 4.22, 4.25, 4.49, 4.50, 4.51].

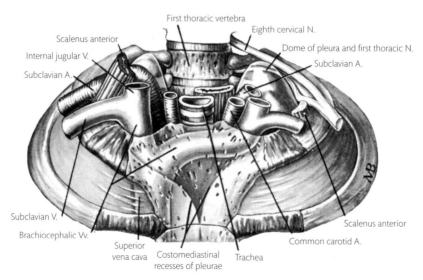

First thoracic vertebra

Eighth cervical N.

Scalenus anterior

Dome of pleura and first thoracic N.

Internal jugular V.

Subclavian A.

Subclavian A.

Subclavian V.

Scalenus anterior

Brachiocephalic Vv.

Common carotid A.

Superior vena cava

Costomediastinal recesses of pleurae

Trachea

Fig. 4.49 The superior aperture of the thorax. The anterior margins (costomediastinal recesses) of the pleural sacs and the great veins are shown through the sternum.

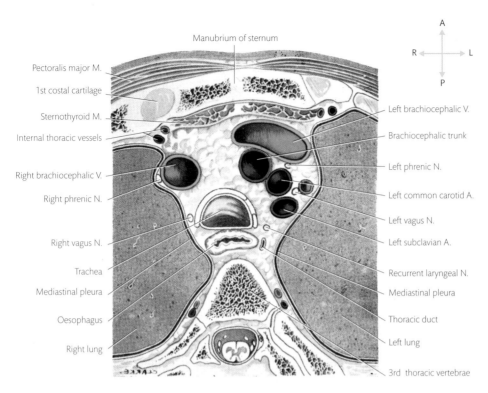

Manubrium of sternum

Pectoralis major M.

1st costal cartilage

Sternothyroid M.

Internal thoracic vessels

Right brachiocephalic V.

Right phrenic N.

Right vagus N.

Trachea

Mediastinal pleura

Oesophagus

Right lung

Left brachiocephalic V.

Brachiocephalic trunk

Left phrenic N.

Left common carotid A.

Left vagus N.

Left subclavian A.

Recurrent laryngeal N.

Mediastinal pleura

Thoracic duct

Left lung

3rd thoracic vertebrae

A

R ←→ L

P

Fig. 4.50 A horizontal section through the thorax at the level of the third thoracic vertebra.

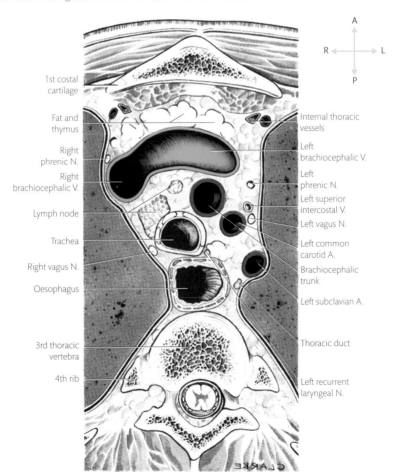

1st costal cartilage

Fat and thymus

Right phrenic N.

Right brachiocephalic V.

Lymph node

Trachea

Right vagus N.

Oesophagus

3rd thoracic vertebra

4th rib

Internal thoracic vessels

Left brachiocephalic V.

Left phrenic N.

Left superior intercostal V.

Left vagus N.

Left common carotid A.

Brachiocephalic trunk

Left subclavian A.

Thoracic duct

Left recurrent laryngeal N.

A

R ←→ L

P

Fig. 4.51 A horizontal section through the thorax at the level of the third thoracic vertebra (at a slightly lower level than the one in Fig. 4.50).

Tributaries of brachiocephalic veins

(1) Venous tributaries: the inferior thyroid, internal thoracic, vertebral, highest intercostal, and left superior intercostal veins drain into the brachiocephalic veins [Fig. 4.22].

(2) Lymphatic tributaries: the brachiocephalic veins receive all the lymph from the body. The left brachiocephalic vein drains lymph from almost all of the body through the thoracic duct. The right brachiocephalic vein drains lymph from the right side of the head, neck, upper limb, and mediastinum. The lymph trunks draining into the right brachiocephalic vein combine in different ways before entering the vein.

Arch of the aorta

The arch of the aorta begins posterior to the right half of the sternal angle as a continuation of the ascending aorta. It passes posteriorly with a slight inclination and convexity to the left, arching through the lower half of the superior mediastinum [Figs. 4.22, 4.29, 4.52]. It continues as the descending aorta on the left side of the intervertebral disc between the fourth and fifth thoracic vertebrae, in the same horizontal plane as its origin [Figs. 4.14B, 4.22]. Anteriorly, it is in contact with remnants of the thymus and with the left brachiocephalic vein. Further posteriorly, the left phrenic nerve, the cervical cardiac branches of the left vagus, the cervical cardiac branch of the left sympathetic trunk, the left vagus, and the left superior intercostal vein cross the left surface of the arch [Fig. 4.14B]. On the right side are the trachea and oesophagus, with the left recurrent laryngeal nerve between them [Fig. 4.53].

Inferior to the arch are the structures passing to the root of the left lung—the bifurcation of the pulmonary trunk, the left pulmonary artery, and the left principal bronchus [Figs. 4.22, 4.48]. The

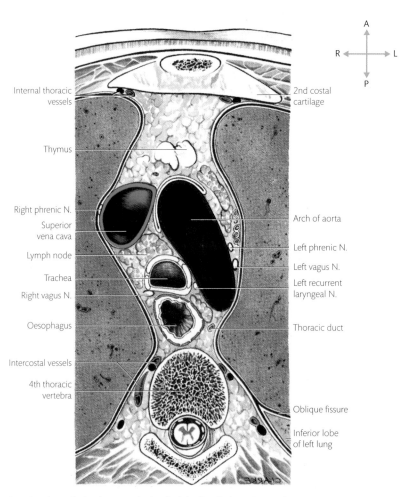

Fig. 4.52 A horizontal section through the thorax at the level of the fourth thoracic vertebra.

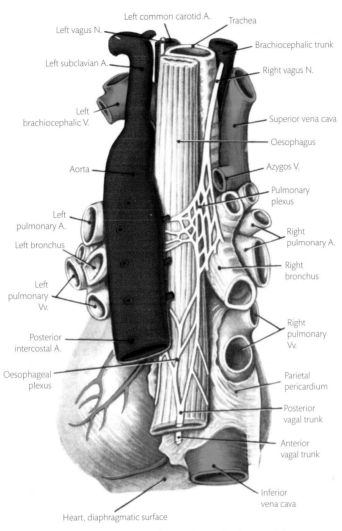

Labels on figure:

Left vagus N.
Left common carotid A.
Trachea
Brachiocephalic trunk
Left subclavian A.
Right vagus N.
Left brachiocephalic V.
Superior vena cava
Oesophagus
Aorta
Azygos V.
Pulmonary plexus
Left pulmonary A.
Right pulmonary A.
Left bronchus
Right bronchus
Left pulmonary Vv.
Right pulmonary Vv.
Posterior intercostal A.
Oesophageal plexus
Parietal pericardium
Posterior vagal trunk
Anterior vagal trunk
Inferior vena cava
Heart, diaphragmatic surface

Fig. 4.53 The posterior aspect of the heart and of the structures in the superior mediastinum and the upper part of the posterior mediastinum.

ligamentum arteriosum is a fibrous band which joins the arch of the aorta to the root of the left pulmonary artery [Figs. 4.22, 4.27]. The left recurrent laryngeal nerve passes under the ligamentum arteriosum to reach the groove between the trachea and oesophagus, on the right side of the arch [Figs. 4.14B, 4.22]. The superficial cardiac plexus lies on the ligamentum arteriosum.

Branches of the arch of the aorta

The **brachiocephalic trunk** is the first and largest of the three branches of the arch. It arises behind the centre of the manubrium sterni [Figs. 4.22, 4.50, 4.51], anterior to the trachea, and posterior to the left brachiocephalic vein. It passes superolaterally to reach the right side of the trachea. It ends posterior to the right sternoclavicular joint and anterior to the dome of the pleura by dividing into the right subclavian and right common carotid arteries. The small, inconsistent **thyroidea ima artery** may arise from it and supply the isthmus of the thyroid gland.

The **left common carotid artery** arises immediately to the left of the brachiocephalic trunk and follows a similar course, but on the left side. It is anterior to the left subclavian artery [Figs. 4.22, 4.49, 4.50], with the left vagus and phrenic nerves between them. It enters the neck posterior to the left sternoclavicular joint.

The **left subclavian artery** arises from the arch of the aorta further to the left and more posterior than the other branches. It ascends vertically in contact with the left mediastinal pleura. Thus it passes obliquely across the left side of the trachea, recurrent laryngeal nerve, oesophagus, and thoracic duct as they curve anteriorly on the vertebral column. The left subclavian artery enters the neck some distance posterior to the sternoclavicular joint and arches laterally, grooving the anterior surface of the cervical pleura [Figs. 4.49, 4.50].

Pulmonary arteries

These arteries are branches of the pulmonary trunk. They will be seen more clearly in the next dissection, but their position should be confirmed now.

The **right pulmonary artery** [Figs. 4.19, 4.22] begins in the concavity of the aortic arch, anterior to the left bronchus. It passes to the right and slightly downwards, anterior to the oesophagus and right principal bronchus, and posterior to the ascending aorta and superior vena cava. Close to the root of the lung, it gives off the branch which accompanies the right superior lobar bronchus.

The **left pulmonary artery** lies inferior to the posterior part of the aortic arch [Fig. 4.22]. It passes posteriorly and to the left, anterior to the left principal bronchus and the descending thoracic aorta [Fig. 4.14A].

Ligamentum arteriosum

The **ligamentum arteriosum** is a short fibrous band which connects the superior surface of the left pulmonary artery to the inferior surface of the arch of the aorta. It reaches the aorta distal to the origin of the left subclavian artery [Figs. 4.22, 4.27]. The left recurrent laryngeal nerve lies posterior to the ligament and the superficial cardiac plexus lies anterior to it. The ligament is the remnant of a wide channel—the **ductus arteriosus**—an important vessel in fetal life.

➲ If the ductus arteriosus fails to close soon after birth, the pressure in the pulmonary circulation remains high. As a result, the right ventricular wall hypertrophies. The heart therefore becomes globular in shape, and the persistent high pulmonary pressure (pulmonary hypertension) has serious effects on the functions of the heart and lungs.

Thoracic part of the trachea

The trachea is a wide tube, 10–12 cm long. It is kept patent by a series of U-shaped bars of **car-** **tilage** embedded transversely in its fibro-elastic wall. The posterior surface is flat [Fig. 4.50] where the ends of the cartilages are united by smooth muscle (trachealis) and fibro-elastic tissue. This surface is applied to the oesophagus. The thoracic part of the trachea is 5–6 cm long and lies in the median plane of the superior mediastinum [Fig. 4.52]. It bifurcates approximately at the level of the sternal angle (level of the third to fourth thoracic spines), but this level moves as the elastic trachea stretches on inspiration. The bifurcation may descend even to the level of the sixth thoracic vertebra.

The thoracic part of the trachea is nearly surrounded by blood vessels. Inferiorly, the **arch of the aorta** lies on the anterior and left surfaces of the trachea [Figs. 4.20, 4.52]; the azygos vein arches forwards on the right surface [Fig. 4.13A]. Superiorly, the anterior surface of the trachea is in contact with the **brachiocephalic trunk** and the **left common carotid artery** [Fig. 4.51]. More superiorly, the inferior thyroid veins and thyroidea ima artery lie in front of the trachea. The left surface is in contact with the left subclavian and left common carotid arteries, with the left vagus and phrenic nerves between them [Fig. 4.14A]. The right surface is covered with pleura, except where the right vagus nerve intervenes [Fig. 4.13B]. The posterior surface of the trachea lies on the oesophagus and left recurrent laryngeal nerve. The nerve sends branches to both the oesophagus and trachea.

Dissection 4.17 describes the dissection of the remaining structures in the superior mediastinum.

Structures passing through the superior mediastinum and posterior mediastinum

A number of important structures pass through the superior and posterior mediastina. They are: (1) the oesophagus which extends from the pharynx in the neck to the stomach in the abdomen; (2) the thoracic duct from the cisterna chyli in the abdomen to the veins in the neck; (3) the right and left vagi; and (4) the right and left sympathetic trunks. These structures are common to superior and posterior mediastinum and are described in the posterior mediastinum.

Objectives

I. To identify the tracheal bifurcation.   II. To trace the elements of the cardiac plexus where possible.

Instructions

1. Divide the ligamentum arteriosum and then remove the pulmonary arteries by separating them from the pleura. This exposes the tracheal bifurcation and the right and left principal bronchi.

2. Follow the **left recurrent laryngeal nerve** to the right side of the arch of the aorta. Note the branches given to the **deep cardiac plexus** on the anterior aspect of the tracheal bifurcation.

3. As the recurrent laryngeal nerve turns superiorly, medial to the aortic arch, it runs close to, or even in the same sheath as, the superior cervical cardiac branch of the left vagus and the middle and inferior cervical cardiac branches of the left sympathetic trunk. These branches descend to the deep cardiac plexus.

4. Expose the bronchi and the inferior part of the trachea.

The posterior mediastinum

Dissection 4.18 describes the dissection of some of the structures in the posterior mediastinum.

Thoracic parts of the vagus nerves

Right vagus

As it enters the thorax from the neck, the **right vagus** runs postero-inferiorly on the right surface of the trachea [Fig. 4.13B]. It is at first medial to the mediastinal pleura and then to the arch of the azygos vein. Posterior to the right bronchus, it divides into a number of branches—the **posterior part of the pulmonary plexus**. Fibres from the plexus pass laterally towards the lung and also to the left pulmonary plexus, anterior and posterior [Fig. 4.53] to the oesophagus.

The right vagus gives a **cardiac branch** which arises on the right of the trachea and descends on it to the deep cardiac plexus. It gives nerves to the heart, bronchi, and lung through the **pulmonary plexus** and to the oesophagus and pericardium through the **oesophageal plexus**.

Left vagus

The left vagus descends to the left side of the arch of the aorta between the left common carotid and subclavian arteries [Fig. 4.14A]. At the inferior border of the arch, it curves medially, gives off the left

Objective

I. To identify and examine the oesophagus, vagus, azygos vein, thoracic duct, and descending aorta.

Instructions

1. Remove the parietal pericardium between the right and left pulmonary veins. This uncovers the anterior surface of the oesophagus in the posterior mediastinum.

2. On each side of the oesophagus and posterior to the corresponding bronchus, find a vagus nerve leaving the pulmonary plexus as one or more trunks [Fig. 4.53]. Follow the vagi on to the oesophagus where their branches unite to form the oesophageal plexus.

Follow the plexus anterior and posterior to the oesophagus.

3. To the right of the oesophagus, find the azygos vein and its tributaries on the vertebral column.

4. To the left of this vein, find and follow the thoracic duct.

5. Lift the left side of the oesophagus forwards and uncover the anterior surface of the descending aorta. As far as possible, follow all these structures upwards and downwards.

6. Turn the trachea upwards to expose the oesophagus in the superior mediastinum, and lift the diaphragm forwards to expose the aorta in the inferior part of the posterior mediastinum.

recurrent laryngeal nerve [Figs. 4.22, 4.52], and breaks up into the left pulmonary plexus posterior to the left bronchus [Fig. 4.53]. It continues as several branches which pass on to the oesophagus (the **oesophageal plexus**).

The **left recurrent laryngeal nerve** curves medially round the inferior surface of the aortic arch, posterior to the ligamentum arteriosum. It sends branches to the deep cardiac plexus. The nerve then ascends in the groove between the left sides of the trachea and oesophagus, giving branches to both.

Pulmonary plexus

The major, posterior part of this plexus lies behind each lung root. Nerve fibres enter it from both vagi and from the second to fourth thoracic ganglia of the sympathetic trunks. The smaller, anterior part of the pulmonary plexus is an extension of the cardiac plexus. It receives branches from the corresponding vagus nerve above the lung root. Both anterior and posterior parts of the pulmonary plexus supply the lung root, the lung (including the smooth muscle of the bronchi), and the visceral pleura.

Oesophageal plexus

This nerve plexus surrounds the oesophagus. It contains nerve fibres from both vagi and sympathetic fibres which join it from the **greater splanchnic nerve**. It supplies the oesophagus, the pericardium, and the adjacent parietal pleura. Inferiorly, the nerves in the plexus come together to form the **anterior** and **posterior vagal trunks**. The two vagal trunks descend on the oesophagus and become the anterior and posterior gastric nerves on the stomach (each of the vagal trunks contains fibres from both vagi and from the sympathetics) [Fig. 4.53].

Oesophagus

The oesophagus extends from the pharynx in the neck through the superior and posterior mediastina to the abdomen. It pierces the diaphragm at the level of the tenth thoracic vertebra (ninth thoracic spine), 2–3 cm to the left of the median plane. In the superior mediastinum, it lies between the trachea and the vertebral column, slightly to the left of the median plane. It enters the posterior mediastinum behind the left principal bronchus and right pulmonary artery, and descends posterior to the left atrium. It is separated from the left atrium by the oblique sinus of the pericardium [Fig. 4.22].

The oesophagus then inclines to the left behind the posterior part of the diaphragm in front of the descending thoracic aorta. (The aorta passes to the median plane before entering the abdomen.)

The oesophagus is separated from the vertebral column sequentially by the longus colli muscle [Fig. 4.4], the thoracic duct, the azygos vein, the upper six or seven right posterior intercostal arteries, and the descending thoracic aorta.

The right side of the oesophagus lies adjacent to the right pleura, and the arch of the azygos vein in the upper part. Lower down, the oesophagus deviates to the left and indents the left pleura and lung [Fig. 4.11].

The left side of the oesophagus lies adjacent to the left pleura above the arch of the aorta, but the thoracic duct and upper part of the left subclavian artery intervene. The arch and the descending part of the aorta lie to the left of the oesophagus from the fourth to the seventh thoracic vertebrae. The left recurrent laryngeal nerve is anterior to the oesophagus in the superior mediastinum.

The oesophageal plexus surrounds the oesophagus in the posterior mediastinum.

The oesophagus is compressed and narrowed at three sites by: (1) the arch of the aorta; (2) the left principal bronchus; and (3) the diaphragm. These sites may be identified as narrowings of the lumen in a barium swallow (an oblique radiograph taken while radio-opaque barium is being swallowed). ➲ If the left atrium is dilated, it produces a large, smooth indentation on the oesophagus, inferior to that produced by the left principal bronchus [Figs. 4.13A, 4.14A, 4.19, 4.43, 4.46, 4.48, 4.49, 4.50, 4.51, 4.52, 4.53, 4.54].

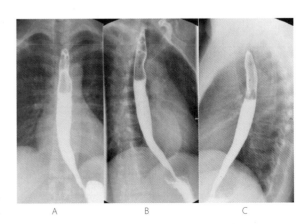

A   B   C

Fig. 4.54 Barium swallow. (A) Anteroposterior view. (B) Oblique view. (C) Lateral view.

Descending aorta

The descending aorta begins on the left side of the fourth thoracic intervertebral disc and descends through the posterior mediastinum [Fig. 4.14A]. The left pleura is on the left side of the aorta. The thoracic duct and azygos vein are on the right. Initially the descending aorta is posterior to the left lung root and the pericardium. Lower down, it inclines anteriorly and to the right behind the oesophagus to reach the anterior surface of the vertebral column behind the inferior part of the diaphragm. It enters the abdomen posterior to the **median arcuate ligament** of the diaphragm at the level of the twelfth thoracic vertebra. Posteriorly, the aorta lies on the vertebral column and the hemiazygos vein [Figs. 4.22, 4.29, 4.46, 4.50, 4.53].

Branches of descending aorta

From the anterior surface: (1) two **left bronchial arteries**. The superior of these may give rise to the right bronchial artery; (2) several **oesophageal branches**; (3) small branches to the fat and lymph nodes of the mediastinum, pericardium, and diaphragm; (4) superior phrenic arteries. From the posterior surface: nine pairs of **posterior intercostal arteries** [Fig. 4.53] and one pair of **subcostal arteries**.

Thoracic duct

This narrow, thin-walled tube conveys lymph from most of the body to the bloodstream. It drains the lower limbs, pelvis, abdomen, posterior thorax and frequently, near its termination, receives lymph from the left side of the head, neck, and left upper limb. The lymph in the thoracic duct often has a milky appearance because of the fine droplets of fat which enter it in the intestinal lymph trunk (**chyle**).

Using Dissection 4.19 follow the thoracic duct to its termination.

The thoracic duct arises from an elongated lymph sac—the **cisterna chyli**—which lies on the first and second lumbar vertebrae [Fig. 4.55]. At its origin, it lies between the aorta and the right crus of the diaphragm. It enters the thorax on the right of the aorta. In the posterior mediastinum, the thoracic duct lies between the aorta and the azygos vein, at first posterior to the diaphragm and then to the oesophagus. At the level of the arch of the aorta, the thoracic duct passes obliquely from right to left behind the oesophagus. The duct then ascends between the oesophagus and the left pleu-

ra to the root of the neck. Here it arches laterally and downwards to enter the junction of the left internal jugular vein and left subclavian vein.

The thoracic duct is frequently double in part of its course. It contains many valves. The last valve is a short distance from the end of the duct, so the terminal part of the duct may be filled with blood.

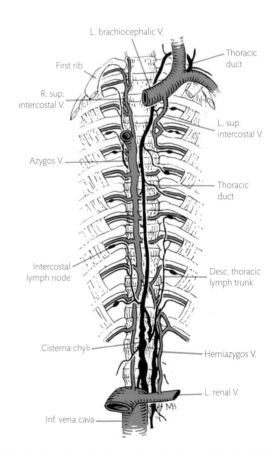

Fig. 4.55 The thoracic duct and posterior intercostal veins. In this case, no accessory hemiazygos vein is present and the number of venous communications across the midline is greater than usual.

Tributaries

The cisterna chyli receives: (1) the right and left **lumbar lymph trunks** which drain the lower limbs, the lower part of the anterior abdominal wall, the pelvis, and the posterior abdominal wall (including the gonads, kidneys, and suprarenal glands); (2) the **intestinal lymph trunks** which drain the abdominal part of the gut tube (except the superior part of the liver which drains through the diaphragm to mediastinal or parasternal lymph nodes); and (3) the lower **posterior intercostal lymph vessels**.

The thoracic duct receives: (1) the remaining posterior intercostal lymph vessels; (2) lymph vessels from the oesophagus, posterior parts of the diaphragm, and pericardium; (3) the left jugular and left subclavian lymph trunks which drain the left side of the head and neck and the left upper limb (though these may enter the left brachiocephalic vein independently); and (4) the **left bronchomediastinal trunk** which drains the left lung, the left side of the heart, and a large part of the mediastinum to the left of the brachiocephalic vein [Fig. 4.55].

Right lymph duct

The right lymph duct, when present, is formed by the union of the right jugular, right subclavian, and right bronchomediastinal lymph trunks. It is more usual for the right jugular and right subclavian lymph trunks to unite and drain into the junction of the right subclavian and right internal jugular veins.

The **right bronchomediastinal trunk** usually enters the right brachiocephalic vein. Like the corresponding vessel on the left side, it drains the right lung, the right side of the heart, the right mediastinum, and, in addition, the upper part of the right lobe of the liver.

Lymph nodes of the thorax

A number of named lymph nodes drain the thorax (and the upper part of the liver).

1. The **parasternal nodes** lie along the internal thoracic vessels. They drain an area corresponding to the distribution of the internal thoracic artery, with the addition of lymph from the upper part of the liver.
2. **Intercostal lymph nodes** lie in the posterior parts of the intercostal spaces and drain to the thoracic duct or cisterna chyli [Fig. 4.55].

3. **Phrenic nodes**. Some phrenic nodes lie on the diaphragm near the entry of the phrenic nerves. Others lie near the attachment of the diaphragm to the anterior thoracic wall.
4. **Posterior mediastinal lymph nodes** lie along the descending aorta. They drain the posterior mediastinum (including the diaphragm, pericardium, and oesophagus) to the thoracic duct.
5. **Tracheobronchial lymph nodes** lie on the thoracic part of the trachea and principal bronchi. They drain these structures and receive lymph from the lungs.
6. **Bronchopulmonary lymph nodes** lie in the hilus of the lung and at the bifurcation of the larger bronchi. They drain the lung and visceral pleura. (Pulmonary nodes lie in the substance of the lung.)
7. **Anterior mediastinal lymph nodes** lie beside the left brachiocephalic vein. They drain the heart, pericardium, and thymus.

The **bronchomediastinal lymph trunks** receive efferent vessels from the bronchopulmonary, tracheobronchial, parasternal, and anterior mediastinal lymph nodes. It ascends over the arch of the aorta on the left side or over the azygos vein on the right.

Lymph from the lungs contains phagocytes which have ingested inspired carbon particles. Many of these phagocytes remain in the interlobular septa of the lung, giving it a mottled appearance. Others reach the lymph nodes which become black with the carbon.

Dissection 4.20 describes the dissection of the remaining structures in the posterior mediastinum.

DISSECTION 4.20 Posterior mediastinum-2

Objectives

I. To identify and trace the posterior intercostal vessels and intercostal nerves.   II. To identify and trace the hemiazygos and accessory hemiazygos veins.

Instructions

1. Complete the exposure of the posterior intercostal vessels and the intercostal nerves. Follow the left posterior intercostal veins to the hemiazygos and accessory hemiazygos veins. Expose these veins and their communications with the azygos vein.

Posterior intercostal arteries

One posterior intercostal artery is present in each intercostal space [Figs. 4.13, 4.14, 4.53]. The posterior intercostal arteries to the first two spaces arise from the **highest intercostal branch** of the costocervical trunk—a branch of the subclavian artery. The highest intercostal artery descends anterior to the necks of the first two ribs.

The remaining posterior intercostal and subcostal arteries arise from the descending thoracic aorta. Because the aorta is displaced down and to the left, the right vessels are longer than the left, and the arteries going to the third to sixth spaces ascend to reach these spaces. The third right posterior intercostal artery usually gives the **right bronchial artery**. The posterior intercostal arteries lie on the periosteum of the vertebral bodies and are posterior to the azygos or hemiazygos vein, the sympathetic trunk, and the thoracic duct on the right side. Each artery enters the intercostal space between the vein (which lies superior to it) and the intercostal nerve (which lies inferior to it). It reaches the costal groove near the angle of the rib.

The **dorsal branch** of the posterior intercostal artery passes posteriorly with the dorsal ramus of the spinal nerve to supply the muscles and skin of the back. A **spinal branch** from it passes through each intervertebral foramen to supply the spinal cord and other contents of the spinal canal.

The **subcostal arteries** accompany the ventral rami of the twelfth thoracic (subcostal) nerves. They pass along the inferior borders of the twelfth ribs and enter the abdomen, posterior to the lateral arcuate ligaments of the diaphragm.

Intercostal nerves

The intercostal nerves are the ventral rami of the upper 11 thoracic spinal nerves. They pass laterally, posterior to the sympathetic trunk, to enter the intercostal spaces inferior to the intercostal vessels. (The course of the intercostal nerves is shown in Fig. 3.10.)

The greater part of the **first thoracic ventral ramus** passes up across the neck of the first rib to join the eighth cervical ventral ramus in the brachial plexus. The small **intercostal branch** runs across the inferior surface of the first rib to enter the first space close to the costal cartilage. It has no cutaneous branches. (The ventral ramus of the **second thoracic nerve** usually sends a small branch to the brachial plexus.)

The **subcostal nerve** passes into the abdominal wall with the subcostal artery. The lateral cutaneous branch of the subcostal nerve crosses the iliac crest to supply the skin in the gluteal region.

Posterior intercostal veins

The **highest**, or **first**, intercostal vein crosses the neck of the first rib to join the corresponding brachiocephalic vein. The second and third posterior intercostal veins unite to form the **right** and **left superior intercostal veins**. The right superior intercostal vein descends to enter the azygos vein. The left passes anterosuperiorly across the arch of the aorta to the left brachiocephalic vein [Figs. 4.13, 4.14, 4.55].

Of the remaining posterior intercostal veins (fourth to eleventh), those on the right side enter the azygos vein [Fig. 4.55]. On the left, the arrangement is variable. Commonly, the fourth to eighth left posterior intercostal veins enter the **accessory hemiazygos vein**. This descends with the aorta, crosses the midline, and enters the azygos vein at the eighth thoracic vertebra. It may be replaced by a number of veins entering the azygos vein separately [Fig. 4.55].

The ninth to eleventh left posterior intercostal veins and the subcostal vein drain into the **hemiazygos vein**. The hemiazygos arises in the abdomen from the posterior surface of the left renal vein. It pierces the left crus of the diaphragm, ascends to the ninth thoracic vertebra, crosses the vertebral column posterior to the aorta and thoracic duct, and joins the azygos vein.

Azygos vein

The azygos vein arises in the abdomen from the posterior surface of the inferior vena cava. It enters the thorax immediately to the right of the aorta and thoracic duct. It ascends in that position to the level of the fourth thoracic vertebra. It then arches anteriorly and empties into the superior vena cava [Fig. 4.55]. It lies at first posterior to the diaphragm and then to the oesophagus, on the anterior surface of the vertebral bodies. The arch of the azygos vein lies superior to the root of the right lung and lateral to the oesophagus, vagus, and trachea. At its termination into the superior vena cava, it lies medial to the phrenic nerve [Fig. 4.13].

➲ Occasionally, a part of the right lung—the **azygos lobe**—extends upwards between the arch of the azygos vein and the structures medial to it. When present, the azygos lobe is surrounded by visceral and parietal layers of pleura and is recognizable on X-rays.

Tributaries of the azygos vein

The azygos vein receives the **right superior intercostal vein**, the fourth to eleventh right **posterior intercostal veins**, the right **subcostal vein**, and blood from the posterior abdominal wall through the **ascending lumbar vein** on the right side. It also drains the same territory on the left side through the **hemiazygos** [Fig. 4.55] and **accessory hemiazygos veins**, except for the area drained by the left superior intercostal vein. **Bronchial veins** and some **oesophageal veins** also enter the azygos vein. The oesophageal tributaries of the azygos vein communicate through the oesophageal orifice in the diaphragm with **gastric veins**. This is one communication between the systemic (body wall) system of veins and the portal (gastro-intestinal) system of veins in the abdomen. (The clinical importance of this porto-systemic anastomosis is discussed later.) The azygos vein also forms anastomosis channels between the superior and inferior venae cavae through: (1) its connection with both venae cavae; (2) the origin of the hemiazygos vein from the left renal vein; and (3) the communications of the tributaries of the inferior vena cava and azygos veins in the valveless **internal vertebral venous plexus**.

The autonomic nervous system

The thoracic part of the sympathetic trunk consists of approximately 11 ganglia joined by longitudinal bundles of preganglionic and post-ganglionic fibres. In the superior part of the thorax, the trunk lies on the neck or head of the ribs. Inferiorly, it passes on to the bodies of the vertebrae as the bodies increase in width. The **first thoracic ganglion** is frequently fused with the inferior cervical ganglion to form the **cervicothoracic** (stellate) **ganglion** on the neck of the first rib. This ganglion may also include the second thoracic ganglion.

Branches of the sympathetic trunk in the thorax

1. **Grey** and **white rami communicantes** are nerves which join each ganglion to one (or two) intercostal nerves. The white rami are preganglionic fibres from the intercostal nerves to the sympathetic trunk. (These fibres have their cell bodies in the lateral horn of the spinal cord.) The grey rami are post-ganglionic fibres from the ganglion cells in the trunk to the intercostal nerves. They are distributed with the branches of the intercostal nerve.

2. **Visceral branches**:

   (i) From the upper five thoracic ganglia, **aortic** and **oesophageal branches** pass to these organs.

   (ii) From the third and fourth ganglia, **cardiac** and **pulmonary nerves** run antero-inferiorly on the vertebral bodies to the corresponding plexuses.

   (iii) The **greater splanchnic nerve** is formed by branches from the fifth to ninth ganglia. They give branches to the aortic and oesophageal plexuses and run antero-inferiorly on the vertebral bodies, pierce the crus of the diaphragm, and enter the abdomen.

   (iv) The **lesser** and **lowest** or **least splanchnic nerves** are formed by similar branches, respectively, from the ninth and tenth, and the last (eleventh) thoracic ganglia. They enter the abdomen together through the crus of the diaphragm.

See Clinical Applications 4.1–4.8 for the practical implications of the anatomy discussed in this chapter.

CLINICAL APPLICATION 4.1 Pneumothorax

Pneumothorax refers to a pathological accumulation of air in the pleural cavity. Symptoms: a small pneumothorax is mostly asymptomatic with minimal physical signs. A large pneumothorax presents with sudden onset of chest pain and breathlessness. Signs: percussion in intercostal spaces yields a typical hyperresonant note due to the underlying air in the pleural cavity. Auscultation reveals absent breath sounds over the affected hemithorax. Causes: spontaneous or primary pneumothorax occurs due to rupture of congenital subpleural blebs at the apices of the lung. Secondary pneumothorax occurs as a complication of an underlying lung disease such as asthma, tuberculosis, or lung abscess. Traumatic pneumothorax occurs from blunt or penetrating injuries of the thorax. Iatrogenic pneumothorax may occur following procedures such as pleural biopsy, positive pressure ventilation, and faulty placement of internal jugular or subclavian vein catheters. Tension pneumothorax results from an abnormal communication between the pleural cavity and the underlying lung acting as a one-way valve, allowing air to enter the pleural space during inspiration but not allowing it to escape during expiration. The accumulation of large amount of air in one pleural cavity causes compression of the lung and a gross shift of the mediastinum to the opposite side, resulting in significant compression of the opposite lung. Treatment: a small pneumothorax may resolve sponta-neously as air in the pleural cavity is absorbed. A large pneumothorax or tension pneumothorax will require the placement of a chest tube. The chest tube is placed within the pleural cavity, connected to an underwater seal drainage, and suction is applied till the air in the pleural cavity is removed, the lung expands, and the air leak subsides.

CLINICAL APPLICATION 4.2 Collapsed lung

When a bronchus is blocked, the air in the lung tissue distal to the block is absorbed into the pulmonary blood vessels, and that part of the lung collapses. Continuing respiratory movements will cause the remainder of the lung to expand and fill the space vacated by the shrinking lobe. If a large segment of the lung is collapsed, the mediastinum will shift towards the affected side as the opposite lung expands. Movement of the chest wall overlying a collapsed segment of the lung may be visibly or palpably reduced.

CLINICAL APPLICATION 4.3 Bronchogenic carcinoma

A 65-year-old chronic smoker presents with a history of cough, haemoptysis (coughing up of blood), dyspnoea (difficulty in breathing), and significant loss of weight and appetite. On examination, his respiratory rate is slightly increased and he has a palpable supraclavicular lymph node. Auscultation reveals decreased breath sounds over the right lung. Chest X-ray and computerized tomography (CT) of the thorax reveal a large mass in the right lung. Biopsy of the mass confirms a diagnosis of bronchogenic carcinoma.

Study question 1: what is the most common risk factor for bronchogenic carcinoma? (Answer: the most common risk factor worldwide is cigarette smoking.)

Study question 2: what is the possible cause for haemoptysis in this patient? (Answer: in lung cancer, haemoptysis indicates a malignant infiltration of bronchial vessels.)

Study question 3: what is the significance of an enlarged supraclavicular lymph node? (Answer: lymph from the lung drains to the lower cervical lymph nodes, which lie in the supraclavicular fossa. The clinical finding of an enlarged supraclavicular lymph node is known as the 'Troisier's sign'. It usually indicates an advanced stage of malignancy.) The supraclavicular node itself is called the 'Virchow's node'.

CLINICAL APPLICATION 4.4 Metastatic lung tumours

Metastatic lung tumours are malignancies that have spread to the lung from a primary tumour at another site—commonly the breast, colon, or urinary bladder. Fig. 4.56 is a radiograph of a 55-year-old woman with metastatic lung cancer.

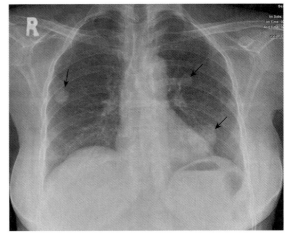

Fig. 4.56 Chest X-ray of a 55-year-old woman with metastatic lung tumours (arrows).

CLINICAL APPLICATION 4.5   Pericarditis

A 40-year-old man presents with a history of low-grade fever and sharp, stabbing chest pain behind the sternum. The pain typically increases with cough and deep breathing and is partially relieved on sitting up and leaning forwards. Auscultation of the chest reveals an audible friction rub heard over the region of the heart. An echocardiogram reveals a mild pericardial effusion.

Study question 1: what is pericarditis? (Answer: pericarditis is inflammation of the pericardium. It commonly occurs as a complication of viral infections or tuberculosis. Other common causes include connective tissue disorders, post-myocardial infarction, malignancy, and uraemia. A friction rub over the pericardium is a typical extra heart sound heard in pericarditis.)

Study question 2: what is pericardial effusion? (Answer: pericardial effusion is a pathological collection of fluid in the pericardial cavity. Large effusions (>1000 ml) that develop gradually over a long period of time may not cause significant haemodynamic changes as the per-

icardium stretches to accommodate the fluid. However, rapidly developing effusions (even 300 ml) can cause severe haemodynamic changes requiring urgent medical treatment.)

Study question 3: what is cardiac tamponade? (Answer: a rapidly developing pericardial effusion that compresses the heart is called cardiac tamponade. Diastolic filling of atria is significantly compromised due to external pressure on the heart. Jugular venous pressure is elevated and systolic blood pressure often low. Heart sounds seem distant and muffled on auscultation. Pericardial tamponade is a medical emergency requiring urgent surgical drainage.)

Study question 4: how is pericardiocentesis done? (Answer: an aspiration needle is introduced into the fifth left intercostal space near the sternum. This approach to the pericardial sac avoids going through the pleura or lung—both of which deviate to the left in this location, leaving the pericardium bare [Fig. 4.23].)

CLINICAL APPLICATION 4.6   Valvular heart disease

A 33-year-old man presents in the clinic with a history of fatigue, palpitations, and gradually increasing breathlessness over the past year. His blood pressure was 120/70 mmHg and pulse rate 80/minute. Examination of the cardiovascular system revealed a forceful apex beat in the seventh left intercostal space, 3 cm lateral to the midclavicular line. On auscultation, a pansystolic murmur was heard loudest at the mitral area and radiated to the left axilla. A diagnosis of mitral regurgitation was made.

Study question 1: what is the function of heart valves? (Answer: heart valves permit unidirectional blood flow and prevent retrograde flow of blood.)

Study question 2: what would be the result of an incompetent mitral valve? (Answer: an incompetent mitral valve causes regurgitation of left ventricular blood into the left atrium during ventricular systole.)

Study question 3: what is the normal position of the apex beat? (Answer: fifth left intercostal space, 1 cm medial to the mid-clavicular line.)

Study question 4: what is the probable cause for the apex beat being grossly displaced in this patient? (Answer: the apex beat is shifted downwards and outwards, indicating a grossly enlarged left ventricle.)

Study question 5: list the components of the mitral valve complex. (Answer: the mitral valve complex includes the mitral valve, chordae tendineae, papillary muscles of the left ventricle, and surrounding myocardium. Dysfunction of any of these components can cause regurgitation of blood.)

Study question 5: can damaged heart valves be repaired or replaced? (Answer: damaged heart valves cannot be repaired, but they can be replaced by prosthetic valves. Prosthetic valves are of two types: (1) mechanical valves are made of pyrolytic carbon and titanium; and (2) bioprosthetic valves are made of animal tissue. Tissue valves are again of two types: (1) xenografts—made from porcine valves or bovine pericardium; and (2) homografts—from human cadavers.)

CLINICAL APPLICATION 4.7 Myocardial infarction

A 65-year-old man was admitted with sudden onset of severe chest pain, nausea, vomiting, and breathlessness. His pulse was weak and rapid, blood pressure low, and breath sounds were harsh. An electrocardiogram (ECG) confirmed that he had had a myocardial infarction—a heart attack. A CT coronary angiogram revealed marked narrowing of the coronary arteries and many of their branches due to atherosclerosis. (Atherosclerosis is a pathological condition resulting in narrowing and hardening of arteries. Myocardial infarction is the death of cardiac muscle, which has been deprived of blood due to sudden blockage of one or both of the coronary arteries or their branches.)

Study question 1: what is the arterial supply of the heart? From where do these arteries arise? (Answer: the heart is supplied by the left and right coronary arteries. They are branches of the ascending aorta and arise from the right and left posterior aortic sinuses, respectively.)

Study question 2: what arteries supply the interventricular septum? (Answer: the anterior interventricular branch of the left coronary artery and the posterior interventricular branch of the right coronary artery supply the interventricular septum. The anterior interventricular artery supplies a larger area of the septum.)

Study question 3: what is the arterial supply to the sino-atrial node? (Answer: the sino-atrial node is supplied by a branch of the right coronary artery.)

CLINICAL APPLICATION 4.8 Pacemaker

The normal heartbeat is controlled by the sinus node. The electrical signal generated by the sinus node spreads throughout the heart, causing it to beat. The most common reason for pacemaker implantation is because the sinus node function becomes too slow. The artificial pacemaker is implanted subcutaneously below the left clavicle. Fig. 4.57 is an X-ray of a patient with a cardiac pacemaker. The pacemaker is in the subcutaneous tissue of the anterior chest wall.

Study exercise 1: follow the wire from the pacemaker through the large veins and chambers of the heart, naming the structures it lies in sequentially. (Answer: the wire from the pacemaker runs through the left subclavian vein, left brachiocephalic vein, superior vena cava, and right atrium, through the right atrioventricular valve to the right ventricle.)

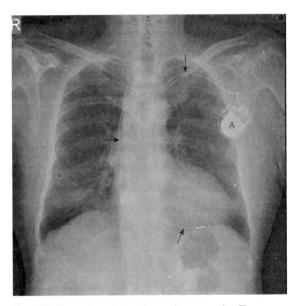

Fig. 4.57 X-ray of a patient with a cardiac pacemaker. The pacemaker is in the subcutaneous tissue of the anterior chest wall (A). Arrows = pacemaker wire.

CHAPTER 5
The joints of the thorax

Introduction

The joints on the anterior wall of the thorax are the sternal joints (between the parts of the sternum), the sternocostal joints (between the sternum and costal cartilages), the costochondral joints (between the ribs and costal cartilages), and the interchondral joints (between adjacent costal cartilages).

Posteriorly are the joints between the ribs and the thoracic vertebrae. The joints between adjacent vertebrae are described in Chapter 1 and will be dissected here.

Dissection 5.1 provides instructions for dissecting the joints between the sternum, the costal cartilages, and the ribs.

DISSECTION 5.1 Joints between the sternum, costal cartilages, and ribs

Objective

I. To study the sternal, sternocostal, interchondral, and costochondral joints.

Instructions

1. Identify the manubriosternal, xiphisternal, sternocostal, interchondral, and costochondral joints in the anterior chest wall which was reflected downwards.

2. Identify the ligaments on the surfaces of these joints, and then remove a thin slice from the anterior surface of each to expose the interior.

Sternal joints

The three parts of the sternum are united by the **manubriosternal** and **xiphisternal joints**. The manubriosternal joint lies at the sternal angle. The articular surfaces of the manubrium and the body of the sternum are covered with cartilage and united by a **fibrous disc**. There may be a small cavity in the disc. The joint is strengthened anteriorly and posteriorly by extensions from the periosteum. This manubriosternal joint moves with respiration and so rarely ossifies, even in old age.

The hyaline cartilages uniting the four sternebrae ossify between childhood and 21 years of age.

The cartilaginous xiphisternal joint between the body of the sternum and the xiphoid process ossifies in middle life.

Sternocostal joints

The first seven pairs of costal cartilages articulate with the margins of the sternum. The **first costal cartilages** begin to ossify at the end of growth and are fused with the manubrium. As such, the two first ribs, their costal cartilages, and the manubrium become a rigid structure which moves as one piece on the first costovertebral joints.

The **second** to **seventh** sternocostal joints are synovial in type. Each has a fibrous capsule which is strengthened anteriorly and posteriorly by a **radiate sternocostal ligament**. The ligament passes from the costal cartilage to the sternum. The joint cavity of the second sternocostal joint is divided into two by the **intra-articular sternocostal ligament**. This ligament passes from the costal cartilage to the

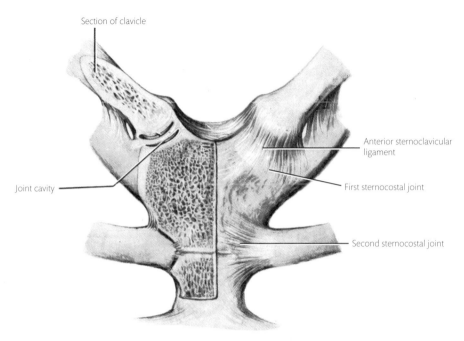

Section of clavicle

Anterior sternoclavicular ligament

First sternocostal joint

Joint cavity

Second sternocostal joint

Fig. 5.1 Sternocostal joints. A coronal section has been made through the anterior surface of the sternum and the costal cartilages on the left side to open the sternocostal joint.

fibrous disc in the manubriosternal joint. Some of the other joints may also be double [Fig. 5.1].

Costochondral joints

At the anterior end of each rib, the corresponding costal cartilage fits into a conical pit on the rib. These articulations form the **costochondral joints**.

Interchondral joints

There are small synovial **interchondral joints** between the adjacent margins of the costal cartilages of the sixth and seventh, seventh and eighth, and eighth and ninth ribs. Between the ninth and tenth costal cartilages, there is a fibrous joint. These interchondral joints increase the strength of the costal margin, while maintaining its flexibility.

Dissection 5.2 provides instructions for dissecting the costovertebral joints.

Costovertebral joints

The costovertebral joints are complex synovial joints between the ribs and the vertebrae.

DISSECTION 5.2 Costovertebral joints

Objective

I. To study the costovertebral joints.

Instructions

1. Expose the ligaments which unite the heads of the ribs to the vertebral bodies and the intervertebral discs [Fig. 5.2].

2. Expose the ligaments that join the tubercles of the ribs to the transverse processes of the vertebrae.

3. Remove the anterior parts of the capsules of the joints of one or more heads of the middle ribs, and identify the intra-articular ligament, if present.

1. Articulation of the head of the rib with the vertebral column. The **head of the rib** has two bevelled facets, the lower one for articulation with the posterolateral surface of its own vertebral body, and the upper one for articulation with the body of the vertebra above [see Fig. 3.3]. The two joints are separated by the intra-articular ligament attached from the head of the rib to the intervertebral disc between the vertebrae. The joints are surrounded by an articular capsule and are strengthened anteriorly by the **radiate ligament** of the head [Fig. 5.2].

2. Articulation of the tubercle of the rib with the transverse process of the vertebra. The articular

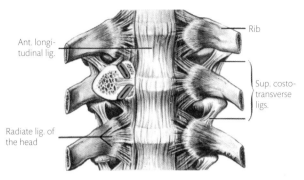

Ant. longi-
tudinal lig.

Rib

Sup. costo-
transverse
ligs.

Radiate lig. of
the head

Fig. 5.2 The anterior longitudinal ligament and costovertebral joints from in front. One joint has been opened by an oblique slice through the head of the rib.

part of the **tubercle of the rib** articulates with the transverse process of its own vertebra.

The presence of these two separate articulations between the rib and the vertebra forces the rib to move round an axis which passes posteriorly, laterally, and downwards through both articulations. The **costotransverse joint** is surrounded by an articular capsule. This is strengthened laterally by: (i) the **lateral costotransverse ligament** passing from the non-articular part of the tubercle to the tip of the transverse process; (ii) the **costotransverse ligament** uniting the neck of the rib to the anterior surface of the transverse process; and (iii) the **superior costotransverse ligament** joining the neck of the rib to the transverse process of the vertebra above. The gap between this superior costotransverse ligament and the vertebral column transmits the dorsal ramus of the spinal nerve and the dorsal branch of the posterior intercostal artery.

There are two exceptions to this general arrangement: (1) the heads of the first and of the last three ribs articulate only with their own vertebral bodies; and (2) the last two ribs do not articulate with the transverse process and so have a much greater range of movement.

Movements of ribs

These have been described already [Chapters 2 and 3]. Note that during inspiration: (1) the **two first ribs**, together with the manubrium sternum, move up as one piece on the first thoracic vertebra. These ribs slope downwards and forwards, so that raising the ribs and manubrium increases the anteroposterior diameter of the superior aperture of the thorax. (The pure vertical movement does not put pressure

on the structures which pass laterally over the first rib.); (2) raising the **true ribs** carries the body of the sternum anteriorly (as in the movements of the first ribs) and increases the anteroposterior diameter of the thorax. The true ribs also move outwards on their obliquely placed posterior hinge [see Fig. 3.7] and so increase the transverse diameter of the thorax; (3) the **false ribs** also move upwards and outwards. By this movement the tendency of the diaphragm to draw the costal margin inwards is resisted; and (4) the **eleventh** and **twelfth ribs** are held down by the muscles of the abdominal wall (posterior part of the external oblique and quadratus lumborum). As such, they increase the efficiency of the diaphragmatic contraction and prevent it from raising the costodiaphragmatic recess of the pleura.

Joints and ligaments of the vertebral column

The intervertebral discs, facet joints, and ligaments of the vertebral column are described in Chapter 1. If the head and neck have been dissected and the spinal cord removed, it is possible to see all the features of the vertebral ligaments now. If this has not been done, display of these structures should be delayed. A clear picture can be obtained from the following description, illustrations, and study of the appropriate vertebrae.

Dissection 5.3 provides instructions for dissecting the intervertebral joints.

DISSECTION 5.3 Intervertebral joints

Objective

I. To study the intervertebral discs.

Instructions

1. If the spinal cord has been removed, cut out a length of the thoracic vertebral column. Split it in the median plane with a saw. Identify the parts of the intervertebral discs and their relation to the vertebral canal and intervertebral foramina.

2. If the spinal cord is *in situ*, expose the anterior part of the intervertebral disc by removing a segment of the anterior longitudinal ligament.

3. Note the positions and orientation of the articular facets.

CHAPTER 6
MCQs for part 2: The thorax

The following questions have four options each. You are required to choose the most correct answer.

1. **The suprapleural membrane extends from the transverse process of the**
   A. seventh cervical vertebra to the inner margin of the first rib
   B. seventh cervical vertebra to the outer margin of the first rib
   C. first thoracic vertebra to the inner margin of the first rib
   D. first thoracic vertebra to the outer margin of the first rib

2. **The muscle fibres present in the suprapleural membrane are the**
   A. scalenus anterior
   B. scalenus posterior
   C. scalenus medius
   D. scalenus minimus

3. **Tributaries of the azygos vein include the**
   A. highest intercostal vein
   B. internal thoracic vein
   C. left superior intercostal vein
   D. right superior intercostal vein

4. **All the cardiac veins drain into the coronary sinus, EXCEPT**
   A. anterior cardiac vein
   B. great cardiac vein
   C. middle cardiac vein
   D. small cardiac vein

5. **The oesophagus is indented by the adjacent**
   A. right atrium
   B. right principal bronchus
   C. arch of the aorta
   D. trachea

6. **The highest intercostal artery arises from the**

   A. descending thoracic aorta
   B. costocervical trunk
   C. thyrocervical trunk
   D. internal thoracic artery

7. **The fibrous pericardium is innervated by the**

   A. vagus
   B. greater splanchnic nerve
   C. phrenic nerve
   D. superficial cardiac plexus

8. **The greater splanchnic nerve enters the abdomen by**

   A. piercing the crus of the diaphragm
   B. piercing the central tendon
   C. passing posterior to the median arcuate ligament
   D. passing posterior to the medial arcuate ligament

9. **The right border of the heart is formed by the**

   A. right ventricle only
   B. right atrium only
   C. right ventricle and right atrium
   D. right atrium, right ventricle, and pulmonary trunk

10. **The base of the heart is separated from the diaphragmatic surface by the**

    A. anterior part of the coronary sulcus
    B. posterior part of the coronary sulcus
    C. anterior interventricular sulcus
    D. posterior interventricular sulcus

11. **All the following muscles are innervated by the intercostal nerves, EXCEPT**

    A. intercostal
    B. subcostal
    C. serratus anterior
    D. serratus posterior

12. **The second sternocostal joint is a**

    A. fibrous joint
    B. primary cartilaginous joint
    C. secondary cartilaginous joint
    D. synovial joint

13. **In the posterior mediastinum, the thoracic duct lies between the**
    A. aorta and oesophagus
    B. aorta and azygos vein
    C. aorta and hemiazygos vein
    D. oesophagus and azygos vein

14. **All the following arteries are branches of the descending thoracic aorta, EXCEPT**
    A. superior left bronchial
    B. inferior left bronchial
    C. right bronchial
    D. subcostal

15. **All the following plexuses receive contribution from the right vagus nerve, EXCEPT**
    a. superficial cardiac plexus
    B. deep cardiac plexus
    C. oesophageal plexus
    D. pulmonary plexus

Please go to the back of the book for the answers.

PART 3

The abdomen

CHAPTER 7
Introduction to the abdomen

Before starting dissection of the abdomen, it is important to appreciate the position of the abdomen in relation to the other parts of the body. This is best achieved by examining the bony points in a living individual and relating these to the bones on a mounted skeleton.

Anteriorly, the **abdominal wall** extends from the **xiphoid process** to the **pubic symphysis**, from the level of the ninth thoracic vertebra to the **coccyx**. Laterally and posteriorly, the abdominal cavity is overlapped by: (1) the thorax superiorly and (2) the gluteal region of the lower limb inferiorly. Due to the overlap of the abdominal and thoracic cavities, the upper abdominal contents fill the concavity of the **diaphragm**. They lie internal to the lower parts of the thoracic cage, pleura, and lungs and are separated from them by the diaphragm. Some abdominal contents reach as high as the level of the eighth thoracic vertebra in the median plane and the fifth rib in the right mid-clavicular line in full expiration. The **costal margin** lies at the level of the first lumbar vertebra in the mid-clavicular line (ninth costal cartilage) and the third lumbar vertebra in the mid-axillary line (eleventh costal cartilage) [Fig. 7.1]. (Note: the **mid-clavicular**, **mid-axillary**, and **paravertebral lines** are three imaginary vertical lines which pass, respectively, through the middle of the clavicle, midway between the anterior and posterior axillary folds, and at the sides of the vertebral column. They are used for descriptive purposes.)

⮕ The overlapping of the abdominal cavity by the lower thorax and gluteal regions means that penetrating wounds of these regions frequently involve the abdominal contents. Also because the mobile diaphragm forms the upper limit of the abdominal cavity, the abdominal contents descend with it on inspiration. This fact is made use of in the clinical examination of organs such as the liver and the enlarged spleen, which may be palpated below the costal margin on deep inspiration. (They are within the thoracic cage in quiet respiration.) The kidney also moves with respiration and can be palpated in the lower back on deep inspiration.

Bones of the abdomen and pelvis

The skeleton of the abdomen and pelvis are formed by: (1) the lower ribs and costal cartilages; (2) the lumbar vertebrae; (3) the sacrum and coccyx; and (4) the hip bones [Fig. 7.1].

Lower ribs

The ribs and costal cartilages are described in Chapter 3. The eleventh and twelfth ribs are short and do not articulate either with the transverse processes of the vertebrae or with other costal cartilages. As such, they are capable of moving independently of the other ribs.

Lumbar vertebrae

The lumbar vertebrae have the same elements as the thoracic vertebrae but are more massive, in keeping with the greater load they bear. The large kidney-shaped **bodies** have flat upper and lower surfaces. As in other vertebrae, on the dry bones, these surfaces show a large, centrally placed, rough area surrounded by a raised, smooth margin. This

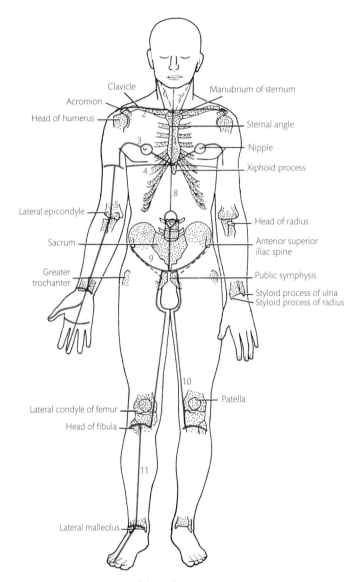

Fig. 7.1 Landmarks and incisions on the anterior aspect of the body.

margin is formed by the **ring epiphysis** which has fused with the upper and lower surfaces of the body [Figs. 7.2, 7.3]. These surfaces are nearly parallel to each other, except in the fifth lumbar vertebra where the body has a greater vertical height anteriorly than posteriorly. This height difference between the anterior and posterior surfaces of the body of the fifth lumbar vertebra, together with the wedge shape of the **lumbosacral intervertebral disc**, contributes to a sharp angulation between the anterior surface of the fifth lumbar vertebra and the first piece of the sacrum. This is the **lumbosacral angle** [see Fig. 1.2B].

The body of the lumbar vertebrae is narrow in the centre and wide close to the intervertebral discs. It is perforated by a number of vascular foramina. These foramina are particularly large on the posterior surface where one or two veins—the **basivertebral veins**—emerge from the body, pass lateral to the posterior longitudinal ligament, and drain into the internal vertebral venous plexus [see Fig. 13.8]. These basivertebral veins drain the **red marrow** in the vertebrae.

The thick **pedicles** of the lumbar vertebrae arise from the upper two-thirds of the posterolateral surface of the body, superior to a deep **inferior**

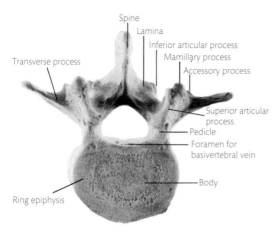

Fig. 7.2 The superior surface of the third lumbar vertebra.

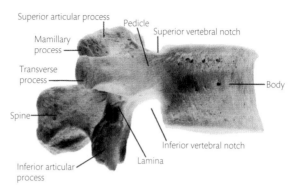

Fig. 7.3 The right surface of the third lumbar vertebra.

vertebral notch. The pedicles join the relatively narrow **laminae**. The laminae pass downwards and backwards to meet each other in a thick rectangular **spine**. The spine projects backwards, posterior to the lower two-thirds of the vertebral body and the intervertebral disc inferior to it. The **vertebral foramen** in the lumbar region is large and triangular and lies between the laminae and pedicles [Fig. 7.2].

The **inferior articular processes** project inferiorly from the lateral aspects of the laminae. Note the V-shaped gap between them. This gap is wider in the lower vertebrae. The **superior articular processes** project upwards from the junction of the pedicle and lamina. The curved facets on the anterolateral surface of the inferior articular processes fit between the blunt superior articular processes [Fig. 7.2]. This interlocking of the articular processes effectively prevents rotation in the lumbar region [see Fig. 1.6]. When two adjacent lumbar vertebrae are articulated, the V-shaped gap between the inferior articular processes is directed towards a similar gap between the laminae of the vertebrae below. Together they form a diamond-shaped interval in the posterior wall of the vertebral canal. This gap is filled by the **ligamentum flava** through which a needle may be introduced into the lumbar vertebral canal—the lumbar puncture. (Compare with the overlapping laminae in the thoracic region.)

The **transverse processes** of the lumbar vertebrae are thin and spatula-shaped in the upper lumbar vertebrae, but thick in the fourth and fifth vertebrae. In the fifth vertebra, the base of the transverse process extends forwards on to the vertebral body, further thickening the pedicles. In an articulated skeleton, the lumbar transverse processes can be seen to lie in series with the ribs. They represent rudimentary lumbar ribs fused to the vertebrae. The extension of the transverse process forwards in the fourth and fifth lumbar vertebrae represent an increase in size of these costal elements which reach the maximum size in the fused vertebrae of the sacrum. The true lumbar transverse process is represented by the small **accessory process** on the base of the dorsal surface of the transverse process. The accessory process is immediately inferior to the rounded **mamillary process** which projects posteriorly from the superior articular process [Fig. 7.2]. The accessory and mamillary processes give attachment to the erector spinae muscle.

Sacrum

The sacrum consists of five fused sacral vertebrae. The bodies of the sacral vertebrae are separated on the pelvic surface by transverse ridges which have the remnants of intervertebral discs between them. Lateral to each ridge is a **pelvic sacral foramen** [Fig. 7.4]. The pelvic sacral foramen is continuous posteriorly with a dorsal sacral foramen and medially with a sacral intervertebral foramen which leads into the sacral canal. The **sacral canal** is the continuation of the vertebral canal, posterior to the sacral vertebral bodies. It contains the caudal parts of the coverings of the spinal cord (the meninges) and the internal vertebral venous plexus. It transmits the sacral nerves to the sacral intervertebral foramina. At the sacral intervertebral foramen, the sacral nerves divide into ventral and dorsal rami which emerge through the pelvic and dorsal sacral foramina, respectively.

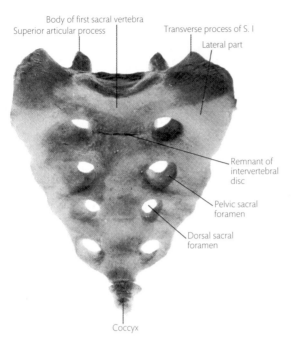

Fig. 7.4 The pelvic surface of the sacrum and coccyx.

The sacrum is wedge-shaped supero-inferiorly and anteroposteriorly. The broad **base** lies antero-superiorly at the marked lumbosacral angle. Here the anterior margin of the first sacral vertebral body projects forwards as the **sacral promontory**. The curved, concave pelvic surface of the sacrum forms the superior and posterior walls of the lesser pelvis. Inferiorly the sacrum ends in a blunt **apex** which articulates with the coccyx [Figs. 7.4, 7.5]. (The sacrum, the two hip bones, and the coccyx together form the skeleton of the pelvis.)

The dorsal surface of the sacrum shows three longitudinal crests—the **median, intermediate**, and **lateral sacral crests**. The median sacral crest is formed by the incomplete fusion of the upper three or four sacral spines. The intermediate sacral crests are formed by the fused articular processes. They lie medial to the dorsal sacral foramina. The intermediate crests are in line with the large, widely set superior articular processes of the sacrum. (The superior articular process of the sacrum articulates with the inferior articular process of the fifth lumbar vertebra.) The lateral sacral crests correspond to the transverse processes of the sacral vertebrae. They lie lateral to the dorsal sacral foramina and are a part of the **lateral part** of the sacrum. The lateral part of the sacrum is made up of the costal elements which are greatly expanded in the first two or three sacral vertebrae. On the lateral aspect of the sacrum is the curved

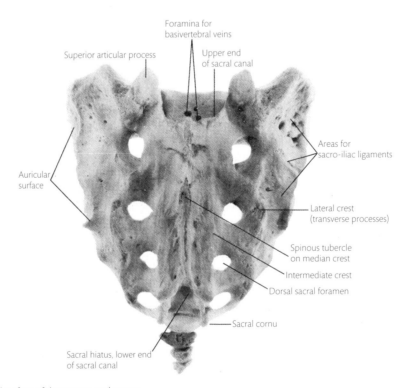

Fig. 7.5 The dorsal surface of the sacrum and coccyx.

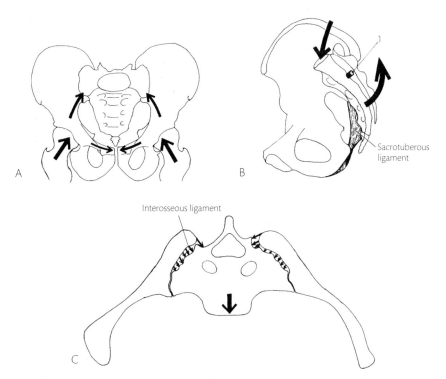

Fig. 7.6 Three diagrams to show the forces acting on the pelvis. (A) shows forces transmitted to the trunk from the lower limbs. (B) and (C) show the effects of the load of the body weight (static and dynamic) on the pelvis. The sacro-iliac joint-1, and sacrotuberous ligament (B) and the interpubic disc of the pubic symphysis (A) provide resilience to the pelvis. In (C), the wedge of the sacrum would appear to permit it to descend into the pelvis when bearing the weight of the trunk (large arrow). But this force is resisted by the posterior and interosseous sacro-iliac ligaments (small arrows) which draw the ilia inwards, and tighten the sacro-iliac joints.

auricular surface which articulates with the sacral surface of the ilium at the sacro-iliac joint [Fig. 7.5]. The fourth and/or fifth sacral spines and medial parts of the laminae are usually absent, leaving a dorsal opening in the lower part of the sacral canal. This opening is the **sacral hiatus** and is of variable length. On the sacrum and both ilia are rough areas, or **tuberosities**, posterior to the auricular surfaces. These tuberosities give attachment to the powerful **interosseous sacro-iliac ligaments**. The upper part of the sacrum lies almost horizontally [Fig. 7.6], wedged between the hip bones and suspended from them by ligaments. The body weight transmitted to the sacrum tends to drive it downwards. This downward movement tightens the posterior sacro-iliac ligaments and draws the two hip bones firmly against the sacrum. It increases the rigidity of the sacro-iliac joints by fitting the irregular surfaces closer together.

The surface of the sacrum which articulates with the lumbosacral intervertebral disc slopes downwards and forwards. The tendency for the fifth lumbar vertebra to slip forwards on the sacrum is prevented, in part, by the large superior articular processes of the sacrum. ➲ Occasionally, the laminae, spine, and inferior articular processes of the fifth lumbar vertebra may be fractured, or ossify separately from the remainder of the bone. When this happens, the fifth lumbar vertebral body may slip forwards and downwards on the sacrum (spondylolisthesis). The large transverse processes of the fifth lumbar vertebra may articulate with, or be fused to, the lateral part of the sacrum. This fusion may be unilateral or bilateral. The fifth lumbar vertebra may be completely fused with the sacrum—**sacralization of the fifth lumbar vertebra**—or the first sacral vertebra may be partly or completely separated from the remainder of the sacrum (**lumbarization of the first sacral vertebra**).

Coccyx

This small triangular bone consists of four partially fused rudimentary vertebrae [Fig. 7.5]. It articulates with the apex of the sacrum and is felt in the natal cleft. The tip of the coccyx lies at the level of the upper border of the pubic symphysis.

Hip bone

The hip bone is made up of the **ilium, ischium**, and **pubis** fused together [Fig. 7.7]. It has the appearance of a two-bladed propeller with a large blade—the ilium—directed upwards, and a smaller blade, made up of the pubis and ischium, directed downwards. The two blades are almost at right angles to one another and meet at a narrow, thick hub where the head of the femur articulates in the **acetabulum**. Inferiorly, the **pubis** lies anteromedially and the **ischium** lies posterolaterally, with a large aperture—the **obturator foramen**—between them. The pubis and ischium are fused at the ischiopubic rami and at the acetabulum. The ischiopubic ramus is a bar of bone formed inferior to the obturator foramen by the union of the **inferior ramus of the pubis** and the **ramus of the ischium**.

The bodies of the two pubic bones articulate with each other at the lowest part of the anterior abdominal wall. The joint between them is the **pubic symphysis**. The anterosuperior margin of the body of the pubis is the **pubic crest**. It extends laterally from the pubic symphysis to a small, blunt projection—the **pubic tubercle**—2.5 cm from the median plane. The pubic crest and tubercle may be palpated, though the tubercle is covered in the male by the soft, cylindrical **spermatic cord**. A sharp ridge—the **pecten pubis**—extends laterally from the pubic tubercle on the **superior ramus of the pubis**. Further laterally is a blunt ridge—the **iliopubic eminence** [Fig. 7.7]. The iliopubic eminence lies on the anterior wall of the acetabulum and marks the line of fusion of the superior ramus of the pubis with the ilium. (A less well-defined ridge on the posterior wall of the acetabulum marks the line of fusion of the ischium with the ilium.)

Lateral to the pubic tubercle, a resilient band is felt in the fold of the groin, between the abdomen and the thigh. This is the **inguinal ligament**. It extends from the pubic tubercle to the anterior superior iliac spine. The inguinal ligament is the inrolled margin of the aponeurosis of the

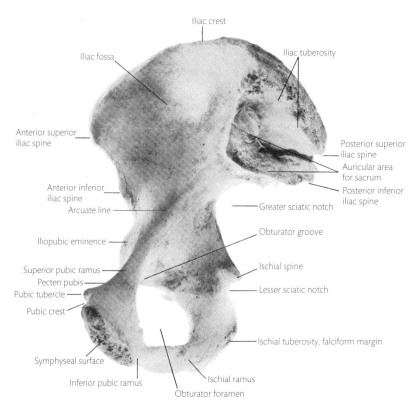

Fig. 7.7 Right hip bone seen from the medial side.

muscle of the anterior abdominal wall—the external oblique. Deep fibres of the inguinal ligament pass posteriorly to the pecten pubis as the **lacunar ligament**. These fibres continue along the superior pubic ramus as the **pectineal ligament**.

The two inferior rami of the pubic bones diverge from the subpubic angle. They form the **pubic arch** together with the rami of the ischia. In the anatomical position, the pubic arch lies horizontally and is palpable between the anterior part of the perineum (the urogenital triangle) medially and the thighs laterally. The ramus of the ischium expands posteriorly into the **ischial tuberosity**. The ischial tuberosity gives attachment to the hamstring muscles of the thigh and the sacrotuberous ligament. Superior to the ischial tuberosity is a shallow depression—the **lesser sciatic notch**. Further superiorly, the **ischial spine** projects posteromedially from the ischium and separates the lesser sciatic notch of the ischium from the **greater sciatic notch** on the posterior margin of the ilium. When the hip bone and sacrum are articulated together, the two notches form the lateral margin of a deep concavity between the bones. This space is converted into two foramina—the greater and lesser sciatic foramina—by the **sacrospinous** and **sacrotuberous ligaments**. The sacrospinous ligament passes from the sacrum to the ischial spine. The sacrotuberous ligament passes from the sacrum to the ischial tuberosity. The greater sciatic foramen leads from the lesser pelvis into the gluteal region, and the lesser sciatic foramen leads from the gluteal region into the perineum [see Figs. 15.4, 15.5].

The **ilium** is a flat, fan-shaped bone which extends superiorly from the acetabulum. The superior margin of the ilium forms the sinuous **iliac crest** at the lower margin of the waist. On yourself, follow the iliac crest forwards and backwards. Anteriorly, it slopes downwards and slightly medially to the **anterior superior iliac spine**. Posteriorly, it turns backwards and downwards to the **posterior superior iliac spine**. The posterior superior iliac spine lies at the bottom of the dimple at the level of the second sacral spine. **Anterior** and **posterior inferior iliac spines** lie on the margins of the ilium, inferior to the corresponding superior spines. The posterior inferior iliac spine lies at the level of the third sacral spine [Fig. 7.7].

The medial aspect of the ilium has three distinct surfaces. (1) The greater part of the medial aspect forms the smooth, concave **iliac fossa**. The iliac fossa lies superiorly and forms the bony wall of the greater pelvis. (2) Posterior to the iliac fossa is the sacral surface, consisting of the auricular surface and tuberosity of the ilium. (The auricular surface articulates with the sacrum.) (3) The part of the ilium medial to the acetabulum forms the superior part of the lateral wall of the lesser pelvis. A thick, curved ridge of bone—the **arcuate line of the ilium**—separates the parts forming the greater and lesser pelvis. The arcuate line crosses the ilium from the antero-inferior part of the auricular surface to the lateral end of the pecten pubis. This strong part of the ilium transmits compression forces from the vertebral column and the auricular surface of the ilium to the acetabulum and lower limb. The pubic crest, pecten pubis, arcuate line of the ilium, and promontory of the sacrum together form the **superior aperture of the (lesser) pelvis**—also called the **linea terminalis** of the pelvis. The internal surfaces of the ilium, pubis, and ischium contribute to the bony wall of the lesser pelvis. The anterosuperior margin of the obturator foramen is notched to form the **obturator sulcus** or **obturator groove**. The obturator foramen is covered by the obturator membrane—a fibrous sheet attached to the sharp margin of the foramen, except at the obturator sulcus. The obturator membrane bridges the sulcus and transforms it into the **obturator canal** which transmits the obturator vessels and nerve.

It is important to understand the orientation of the hip bone. The symphyseal surface of the pubic bones lies in the sagittal plane. The pubic tubercle and anterior superior iliac spine lie in the same coronal plane. The linea terminalis of the pelvis lies at an angle of approximately 70° to the horizontal, entirely superior to the pubic symphysis, with the sacral promontory at the level of the anterior superior iliac spines. As such, the superior aperture of the pelvis faces the lower part of the anterior abdominal wall. The upper border of the ischial tuberosities and the tip of the coccyx lie in the same horizontal plane. The **inferior aperture of the pelvis** is formed by the pubic arch, the ischial tuberosities, the coccyx, and the sacrotuberous ligaments. It is approximately horizontal and is filled by the perineum. In the median plane, the pubic symphysis forms the short antero-inferior wall of the lesser pelvis, and the sacrum and coccyx form the long posterosuperior wall.

CHAPTER 8
The anterior abdominal wall

Surface anatomy of the anterior abdominal wall

Anteriorly, in the midline, the **abdominal wall** extends from the surface of the **xiphoid process** to the **pubic symphysis**. On each side, the wall extends from the costal margin to the inguinal ligament. For purposes of description, the anterior abdominal wall is divided into nine regions by two vertical and two horizontal planes. The right and left vertical planes pass through the **mid-inguinal points**—a point on each inguinal ligament midway between the anterior superior iliac spine and the pubic symphysis. The **transpyloric plane** lies horizontally midway between the jugular notch of the sternum and the pubic symphysis, approximately midway between the xiphoid process and the umbilicus. It lies at the level of the first lumbar vertebra. The **transtubercular plane** passes horizontally through the tubercles of the iliac crests at the level of the fifth lumbar vertebra. The nine regions demarcated by these planes are (1) epigastric, (2 and 3) right and left hypochondrium, (4) umbilical or central, (5 and 6) right and left lumbar, (7) hypogastric or suprapubic, and (8 and 9) right and left iliac fossae [Fig. 8.1].

The mid-inguinal point marks the position where, deep to the inguinal ligament, the external iliac artery leaves the abdomen to become the femoral artery in the thigh. Feel the pulsations of the femoral artery at this point on yourself. On the cadaver, run your finger medially on the inguinal ligament to the pubic tubercle which is covered by the spermatic cord in the male. Immediately superolateral to the tubercle is the **superficial inguinal ring**—an aperture in the aponeurosis of the external oblique muscle of the abdomen. The **spermatic cord** descends to the scrotum in front of the pubis through the superficial inguinal ring [Fig. 8.2]. In the female, the **round ligament of the uterus** descends to the labium majus through the superficial inguinal ring. The margins of the ring are easily felt in the male. Place the tip of your little finger on the loose skin of the upper part of the scrotum in front of the pubis and spermatic cord and invaginate the skin upwards along the line of the cord. Where the cord disappears through the ring, the sharp margins of the superficial inguinal ring can be felt by pressing posteriorly. Pick up the spermatic cord in the scrotum between the finger and thumb. Note the firm, cord-like **vas deferens** buried in its posterior part. This is the duct of the testis. The ring is smaller in the female and more difficult to feel because of the amount of subcutaneous fat in this region.

Note the slight median groove on the anterior abdominal wall between the xiphoid process and the pubic symphysis. Deep to this is the **linea alba**—an extensive fibrous raphe formed by the interlocking of the aponeuroses of the three flat muscles on each side of the abdominal wall. Immediately lateral to the linea alba, the paired **rectus abdominis** muscles run vertically, one on each side of the midline [Fig. 8.3]. The **umbilicus** lies in the linea alba, nearer the pubis than the xiphoid process. It is the scar formed from the remnants of the root of the umbilical cord through which the fetus *in utero* is attached to the placenta. The

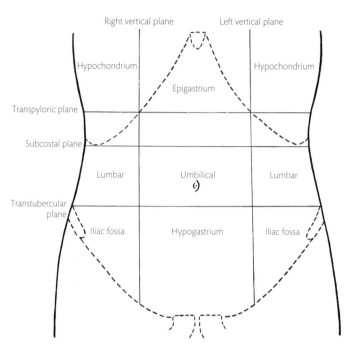

Fig. 8.1 Planes of subdivision of the abdomen, and names of the nine abdominal regions.

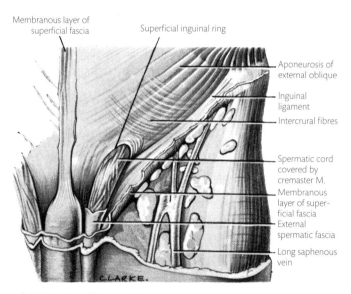

Fig. 8.2 A drawing of the superficial dissection of the inguinal region.

linea alba and umbilical scar are formed of relatively avascular, white fibrous tissue. ➲ Incisions into the abdominal cavity made through the linea alba have the advantage of not causing injury to nerves or blood vessels of any considerable size. But the linea alba has poor healing qualities because of its avascularity, and wounds are liable to break down because of the pull of the abdominal muscles on it.

The lateral edge of each rectus abdominis muscle is marked on the surface by a slight groove—the **linea semilunaris**—which is visible in thin, muscular individuals. It is most obvious where the aponeuroses of the abdominal muscles split to enclose the rectus abdominis [Fig. 8.3] in the upper two-thirds of the abdomen. The linea semilunaris meets the costal margin at the **ninth**

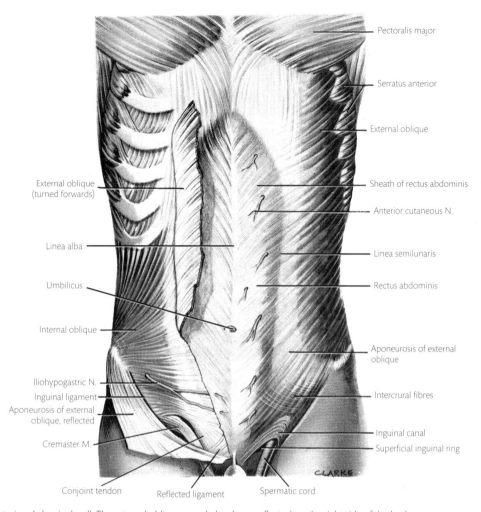

Pectoralis major

Serratus anterior

External oblique

External oblique
(turned forwards)

Sheath of rectus abdominis

Anterior cutaneous N.

Linea alba

Linea semilunaris

Umbilicus

Rectus abdominis

Internal oblique

Aponeurosis of external
oblique

Iliohypogastric N.

Inguinal ligament

Intercrural fibres

Aponeurosis of external
oblique, reflected

Cremaster M.

Inguinal canal

Superficial inguinal ring

CLARKE

Conjoint tendon

Reflected ligament

Spermatic cord

Fig. 8.3 Anterior abdominal wall. The external oblique muscle has been reflected on the right side of the body.

costal cartilage, the position of the **fundus of the gallbladder** on the right. Three transverse grooves may be seen crossing the rectus abdominis between the umbilicus and the xiphoid process. They are formed by tendinous intersections in the rectus abdominis muscles.

The distance between the costal margin and iliac crest is greater in infants and children (where the ribs are more horizontal) than in adults. The distance is still further reduced in old age by the progressive narrowing of the intervertebral discs and by the tendency to stoop. The distance between the costal margin and the iliac crest is also less in the standing position (because of the lower position taken up by the ribs) than while lying supine, and greater in inspiration than in expiration.

Dissection 8.1 describes the skin reflection of the anterior abdominal wall.

DISSECTION 8.1 Anterior abdominal wall–skin reflection

Objective

I. To reflect the skin from the anterior abdominal wall.

Instructions

1. Make skin incisions 8 and 9 [see Fig. 7.1]. Carry incision 8 around each side of the umbilicus and incision 9 posteriorly along the iliac crest. If the thorax has not been dissected, make incision 4 also. Carry it posteriorly at least to the mid-axillary line.

2. Reflect the flaps of skin, leaving the superficial fascia on the anterior abdominal wall intact.

Superficial fascia

The superficial fascia of the abdomen contains a variable amount of fat which is usually greatest over the inferior half of the abdomen. Here the superficial fascia consists of two layers—a **superficial fatty layer** and a **deep membranous layer**. On each side of the midline, it is separated from the underlying muscle (the external oblique) by a loose areolar layer which disappears superiorly and towards the median plane. Inferiorly, the membranous layer of the superficial fascia is attached to deeper structures at certain specific places [Fig. 8.4]. These firm attachments are significant as they form limiting boundaries for potential spaces, for example the superficial perineal space. The membranous layer of the superficial fascia is attached: (1) to the pubic tubercle; (2) laterally from the pubic tubercle to the deep fascia of the thigh, 1 cm below the inguinal ligament; (3) medially from the pubic tubercle, on the front of the body of the pubis and along the corresponding subcutaneous margin of the pubic arch; and (4) posteriorly, in front of the anus, the membranous layer of the superficial fascia fuses with the posterior edge of the **urogenital diaphragm**—a musculofascial sheet stretched across the pubic arch at a deeper level. Thus a pocket-like extension of the areolar tissue, deep to the membranous layer, passes from the abdomen in front of the pubic bones into the anterior part of the perineum. This space is the **superficial perineal space**. The floor of this space is formed by the membranous layer of the superficial fascia, and the roof is formed by the urogenital diaphragm.

In the male, the superficial perineal space contains the root of the penis, and the spermatic cords passing to the testes. Both the penis and scrotum project anteriorly from the space and receive a covering from the membranous layer. This covering forms the **fascia** and **fundiform ligament of the penis** and the smooth muscle—**dartos**—of the scrotum.

In the female, the superficial perineal space is split in the median plane by the vulva. Thus a separate pocket of areolar tissue extends into the base of each labium majus which corresponds to the scrotum. (Further details of the superficial perineal space and its contents are given in Chapter 16.)

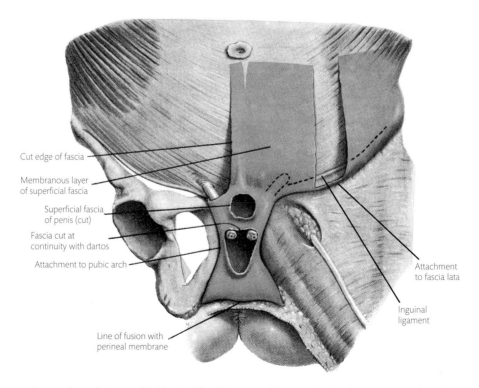

Cut edge of fascia

Membranous layer of superficial fascia

Superficial fascia of penis (cut)

Fascia cut at continuity with dartos

Attachment to pubic arch

Attachment to fascia lata

Inguinal ligament

Line of fusion with perineal membrane

Fig. 8.4 The membranous layer of the superficial fascia of the abdomen and its extension into the perineum in the male.

DISSECTION 8.2 Superficial fascia of the anterior abdominal wall

Objectives

I. To identify the two layers of the superficial fascia.   II. To explore the attachments of the membranous layer of the superficial fascia on the thigh, pubic tubercle, and pubic arch.   III. To identify the superficial inguinal ring and iliohypogastric nerve.

Instructions

1. Make a transverse cut through the entire thickness of the superficial fascia, from the anterior superior iliac spine to the median plane.

2. Raise the lower margin of the cut fascia and identify the fatty and membranous layers.

3. Pass a finger deep to the membranous layer. This layer separates easily from the aponeurosis of the external oblique muscle deep to it until a point just inferior to the inguinal ligament. At this point, the membranous layer fuses with the fascia lata of the thigh.

4. Medial to the pubic tubercle, pass a finger along the side of the spermatic cord (or the round ligament of the uterus), anterior to the body of the pubis, into the perineum. In this position, movement of the finger laterally is limited by the attachment of the membranous layer of the fascia to the pubic bone and arch.

5. Find the **superficial inguinal ring** immediately supe-rolateral to the pubic tubercle. The ring is a triangular aperture in the aponeurosis of the external oblique muscle [Fig. 8.2], and has the spermatic cord (or the round ligament of the uterus) emerging through it.

6. Note the anterior cutaneous branch of the **ilio-hypogastric nerve** piercing the aponeurosis of the ex-ternal oblique muscle a short distance superior to the superficial inguinal ring.

Dissection 8.2 gives instruction to dissect the su-perficial fascia of the anterior abdominal wall.

Cutaneous vessels and nerves of the anterior abdominal wall

The muscles and skin of the abdominal wall are al-most entirely supplied by the ventral rami of the low-er intercostal and subcostal nerves. The most inferior part is supplied by the first lumbar nerve through the **iliohypogastric** and **ilio-inguinal nerves**.

Anterior cutaneous branches

The anterior cutaneous branch of the lower inter-costal and subcostal nerves pierces the deep fascia close to the midline and gives off a small medial and a larger lateral cutaneous branch [Figs. 8.3, 8.5]. They are arranged in sequence with the corre-sponding branches of the upper intercostal nerves and supply skin from the midline to the lateral margin of the rectus abdominis muscle. The ante-rior cutaneous branch of the tenth thoracic nerve emerges close to the umbilicus, and that of the first lumbar nerve (the iliohypogastric nerve) appears above the superficial inguinal ring. The anterior cutaneous branch of the ilio-inguinal nerve passes through the superficial inguinal ring. This branch supplies the skin on the medial side of the upper thigh, the scrotum or labium majus.

Dissection 8.3 gives instructions for dissecting the cutaneous nerves of the anterior abdominal wall.

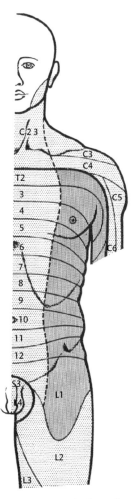

Fig. 8.5 Dermatomal pattern on the front of the trunk. The areas of skin supplied by the ventral rami are illustrated.

Lateral cutaneous branches

The lateral cutaneous branches pierce the deep
fascia in the mid-axillary line after dividing into
anterior and posterior branches. These nerves
emerge through the external oblique muscle. The
subcostal and **iliohypogastric branches** appear close to the iliac crest and descend over it to
supply the skin in the upper lateral part of the gluteal region. The remainder give large anterior and
small posterior branches. The ilio-inguinal nerve
does not have a lateral cutaneous branch.

Cutaneous vessels

Small arteries accompany the cutaneous nerves.
The arteries which accompany the lateral cutaneous nerves arise from the **posterior intercostal
arteries**. Those which accompany the anterior cutaneous nerves arise from the superior and inferior
epigastric arteries.

Below the umbilicus, the skin and superficial
fascia are supplied by three small branches from
the femoral artery. The **superficial external
pudendal arteries** run medially to supply the
scrotum or labium majus, and the penis. The **superficial epigastric arteries** run superome-
dially across the inguinal ligament as far as the
umbilicus. The **superficial circumflex iliac
arteries** run towards the anterior superior iliac
spine supplying the skin of the abdomen and
groin.

Superficial veins

Below the umbilicus, the superficial veins drain
along the superficial arteries to the long saphen-
ous vein in the groin, and eventually to the inferior vena cava. Above the umbilicus, they drain to
the axilla and eventually to the superior vena cava.
Both groups anastomose freely with each other in
the anterior abdominal wall and with small veins
which drain to the umbilicus from the liver along
the obliterated umbilical vein. ↪ In obstruction of
the superior or inferior vena cava, these veins may
be distended to form an alternative route for venous
return. If the venous drainage through the liver is
blocked, backflow may occur to the umbilicus from
the liver. This blood is then drained superiorly and
inferiorly on both sides to the axillary and inguinal
veins. In later stages of liver disease, a pattern of
distended veins radiating from the umbilicus may
be seen. These radiating and distended veins have
been called 'caput medusae' (caput = head; Medusa
= a mythological character who was said to have
living venomous snakes instead of hair).

Muscles of the anterior abdominal wall

Three flat muscles of the anterior abdominal wall—
the **external oblique**, **internal oblique**, and
transversus abdominis—lie in three layers [Figs.
8.3, 8.6]. Each muscle is muscular posterolaterally
and aponeurotic anteromedially. Two other muscles, the **rectus abdominis** and **pyramidalis**
are located close to the midline. As the **aponeuroses** of the three flat muscles approach the midline,
they partially enclose the rectus abdominis muscle
between them to form the **rectus sheath**. Medial
to the rectus abdominis, the three aponeuroses
fuse with each other and with the aponeuroses of
the opposite side in the median raphe—the **linea
alba**. The linea alba extends from the xiphoid process to the pubic symphysis.

The outer two muscles—the external and internal obliques—are approximately fan-shaped. The
external oblique takes origin superiorly from the
external surfaces of the lower eight ribs and radiates
downwards and forwards. It has a long linear insertion into the linea alba, pubic crest, pubic tubercle,
and the anterior two-thirds of the iliac crest. (Fibres
of the external oblique reach the linea alba by passing in front of the rectus abdominis. As such they

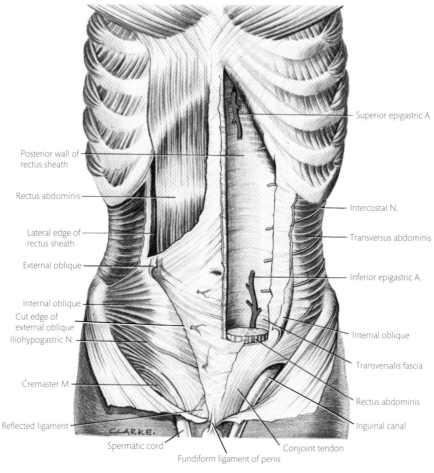

Fig. 8.6 Deep dissection of the anterior abdominal wall. On the left side of the body, the external and internal oblique muscles, the anterior wall of the rectus sheath, and the greater part of the rectus abdominis have been removed. On the right side the external oblique and upper parts of the internal oblique and the upper part of the anterior wall of the rectus sheath have been removed.

contribute to the anterior wall of the rectus sheath). Between the pubic crest and anterior superior iliac spine, the free margin of the external oblique aponeurosis forms the inguinal ligament [Fig. 8.3]. At the pubic tubercle, the deep fibres of the inguinal ligament curve horizontally backwards to the medial part of the pecten pubis as the **lacunar ligament**. Other fibres continue along the pecten pubis to the iliopubic eminence as the **pectineal ligament** [Fig. 8.7]. Over the lateral half of the pubic crest, there is a triangular deficiency in the aponeurosis of external oblique—the **superficial inguinal ring**. The medial and lateral margins of the superficial inguinal ring are also known as the **medial** and **lateral crus**. The spermatic cord in the male and the round ligament of the uterus in the female pass through the superficial inguinal ring [Fig. 8.2].

The **internal oblique** takes origin inferiorly from the thoracolumbar fascia, the iliac crest, and the lateral two-thirds of the inguinal ligament [Fig. 8.7]. It radiates upwards and forwards and is inserted into the costal margin, the linea alba, and the pubic crest [Fig. 8.3]. The lower fibres of the internal oblique fuse with similar fibres of the transversus abdominis to form the **conjoint tendon**. The conjoint tendon turns downwards and is inserted into the pubic crest and the pecten pubis [Figs. 8.6, 8.8]. (Fibres of the internal oblique which are inserted into linea alba have different relations to the rectus abdominis in different regions. In the upper three-fourths the aponeurosis splits into two. The anterior part goes in front of the rectus and fuses with the aponeurosis of external oblique. This part contributes to the formation of the anterior wall of the rectus sheath. The posterior part goes behind the rectus and fuses with the aponeurosis of transversus abdominis. This part contributes to the formation of the posterior wall of the rectus sheath. In the lower one-fourth of the abdomen, the internal oblique aponeurosis passes

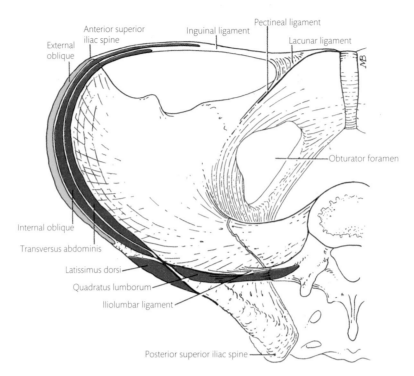

Fig. 8.7 The bony pelvis and fifth lumbar vertebra seen from above.

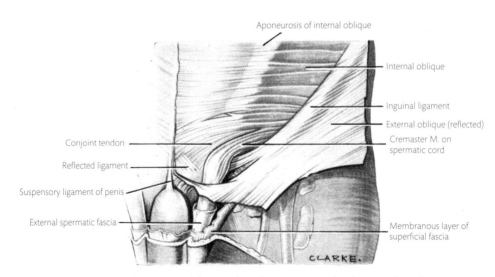

Fig. 8.8 Inguinal region. The external oblique is turned down to show the spermatic cord in the inguinal canal.

in front of the rectus abdominis, contributing only to the anterior wall.)

The posterior fibres of the external oblique and the posterior fibres of the internal oblique are almost vertical and unite the iliac crest and the rib cage. The upper fibres of the external oblique and the lower fibres of the internal oblique are nearly horizontal. The middle fibres of both cross each other at right angles. From the lower margin of the internal oblique, muscle fibres pass over the spermatic cord to form the **cremaster muscle** [Fig. 8.8]. The cremaster loops down around the spermatic cord and turns upwards to be attached to the pubic tubercle.

The innermost muscle—the **transversus abdominis**—is horizontally placed [Fig. 8.6]. It takes origin from the internal surface of the rib cage, the thoracolumbar fascia, the iliac crest, and the lateral one-third of the inguinal ligament. It runs forward to be inserted into the linea alba. (In the upper two-thirds of the abdominal wall, the muscle fibres pass behind the rectus abdominis, and contribute to the posterior wall of the rectus sheath. In the lower one-third the fibres of transversus abdominis pass in front of the rectus abdominis and contribute to the anterior wall of the rectus sheath.) The muscle fibres of the transversus abdominis lie at an angle to the intermediate fibres of both the external and internal obliques but are parallel to those of the external oblique superiorly and to the internal oblique inferiorly. This arrangement gives maximum strength to the abdominal wall and holds the abdominal contents in place when the intra-abdominal pressure is raised by contraction of these muscles.

Nerve supply: these muscles are supplied by the ventral rami of the lower five or six intercostal nerves and the subcostal nerve. In addition, the internal oblique and transversus abdominis are supplied by the iliohypogastric nerve. The cremaster muscle is supplied by the genital branch of the genitofemoral nerve.

Actions of the external oblique, internal oblique, and transversus abdominis muscles

These three flat muscles of the anterolateral abdominal wall have a number of important actions. (1) They rotate the trunk when the internal oblique fibres of one side act with the external oblique of the other. (2) They help to support the abdominal contents. (3) Contraction of the abdominal muscles raises the intra-abdominal pressure and plays an important part in many functions such as: (i) Forced expiration: when the thoracic cage and diaphragm are relaxed, the three muscles produce forced expiration by pulling down the lower ribs (assisted by the rectus abdominis) and by forcing the abdominal contents and diaphragm upwards. When such actions are violent, they produce the force required for coughing, sneezing, and vomiting. (ii) Forced expulsion of pelvic luminal contents: when the ribs and diaphragm are fixed, the contraction of the abdominal muscles raises the pressure inside the abdomen and pelvis. This assists with defecation, micturition, and childbirth (parturition). (iii) Stabilizing the trunk: the contracting muscles turn the trunk into a rigid pillar. During this action, the thoracic expiratory muscles are also contracted, but the inspired air is prevented from leaving the lungs by closure of the glottis [Vol. 3]. This action is used in forced movement such as pushing heavy objects or lifting heavy weights.

➲ In actions such as the lifting of heavy weights, the intra-abdominal pressure rises to very high lev-

els. This increased intra-abdominal pressure may cause: (1) discharge of urine through a weakened sphincter of the urinary bladder (stress incontinence); or (2) the protrusion of abdominal contents through a weak point in the abdominal or pelvic walls. Such a protrusion of abdominal contents is known as a **hernia**.

Actions of the cremaster

Contraction of the cremaster raises the testis in the scrotum towards the superficial inguinal ring. This movement can be produced in the living by stroking the medial side of the upper thigh—the **cremasteric reflex**. The cremasteric reflex tests the integrity of the first and second lumbar spinal nerves as the skin on the medial side of the upper thigh is supplied by the **ilio-inguinal nerve** (afferent limb of the reflex), and the cremaster muscle is supplied by the **genitofemoral nerve** (efferent limb of the reflex).

Transversalis fascia

The deep surface of the transversus abdominis is lined by the transversalis fascia. The transversalis fascia is a part of a continuous fascial lining of the abdominal and pelvic cavities. Each part of the fascial lining of the abdomen is named after the structures on which it lies. The fascia on the inferior surface of the diaphragm is the **diaphragmatic fascia**. The fascia on the iliacus and psoas muscles is the **iliac fascia**. Around the kidneys is the **renal fascia**, and the fascia in the pelvis is the **pelvic fascia**.

Immediately superior to the mid-inguinal point, there is a small defect in the transversalis fascia—the **deep inguinal ring**. In the fetus, the descending testis carries a covering of the transversalis fascia from the deep inguinal ring into the scrotum.

Deep to the transversalis fascia is the serous lining of the abdomen—the **parietal peritoneum**—separated from the fascia by a variable amount of extraperitoneal fat.

Dissection 8.4 describes the dissection of the muscles, vessels, and nerves of the anterior abdominal wall.

Rectus abdominis and rectus sheath

The rectus abdominis muscle arises from the pubic crest, posterior to the conjoint tendon. It runs upward and is inserted into the anterior surfaces of the fifth, sixth, and seventh costal cartilages.

The rectus is enclosed in the rectus sheath. In the upper part of the abdomen—from the costal margin

DISSECTION 8.4 Muscles, vessels, and nerves of the anterior abdominal wall

Objectives

I. To study the muscles of the anterior abdominal wall, the inguinal ligament, and the rectus sheath. II. To identify and trace the course of the abdominal nerves and the superior and inferior epigastric arteries. III. To study the formation of the rectus sheath. IV. To identify the contents of the rectus sheath.

Instructions

1. Remove any fascia from the surface of the external oblique muscle and its aponeurosis. Take special care superiorly where the aponeurosis is thin and easily destroyed, and also antero-inferiorly where the **superficial inguinal ring** forms a triangular deficiency immediately superolateral to the pubic tubercle.

2. In the male, identify the **spermatic cord** emerging from the superficial inguinal ring. Note the extension of the fascia from the margins of the ring over the spermatic cord. This is the **external spermatic fascia**. In the female, the fatty, fibrous structure emerging from the superficial inguinal ring is the **round ligament of the uterus**. In both sexes, define the margins of the ring by blunt dissection.

3. Identify the origin of the **external oblique** muscle from the lower eight ribs. Here it interdigitates with the serratus anterior and latissimus dorsi. Separate the upper six digitations from the ribs. Cut vertically through the muscle down to the iliac crest, posterior to the sixth digitation. Separate the external oblique from the iliac crest in front of this, but avoid injury to the lateral cutaneous branches of the nerves which pierce it close to the crest.

4. Turn the superior part of the external oblique forwards and expose the **internal oblique** and its aponeurosis. Follow the internal oblique medially to the line of fusion with the aponeurosis of the external oblique, anterior to the rectus abdominis.

5. Divide the external oblique aponeurosis vertically, lateral to this line of fusion, and turn the muscle and aponeurosis inferiorly as you do so. The cut should pass to the pubis medial to the superficial inguinal ring [Fig. 8.6]. This exposes the remainder of the internal oblique.

6. Note the inrolled margin of the external oblique aponeurosis between its attachments to the anterior superior iliac spine and the pubic tubercle. This is the **inguinal ligament**. Note that this ligament gives origin to the internal oblique muscle from its lateral part and has the spermatic cord or the round ligament of the uterus lying on its superior surface medially.

7. Lift the cord or round ligament of the uterus and identify the deep fibres of the inguinal ligament passing posteriorly to the pecten pubis. This is the **lacunar ligament** on which these structures also lie.

8. Follow the lateral margin (**lateral crus**) of the **superficial inguinal ring** to the **pubic tubercle** and note the relationship of this crus and the tubercle to the spermatic cord. The **medial crus** may be followed to the pubic crest.

9. Remove the fascia from the surface of the internal oblique and its aponeurosis. Identify the lower fibres of the internal oblique which pass around the spermatic cord. These are the **cremaster muscles** which loop down on the cord and turn upwards to be attached to the pubic tubercle.

10. Lift the internal oblique and cut carefully through its attachments to the inguinal ligament, iliac crest, and costal margin. Do not cut deeply or the nerves of the anterior abdominal wall which lie deep to the internal oblique will be divided. Cut vertically through the internal oblique from the twelfth costal cartilage to the iliac crest. Attempt to strip the muscle forwards from the transversus abdominis and the nerves. The separation of the internal oblique and the transversus abdominis is difficult superiorly because of the dense fascia between the muscles. The separation of the internal oblique and the transversus is impossible inferiorly where the aponeuroses of the two muscles fuse in the **conjoint tendon** [Fig. 8.6].

11. Superior to a horizontal line, midway between the umbilicus and the symphysis pubis, the aponeurosis of the internal oblique splits at the lateral edge of the rectus abdominis to enclose that muscle. The part of the internal oblique aponeurosis which passes anterior to the rectus abdominis fuses with the aponeurosis of the external oblique. The part of the internal oblique aponeurosis which passes posterior to the rectus fuses with the underlying aponeurosis of the transversus abdominis. The three aponeuroses enclose the rectus abdominis to form the **rectus sheath** [Fig. 8.9].

12. Inferior to a horizontal line midway between the umbilicus and the symphysis pubis, the aponeuroses of all three muscles pass anterior to the rectus abdominis. The rectus then lies on the transversalis fascia posteriorly. The inferior edge of the posterior layer of the rectus sheath often forms a sharp margin—the **arcuate line**. This will be seen when the rectus sheath is opened.

13. Remove the fascia from the surface of the transversus abdominis and from the nerves and vessels which lie on it. Confirm the continuity of the lateral cutaneous branches of these nerves.

14. Define the origins of the transversus. Follow its aponeurosis medially. Above the arcuate line, it fuses with the aponeurosis of the internal oblique, posterior to the rectus abdominis. Below the arcuate line also, it fuses with the aponeurosis of the internal oblique, but anterior to the rectus [Fig. 8.9].

15. Note that, below the arcuate line, the aponeurosis of the external oblique is less firmly fused with that of the internal oblique.

16. Open the rectus sheath by a vertical incision along the middle of the muscle. Reflect the anterior layer of the sheath medially and laterally, cutting its attachments to the **tendinous intersections** in the anterior part of the rectus muscle. Lift the rectus muscle and identify the intercostal and subcostal nerves entering the sheath and piercing the muscle. Confirm the mode of formation of the rectus sheath.

17. On the lower part of the rectus, identify the **pyramidalis muscle**, if present. This small triangular muscle arises from the upper surface of the pubic crest and symphysis. It lies anterior to the rectus and is inserted into the lowest part of the linea alba. It is supplied by a small branch of the subcostal nerve.

18. Divide the rectus abdominis transversely at its middle. Identify its attachments. Expose the posterior wall of the rectus sheath by turning its parts superiorly and inferiorly, cutting the nerves as they enter it. Identify and follow the superior and inferior **epigastric arteries** running longitudinally deep to the muscle within the rectus sheath [Fig. 8.6]. The tendinous intersections are only in the anterior part of the rectus abdominis, so they do not interfere with this longitudinal **anastomosis** between the superior and inferior epigastric arteries. Try to define the **arcuate line** on the posterior wall of the rectus sheath. The inferior epigastric artery enters the sheath by passing anterior to this line.

117

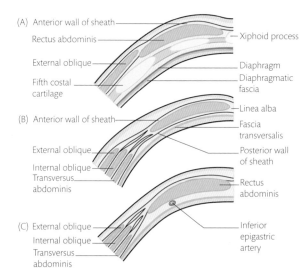

(A) Anterior wall of sheath
Rectus abdominis
External oblique
Fifth costal cartilage
Xiphoid process
Diaphragm
Diaphragmatic fascia
(B) Anterior wall of sheath
External oblique
Internal oblique
Transversus abdominis
Linea alba
Fascia transversalis
Posterior wall of sheath
Rectus abdominis
(C) External oblique
Internal oblique
Transversus abdominis
Inferior epigastric artery

Fig. 8.9 Transverse sections of the anterior abdominal wall to show the formation of the rectus sheath at different levels. (A) Above the costal margin. (B) Upper two-thirds of the abdominal wall. (C) The lower one-third of the wall.

to a point midway between the umbilicus and pubic symphysis—the anterior wall of the rectus sheath is formed by the aponeurosis of the external oblique and the anterior part of the aponeurosis of internal oblique. The posterior wall is formed by the posterior part of internal oblique aponeurosis and the aponeurosis of the transversus abdominis. In the lower part—below the line midway between the umbilicus and pubis symphysis—the anterior wall is formed by the aponeurosis of all three muscles, and the posterior wall is deficient. The rectus lies directly on the transversalis fascia. The lower border of the posterior wall of the rectus sheath is called the arcuate line. On the anterior surfaces of the costal cartilages, the posterior layer of the sheath is lost, as the transversus abdominis passes internal to the costal cartilages. (The internal oblique is attached to the costal margin and does not extend posterior to the rectus abdominis.) At this level, the aponeurosis of the external oblique continues anterior to the rectus and gives attachment to the lowest fibres of the pectoralis major [Fig. 8.9].

Three horizontal **tendinous intersections** present in the anterior part of the rectus abdominis attach the muscle to the anterior layer of the rectus sheath. They are at the level of the umbilicus, at the tip of the xiphoid process, and midway between these two. Occasionally, a fourth intersection is present between the umbilicus and the pubis.

Nerve supply: the lower five or six intercostal nerves and the subcostal nerve. **Action**: the rectus abdominis is a powerful flexor of the vertebral column. It may be made to stand out when attempting to raise the head and shoulders (or lower limbs and pelvis) from the floor when lying on the back (supine position). When the extensors of the vertebral column (erector spinae) contract at the same time, the rectus muscles tighten the anterior abdominal wall against blows, provided the ribs are fixed by inspiratory muscles. When the ribs are not fixed, the rectus acts as an expiratory muscle.

Pyramidalis

When present, this small muscle is found in front of the lower part of the rectus abdominis. It arises from the front of the pubis and pubic symphysis. It tapers as it ascends and is inserted into the linea alba.

Nerve supply: the subcostal nerve. **Action**: the pyramidalis tenses the lower part of the linea alba.

Dissection 8.5 provides instructions on dissection of the posterior aspect of the anterior abdominal wall.

Umbilical folds and ligaments

The **median umbilical fold** lies in the midline. It overlies the **median umbilical ligament**

DISSECTION 8.5 Posterior aspect of the anterior abdominal wall

Objectives

I. To reflect the anterior abdominal wall inferiorly.   II. To identify the falciform ligament, the umbilical folds and ligaments, and the deep inguinal ring on the posterior aspect of the anterior abdominal wall.

Instructions

1. Cut through the remaining ribs in the mid-axillary line, and carefully turn down the sternum, costal cartilages, and the anterior parts of the ribs.

2. Remove the pleura and fascia from the back of the sternum and the superior surface of the exposed part of the diaphragm. Note the slips by which the diaphragm arises from the xiphoid process and the costal cartilages.

3. Identify the musculophrenic and superior epigastric branches of the **internal thoracic arteries**, the slips of origin of the transversus abdominis beside those of the diaphragm, and the continuity of the transversus abdominis with the transversus thoracis superiorly.

4. Cut through the slips of origin of the diaphragm in front of the mid-axillary line, and cut vertically through the transversus abdominis in the mid-axillary line to the iliac crest. (Avoid injury to the peritoneum deep to the transversalis fascia.)

5. Turn down the remnants of the anterior abdominal wall with the sternum, costal cartilages, and ribs, attempting to strip the peritoneum from the transversalis fascia.

6. Identify the peritoneum. Divide and reflect it with the anterior abdominal wall. Cut the fold of peritoneum which passes from the median part of the supra-umbilical anterior abdominal wall to the liver. This is the **falciform ligament** [see Fig. 11.20]. This fold contains the **ligamentum teres of the liver** (the **obliterated left umbilical vein** [see Fig. 11.12]) in its free posterior border. Identify the ligamentum teres.

7. Examine the posterior surface of the reflected anterior abdominal wall. Identify five ill-defined peritoneal folds on the lower part of the abdominal wall. These folds, one in the midline and two on each side, pass upwards towards the umbilicus. These are the lateral, medial, and median umbilical folds [Fig. 8.10].

8. Strip the peritoneum from the posterior surface of the infra-umbilical abdominal wall to expose these structures. Identify the attachments of the transversus abdominis and the conjoint tendon. Before removing the transversalis fascia from the deep surface of the inguinal ligament, pull on the spermatic cord or round ligament of the uterus from the superficial aspect and confirm the continuity of the transversalis fascia over these structures. The transversalis fascia forms the **internal spermatic fascia** over the spermatic cord.

9. The intrinsic weaknesses in the abdominal wall lie in the region of the groin (femoral and inguinal canals) and at the umbilical scar in the linea alba. Note their positions on the body.

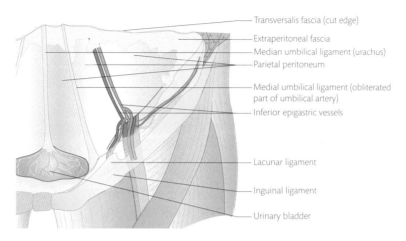

Fig. 8.10 The parietal peritoneum deep to the anterior abdominal wall, with the umbilical folds and ligaments.

119

which is the remnant of the intra-abdominal part of the **allantois**. (The allantois forms the **urachus** which in the fetus, extends from the apex of the bladder to the umbilicus.) The lateral umbilical ligaments are the remnants of the **obliterated umbilical arteries**, which in the fetus, carry blood to the placenta. These ligaments raise the **medial umbilical folds** of the peritoneum. The **lateral umbilical folds** are formed by the inferior epigastric vessels. (Note that there are five folds, but only three ligaments, as the two lateral folds are raised by arteries.)

Arrangement of structures in the groin

The anterior and posterior abdominal walls meet each other at the groin, and their fascial linings—the transversalis fascia and iliac fascia—become continuous [Fig. 8.11]. The muscles of the anterior abdominal wall end at the **inguinal ligament**. The transversalis and iliac fasciae fuse with each other at the lateral part of the inguinal ligament. Structures of the posterior abdominal wall enter the thigh deep to this line of fusion [Figs. 8.7, 8.11,

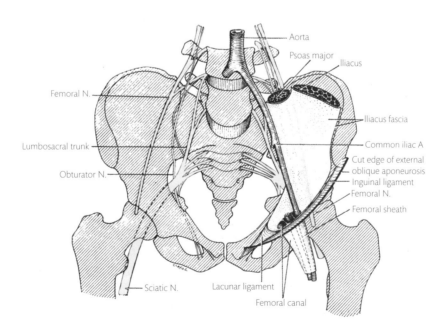

Fig. 8.11 A diagram to show the structures in the inguinal region and the nerves of the lower limb related to the pelvis.

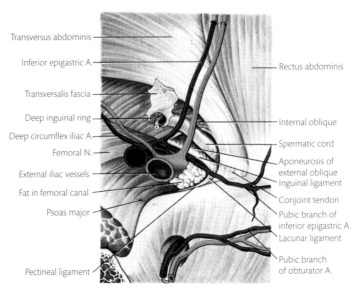

Transversus abdominis

Inferior epigastric A.

Transversalis fascia

Deep inguinal ring

Deep circumflex iliac A.

Femoral N.

External iliac vessels

Fat in femoral canal

Psoas major

Pectineal ligament

Rectus abdominis

Internal oblique

Spermatic cord

Aponeurosis of external oblique

Inguinal ligament

Conjoint tendon

Pubic branch of inferior epigastric A.

Lacunar ligament

Pubic branch of obturator A.

120

Fig. 8.12 Posterior surface of the anterior abdominal wall in the inguinal region. Note the pubic branches of the obturator and inferior epigastric arteries.

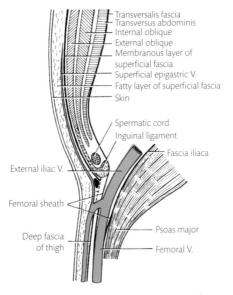

Transversalis fascia
Transversus abdominis
Internal oblique
External oblique
Membranous layer of superficial fascia
Superficial epigastric V.
Fatty layer of superficial fascia
Skin

Spermatic cord
Inguinal ligament

Fascia iliaca

External iliac V.

Femoral sheath

Deep fascia of thigh

Psoas major

Femoral V.

Fig. 8.13 Sagittal section along the external iliac and femoral veins to show the fasciae and muscles of the inguinal region.

8.12, 8.13]. These structures include the **iliacus** and **psoas muscles**, the **femoral nerve**, and the **lateral cutaneous nerve of the thigh**. They lie behind the iliac fascia and descend into the thigh, posterior to the lateral half of the ligament.

Behind the medial part of the inguinal ligament, the external iliac vessels of the abdomen are continuous with the femoral vessels of the thigh. The transversalis and iliac fasciae pass down anterior and posterior to the femoral vessels, forming a sheath around them—the **femoral sheath** [Figs. 8.11, 8.12]. Not

all of the sheath is filled by the femoral vessels. Its medial part is a loose connective tissue space—the **femoral canal**. The femoral canal is filled with fat, some lymph vessels, and an occasional lymph node. The femoral canal allows for distension of the femoral vein. The sharp lateral edge of the lacunar ligament lies medial to the femoral canal.

Inguinal canal

The inguinal canal is an intermuscular passage parallel to, and immediately superior to, the medial half of the inguinal ligament [Figs. 8.14, 8.15]. It is the space through which the **testis** descends from within the abdominal cavity to the scrotum during intrauterine life. The canal therefore contains the duct of the testis (the vas deferens), blood and lymph vessels, and nerves of the testis. Together these structures constitute the **spermatic cord**.

The inguinal canal has an **anterior wall**, a **floor**, a **posterior wall**, and a **roof**. The canal also has two openings through which the contents pass—the **deep** and **superficial inguinal rings**.

The floor of the inguinal canal is formed by the inguinal and lacunar ligaments [Fig. 8.7]. The anterior wall is formed by the aponeurosis of the external oblique and the internal oblique, deep to the external oblique in the lateral 1 cm. The roof is formed by the lower fibres of the transversus abdominis and the internal oblique arching over the spermatic cord [Fig. 8.6]. The posterior wall is

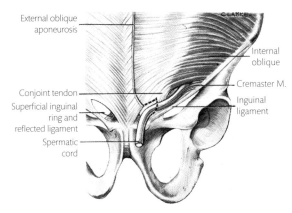

Fig. 8.14 A diagram of the inguinal canal to show the conjoint tendon and the internal oblique muscle. Note that the internal oblique muscle arches over the spermatic cord and sends fibres (the cremaster muscle) on to it.

formed by the transversalis fascia laterally and the conjoint tendon medially.

The deep inguinal ring is an opening or a defect in the transversalis fascia (posterior wall), through which the testis enters the inguinal region in the fetus [Figs. 8.10, 8.12]. It lies immediately superior to the inguinal ligament, at the mid-inguinal point, lateral to the inferior epigastric artery [Figs. 8.10, 8.12]. At this point, the descending testis carries part of the transversalis fascia and the most medial fibres of the internal oblique muscle before it [Fig. 8.8]. These extensions form the coverings for the testis and spermatic cord. The covering derived from the transversalis fascia is the **internal sper-**

matic fascia, and that from the internal oblique is the **cremaster muscle** and **cremasteric fascia**. The superficial inguinal ring is a defect in the external oblique aponeurosis (anterior wall of the canal), through which the testis descends into the scrotum. It lies immediately superolateral to the pubic tubercle [Fig. 8.3]. The **external spermatic fascia** covering the testis and spermatic cord arises from the margins of the superficial inguinal ring. The spermatic cord comes to lie anterior to the pubis, deep to the membranous layer of the superficial fascia, as it descends into the scrotum.

In the female, the ovary remains intra-abdominal and the inguinal canal is small, containing only the round ligament of the uterus, the homologue of the gubernaculum testis in the male. As such, inguinal hernias are much more common in the male than in the female (see also Clinical Application 8.1).

When the muscles of the anterior abdominal wall contract, the aponeurosis of the external oblique is pulled firmly against the taut conjoint tendon. The contraction of the fibres of the internal oblique and transversus which form the conjoint tendon pulls the arched roof of the canal downwards and narrows the deep ring and the canal. Thus the tendency of a hernia to occur through the canal is reduced as the intra-abdominal pressure rises. (A hernia is an abnormal protrusion of abdominal contents through the abdominal wall.)

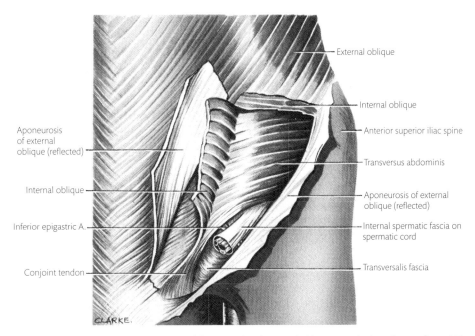

Fig. 8.15 Deep dissection of the inguinal region. Parts of the internal and external oblique muscles have been reflected. The spermatic cord and internal spermatic fascia are cut across.

Nerves of the abdominal wall

Nerves of the anterior abdominal wall are the ventral rami of the lower six **thoracic nerves** and the **first lumbar nerve**. The lower five intercostal nerves leave the intercostal spaces between the slips of origin of the transversus abdominis. They pass either directly (eleventh) or deep to the upturned ends of the costal cartilages to lie between the transversus abdominis and the internal oblique muscles. They run antero-inferiorly between these two muscles and enter the rectus sheath. They supply and pierce the rectus abdominis and emerge through the anterior wall of the rectus sheath as anterior cutaneous branches.

The subcostal, iliohypogastric, and ilio-inguinal nerves also supply the muscles of the abdominal wall. They pierce the transversus abdominis posteriorly to enter the same layer as the lower intercostal nerves but differ from them in that: (1) the **lateral cutaneous branches** of the **subcostal** and **iliohypogastric nerves** pierce the oblique muscles close to the iliac crest and descend over it to the gluteal skin; (2) the iliohypogastric nerve pierces the internal oblique close to the anterior superior iliac spine [Fig. 8.6] and becomes cutaneous by piercing the external oblique 2–3 cm superior to the superficial inguinal ring; (3) the **ilio-inguinal nerve** has no lateral cutaneous branch. It lies in the inguinal canal, and accompanies the spermatic cord or round ligament of the uterus through the superficial inguinal ring to supply the skin on the front of the thigh and the anterior parts of the external genitalia. Although these nerves run an oblique course, the lateral cutaneous branches descend to such an extent that the parts of each dermatome which they supply are much more horizontal than the ventral rami from which these branches arise. (The cutaneous branches are described earlier in this chapter.)

Arteries of the anterior abdominal wall

Most of the skin and superficial tissue of the lower anterior abdominal wall is supplied by superficial branches of the femoral artery—the superficial circumflex iliac, the superficial epigastric, and the superficial external pudendal arteries.

Branches of the internal thoracic artery

(1) The **superior epigastric artery** enters the rectus sheath, deep to the seventh costal cartilage. It lies deep to the rectus abdominis, supplies that muscle, and sends branches through it to the overlying skin. It anastomoses with the inferior epigastric artery.

(2) The **musculophrenic artery** runs along the upper surface of the costal origin of the diaphragm to the eighth intercostal space. It gives branches to the diaphragm and anterior abdominal wall.

Branches of the external iliac artery

(1) The **inferior epigastric artery** arises from the external iliac artery, immediately superior to the inguinal ligament at the mid-inguinal point. It ascends towards the umbilicus in the extraperitoneal tissue. At the lateral border of the rectus abdominis, it pierces the transversalis fascia and runs on the deep surface of the rectus abdominis to anastomose with the superior epigastric artery. It supplies the rectus abdominis and sends branches to the overlying skin. (Through the anastomosis of the superior and inferior epigastric arteries, the subclavian artery is linked to the external iliac artery.)

Branches of inferior epigastric artery

1. The **pubic branch** of the inferior epigastric artery runs inferomedially on the inguinal ligament. It crosses the lacunar ligament and anastomoses with the **pubic branch** of the **obturator artery** on the posterosuperior surface of the body of the pubis [Fig. 8.12]. This small branch may at times replace the proximal part of the obturator artery and form an **abnormal obturator artery**. It is then greatly enlarged and may be damaged in surgical division of the lacunar ligament.

2. A small **cremasteric artery** to the cremaster muscle is given off from the inferior epigastric artery as it passes medial to the deep inguinal ring. This may anastomose with the testicular artery near the testis. In the female, there is a smaller artery of the round ligament of the uterus.

3. The **deep circumflex iliac artery** arises close to the origin of the inferior epigastric artery. It passes to the anterior superior iliac spine, deep to the inguinal ligament, giving an ascending branch between the transversus abdominis and internal oblique muscles. It runs along the iliac crest, pierces the transversus abdominis at about the middle of the crest, and sends branches in

the abdominal wall deep to the internal oblique muscle.

See Clinical Applications 8.1 and 8.2 for the practical implications of the anatomy in this chapter.

CLINICAL APPLICATION 8.1 Hernias

The presence of the femoral and inguinal canals at the lowest part of the abdomen means that there is continuous pressure on these canals from the weight of the abdominal contents. Hernias tend to occur where structures enter or leave the abdominal or pelvic cavities and the wall is either intrinsically weak or has been weakened by surgery. Hernias can also occur more easily when the abdominal wall is stretched by excessive accumulation of fat in the abdomen or following repeated pregnancies. The presence of chronic cough, lifting of heavy weights, or straining to pass urine through a partially obstructed urethra may also cause or aggravate a hernia.

In a **femoral hernia**, the peritoneum overlying the abdominal end of the femoral canal is forced through it into the proximal part of the thigh. This outpocket of peritoneum forms the hernial sac. The hernial sac passes through the **femoral ring**, formed by the inguinal ligament anteriorly, the lacunar ligament medially, and the pectineal ligament posteriorly. The pressure of this ring on the herniating bowel may obstruct the loop of the small intestine in the sac or even cut off its blood supply so that it becomes gangrenous. Relieving the pressure on the femoral ring is usually achieved by dividing the lacunar ligament, a procedure which requires caution so as not to injure an **abnormal obturator artery** which may lie on it.

Protrusion of an abdominal viscus through the abdominal wall of the inguinal region is an **inguinal hernia**. An **indirect inguinal hernia** arises lateral to the inferior epigastric artery and traverses the inguinal canal.

It may be predisposed to by the persistence of the **processus vaginalis**. The processus vaginalis is the tube of peritoneum which extends from the abdomen into the scrotum, along which the testis descends [Chapter 9]. Under normal circumstances, the cavity of the processus is obliterated shortly after birth, leaving only a small part of it around the testis patent. If the processus persists, it forms a ready-made hernial sac, along which a loop of intestine may pass. This is one type of indirect inguinal hernia. The other type occurs when a secondary hernial sac passes through the inguinal canal from deep to superficial inguinal rings. A **direct inguinal hernia** usually occurs from the weakening of the conjoint tendon. The hernial sac pushes through the weakened conjoint tendon and distending the superficial inguinal ring. Direct inguinal hernias arise medial to the **inferior epigastric artery**.

An **umbilical hernia** usually occurs as a result of abdominal distension, e.g. by repeated pregnancies. The umbilical scar in the linea alba tends to stretch and thin. Unlike the muscular parts of the abdominal wall, it does not return to its normal thickness once the distending force is removed and it may subsequently bulge outwards, forming a hernial sac. *In utero*, there is a physiological extension of the peritoneal cavity into the root of the umbilical cord. If this persists, a **congenital umbilical hernia** is present at birth. The presence of a peritoneal dimple at the umbilicus, as at the deep inguinal ring, following obliteration of the peritoneal extension, may also facilitate a hernia at these points.

CLINICAL APPLICATION 8.2 Superficial reflexes

Abdominal reflexes

Superficial reflexes are reflexes that have evolved to protect the viscera from external danger. The abdominal reflex consists of contraction of abdominal muscles in response to sensory abdominal stimulation (in an effort to protect the abdominal viscera). To elicit the reflex, the subject is made to lie down comfortably, with the anterior abdominal wall exposed. Using a blunt object, the abdominal skin is gently stroked from lateral to medial. A normal positive response is the contraction of the underlying abdominal muscles, with the umbilicus moving to the side of the stimulus. The test is done on all four quadrants of the abdomen.

Study question 1: what cutaneous nerves supply the anterior abdominal wall? (Answer: ventral rami of T. 7–T. 12.)

Study question 2: which of these nerves are likely to be affected in a patient who has an absent abdominal reflex in the right lower quadrant? (Answer: from the information given, it is clear that the reflex is normal on the left, so the nerves on the left side are unaffected. The reflex is also normal in the right upper quadrant. As the skin around the umbilicus is supplied by the ventral ramus of T. 10, it is likely that the lower thoracic nerves (T. 10–T. 12) of the right side are affected.)

Cremasteric reflex

Contraction of the cremaster muscle pulls the testis up towards the superficial inguinal ring (in an effort to protect the testis from injury). To elicit the reflex, the skin on the medial side of the upper thigh is lightly stroked. The upward movement of the testis on the same side indicates a positive test.

Study question 1: what is the sensory nerve supply to the medial side of the upper thigh? (Answer: the ilio-inguinal nerve (L. 1)).

Study question 2: what is the nerve supply of the cremaster muscle? (Answer: the genital branch of the genitofemoral nerve (L. 1, L. 2)).

CHAPTER 9
The male external genital organs

The male external genitalia includes the penis, the scrotum, and its contents—the testes and spermatic cords.

Scrotum

The scrotum is a pendulous sac of dark-coloured, rugose (wrinkled) skin, containing the testes, their associated ducts, and the lower parts of the spermatic cords in their coverings. In the median plane, there is a ridge or raphe which indicates the embryological line of fusion of the two halves of the scrotum [Figs. 9.1, 9.2].

The superficial fascia of the scrotum has no fat, is reddish in colour, and contains a layer of involuntary muscle—the **dartos**. When the dartos contracts, it decreases the surface area of the scrotum and helps to decrease the heat loss through the thin, fat-free skin. The dartos also forms an incomplete **septum** between the testes. Each testis is covered by three fascial sheaths—the external spermatic fascia, the cremasteric fascia and muscle, and the internal spermatic fascia. In the scrotum, these layers are fused together and are difficult to differentiate, except by the presence of loops of the cremaster muscle in the middle layer. The testis is

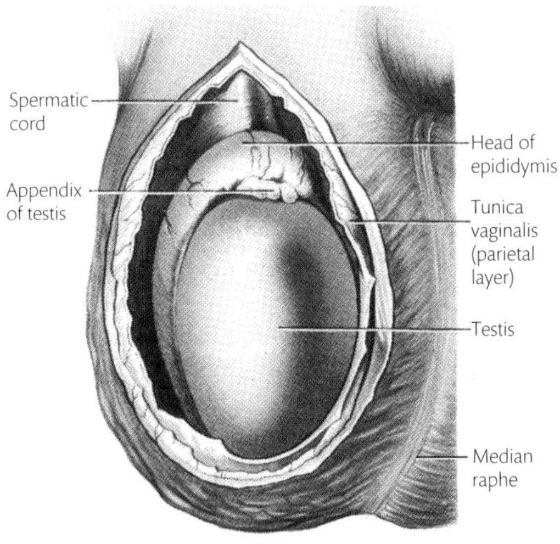

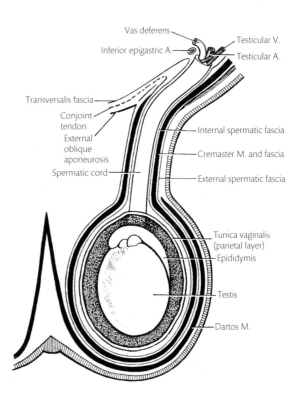

Fig. 9.1 The right testis and epididymis exposed by removal of the anterior wall of the scrotum and tunica vaginalis.

Fig. 9.2 Coronal section through the spermatic cord and scrotum.

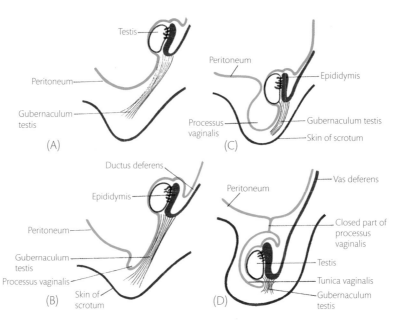

Fig. 9.3 (A, B, C, D) Illustration of the descent of the testis and the formation of the tunica vaginalis.

invaginated into the posterior wall of a serous sac—the **tunica vaginalis testis**. In the fetus, this serous sac is the distal end—the processus vaginalis [Fig. 9.3]—which passes through the inguinal canal into the scrotum.

In early fetal life, the testes are formed in the lumbar region. A fibromuscular band—the **gubernaculum testis**—extends from the caudal pole of each developing testis to the scrotum. This band lies on the posterior abdominal wall, immediately posterior to the peritoneum, and passes through the inguinal canal. As the fetus grows, the gubernaculum shortens, relative to the growing fetus. The peritoneum on the anterior aspect of the gubernaculum is drawn through the inguinal canal to the scrotum as the **processus vaginalis**. The testis being attached to the gubernaculum descends on the posterior abdominal wall, posterior to the processus. As it descends, the testis drags with it the blood vessels, lymphatics, and nerves supplying it. Subsequently, the lumen of the proximal part of the processus is obliterated, and the processus is reduced to a fibrous thread within the spermatic cord [Fig. 9.3]. Occasionally, parts of the processus vaginalis remain patent and form isolated cavities. These cavities can become filled with fluid and form hydroceles of the spermatic cord.

➲ The descent of the testis may be arrested at any stage—in the abdomen, in the inguinal canal, or in the groin. Such undescended testes usually do not produce spermatozoa and commonly develop cancers.

Using the instructions given in Dissection 9.1 complete the superficial dissection of the scrotum.

DISSECTION 9.1 Superficial dissection of the scrotum

Objective

I. To reflect the skin and superficial tissue of the scrotum.

Instructions

1. Begin at the superficial ring and make a longitudinal incision downwards through the skin of the anterolateral aspect of the scrotum. Carefully reflect the skin from the dartos which is attached to it.

2. Reflect the dartos layer from the loose areolar tissue, the external spermatic fascia, deep to it. Towards the median plane, the dartos layer extends superiorly between the testes. Complete the separation through the layer of areolar tissue up to the superficial inguinal ring. Lift the testis and spermatic cord from the scrotum.

Spermatic cord

The spermatic cord is made up of a collection of structures passing from the abdomen to the testis. The spermatic cord begins at the deep inguinal ring and ends at the superior pole of the testis. It is covered by three concentric layers of fascia derived from the layers forming the anterior abdominal wall. The external spermatic fascia is derived from the external oblique aponeurosis at the margins of the superficial inguinal ring. The cremaster muscle and fascia are derived from the internal oblique muscle. The internal spermatic fascia is derived from the transversalis fascia at the margin of the deep inguinal ring.

Structures in the spermatic cord

The following structures lie in the spermatic cord.

1. The vas deferens, which is the duct of the testis.
2. Arteries:

   (i) the artery of the vas deferens;
   (ii) the testicular artery.
      (The cremasteric artery is in the sheath of the spermatic cord and is not a content.)

3. Veins—the pampiniform plexus of veins.
4. Lymph vessels which drain the testis and immediately associated structures, but not the scrotal wall.
5. Nerves—sympathetic fibres on the arteries and pelvic autonomic fibres on the vas deferens [Fig. 9.4].

Dissection 9.2 explores the coverings and contents of the spermatic cord.

Vas deferens

The vas deferens is a thick-walled muscular part of the duct system of the testis. It begins at the lower pole of the testes as a continuation of the epididymis [Figs. 9.5, 9.6, 9.7] and ends by uniting with the duct of the seminal vesicle in the pelvis [see Fig. 17.16]. Initially it is very tortuous but straightens as it ascends along the medial aspect of the epididymis, posterior to the testis. It runs in the posterior part of the spermatic cord and passes through the superficial inguinal ring, inguinal canal, and deep inguinal ring. At the deep inguinal ring, it leaves the other structures of the spermatic cord and turns medially around the lateral side of the inferior epigastric artery to enter the pelvis. It is accompanied by the **artery of the vas deferens**, a branch of the internal iliac artery which anastomoses with the testicular artery at the testis.

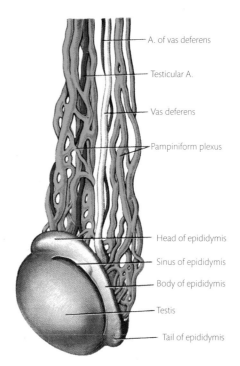

Fig. 9.4 Contents of the left spermatic cord.

DISSECTION 9.2 Coverings and contents of the spermatic cord

Objective

I. To explore the coverings and contents of the spermatic cord.

Instructions

1. Incise and reflect the coverings—the remains of the external spermatic fascia, the cremaster muscle and cremasteric fascia, and the internal spermatic fascia. Begin superiorly, for the layers cannot be differentiated inferiorly.

2. Now separate the various structures in the spermatic cord. The vas deferens—a firm, cord-like structure—and the blood vessels can be easily identified. The nerves and lymph vessels are not visible as separate structures.

Testicular artery

The testicular artery arises from the front of the abdominal aorta at the level of the second lumbar vertebra (the same level as the origin of the testis). It descends on the posterior abdominal wall to

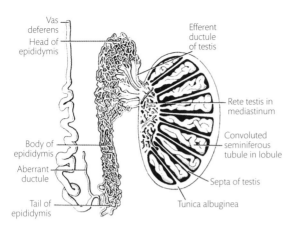

Fig. 9.5 Sagittal section of the testis, epididymis, and vas deferens.

the deep inguinal ring, enters the spermatic cord, and runs through it to the posterior border of the testis [Fig. 9.4]. Small branches enter the posterior border of the testis. Larger branches pass forwards on both sides of the testis and form a vascular layer deep to a dense layer of fibrous tissue—the **tunica albuginea**—which encloses the testis [Fig. 9.7].

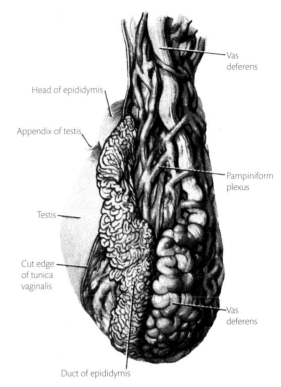

Fig. 9.6 The left testis, epididymis, and lower part of the spermatic cord seen from behind.

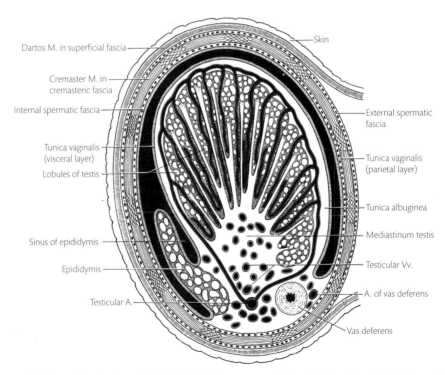

Fig. 9.7 Diagrammatic horizontal section through the left half of the scrotum and left testis. The cavity of the tunica vaginalis (black) is distended to make it obvious.

Veins

Numerous veins leave the posterior border of the testis to form the extensive **pampiniform plexus** of veins [Figs. 9.4, 9.6, 9.7]. The pampiniform plexus makes up a large part of the spermatic cord. At the deep inguinal ring, the veins of the plexus unite to form the testicular vein. The testicular vein ascends over the posterior abdominal wall. The left testicular vein drains into the left renal vein, and the right testicular vein drains into the inferior vena cava. ➲ The venous channels of the pampiniform plexus may be greatly distended to produce a **varicocele** of the spermatic cord.

Lymph vessels

The testicular lymph vessels (but not those of the scrotum) ascend through the spermatic cord. They pass over the posterior abdominal wall and enter the **lumbar lymph nodes** that lie along the side of the aorta between its bifurcation and the level of the renal arteries [see Fig. 13.2].

Nerves

Sympathetic nerves from the renal or aortic plexus run with the testicular artery. Small ganglia may be found along the artery. Sympathetic and parasympathetic nerve fibres from the inferior hypogastric plexus in the pelvis run on the vas deferens (deferential plexus).

Dissection 9.3 is designed to demonstrate the tunica vaginalis testis.

Tunica vaginalis testis

This closed serous sac encloses the testis and epididymis which are invaginated into it from the posterior side. The parietal layer lines the internal spermatic fascia. The visceral layer covers the front and sides of the testis and epididymis and is continuous with the parietal layer near the posterior border of the testis [Fig. 9.7]. On the lateral side, the visceral layer is tucked between the epididymis and testis to form the slit-like **sinus of the epididymis** [Figs. 9.4, 9.7]. Normally there is only a thin film of fluid between the two layers. ➲ In certain pathological conditions, the space may be distended with fluid, a condition called hydrocele. Rarely the tunica vaginalis testis is continuous with the peritoneal cavity through a persistent processus vaginalis.

Testis

The oval-shaped testis is variable in size. It is approximately 4 cm long, 2.5 cm anteroposteriorly, and 2 cm transversely. It is enclosed in a thick, dense layer of white fibrous tissue—the **tunica albuginea**. This fibrous tissue layer is covered by the visceral layer of the **tunica vaginalis**, except superiorly and posteriorly where it is in contact with the epididymis. The testis is made up of approximately 250 lobules which contain fine, highly convoluted, thread-like **seminiferous tubules**. These tubules are lined with a thick epithelium that produces immature spermatozoa. From the superior pole of the testis, 15 to 20 delicate ducts, known as **efferent ductules**, pass to the epididymis [Figs. 9.1, 9.5].

Epididymis

The epididymis is a comma-shaped structure overlying the superior and posterolateral aspects of the testis. The superior extremity of the epididymis is the **head** and the inferior extremity is the **tail**. The intermediate part, partly separated from the testis by the sinus of the epididymis, is the **body** [Figs. 9.1, 9.5, 9.7].

At the head of the epididymis, the efferent ductules of the testis connect the passages of the testis to the epididymis. The epididymis consists almost entirely of a single, complexly convoluted tube—the **duct of the epididymis**—which is 5–7 m in length. This duct is continuous with the vas deferens at the tail of the epididymis [Fig. 9.5].

DISSECTION 9.3 Tunica vaginalis testis

Objective

I. To demonstrate the extent of the tunica vaginalis testis.

Instructions

1. With a syringe and needle, force some air or water into the tunica vaginalis of the testis through the anterior wall. This demonstrates the extent of the cavity which extends upwards in front of the lower part of the spermatic cord.

2. Open the cavity through its anterior wall.

DISSECTION 9.4 Testis and epididymis

Objective

I. To study the cut surface of the testis and epididymis.

Instructions

1. Trace the blood vessels to the testis.

2. Free the tail and body of the epididymis from the testis.

3. Make a longitudinal cut through the testis, and examine its structure with a hand lens. Attempt to unravel some of the seminiferous tubules on the cut surface of the testis by drawing them out with

a needle under water. Only a general idea of the arrangement can be obtained by this method. With the aid of a stream of water and gentle agitation with the needle, remove the tubules from part of the testis and uncover the fibrous septa.

4. At the superior pole of the testis, divide the tunica vaginalis which joins it to the head of the epididymis. Separate the testis and epididymis by gentle blunt dissection. This may demonstrate the efferent ductules passing from the testis to the head of the epididymis.

130

The **appendix of the testis** is a small, sessile body attached to the upper part of the anterior border of the testis. It is thought to be a remnant of the proximal end of the embryonic **paramesonephric duct** [Fig. 9.1]. The **appendix of the epididymis** is a small, pedunculated structure on the superior pole of the epididymis. It represents the remains of the embryonic mesonephric tubules cephalic to the **efferent ductules of the testis**. Caudal to the efferent ductules, other mesonephric tubules may persist. These form small **aberrant ductules** which enter the vas deferens at the tail of the epididymis [Fig. 9.5].

In Dissection 9.4 you will find instructions to study the cut section of the testis and epididymis.

Penis

The penis is described as if it were erect. It consists of three parallel cylindrical bodies—the paired dorsally placed **corpora cavernosa** and the more ventrally placed **corpus spongiosum**. The

relationship of these three structures is best seen in the cut section of the penis [Fig. 9.8]. The **corpora cavernosa** are fused together in the body of the penis but diverge in the perineum to form the **crura** of the penis. Each crus is attached to the sides of the pubic arch. The **corpus spongiosum** enlarges proximally to form the **bulb of the penis**. Here it is attached between the crura to the inferior surface of the urogenital diaphragm (the perineal membrane) [Fig. 9.9]. Distally the corpus spongiosum

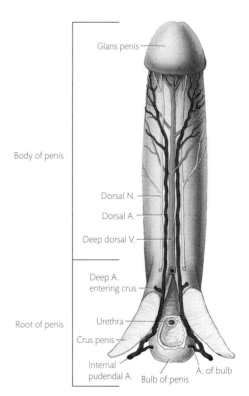

Fig. 9.9 Dorsal view of the body and root of the penis.

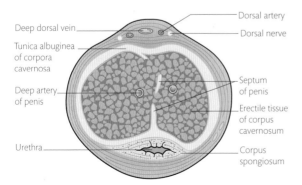

Fig. 9.8 Transverse section through the body of the penis.

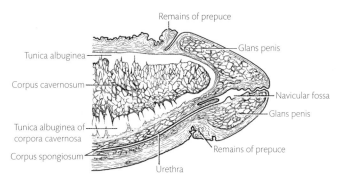

Fig. 9.10 Median section through the terminal part of a circumcised penis.

expands to form the **glans penis** into which the tapered ends of the corpora cavernosa are inserted [Fig. 9.10]. The penile urethra traverses the bulb of the penis, the corpus spongiosum and the glans. It opens at the tip of the glans as a vertical slit—the **external urethral orifice**. The glans penis is more extensive on the dorsal and lateral surfaces than on the ventral surface. The projecting margin of the base of the glans is the **corona glandis**.

The superficial fascia of the penis is composed of loose areolar tissue without fat. The deep fascia forms a close-fitting sheath around the corpora [Fig. 9.8]. The skin of the penis is delicate, elastic, and hairless, except at the base. It is freely movable over the surface of the penis. Distally the skin of the penis forms a tubular fold—the **prepuce** [Fig. 9.10]—which extends over the glans for a variable distance. This skin turns inwards at the distal end of the prepuce, doubles over itself, and becomes continuous with the skin which covers the glans. It is firmly attached on the surface of the glans. In the midline ventrally, a narrow, free fold of skin (the **frenulum of the prepuce**) passes from the glans to the deep aspect of the prepuce. ➲ The greater part of the prepuce is removed in the operation of circumcision [Fig. 9.10].

The ligaments and blood vessels on the dorsum of the penis are dissected in Dissection 9.5.

Dorsal vessels and nerves of the penis

The superficial and deep dorsal veins are both unpaired median structures. The superficial vein lies in the superficial fascia and divides proximally into right and left branches which pass to the external pudendal veins of the thigh. The **deep**

DISSECTION 9.5 Penis-1

Objective

I. To study the ligaments and blood vessels on the dorsum of the penis.

Instructions

1. Cut through, and reflect, the skin along the dorsum of the penis, from the symphysis pubis to the end of the prepuce.

2. Find the extension of the membranous layer of the superficial fascia of the abdomen on to the penis.

3. Remove the fascia on the anterior surface of the pubis in the midline and identify the **fundiform ligament** [see Fig. 8.6].

4. Find the superficial dorsal vein of the penis as it lies in the superficial fascia. Trace it proximally towards the superficial veins of the thighs. Deep to this vein is the deep fascia of the penis.

5. Divide the deep fascia in the same line as the skin incision. Reflect the fascia to uncover the deep dorsal vein of the penis, with the dorsal arteries and nerves on each side of it [Fig. 9.9].

6. The suspensory ligament of the penis is a fibro-elastic structure which spreads out from the anterior surface of the pubic symphysis to the deep fascia on the dorsum and sides of the penis. It lies deep to the fundiform ligament.

dorsal vein lies deep to the deep fascia. It drains to the prostatic plexus of veins by passing below the pubic symphysis into the pelvis. The deep dorsal vein has a thick muscular wall, close to the pubis.

The paired dorsal arteries and nerves are the terminal branches of the internal pudendal arteries and the pudendal nerves, which are described in Chapter 16. On the dorsum of the penis, the nerves are lateral to the arteries. Both supply the skin of the penis and the glans penis.

Dissection 9.6 examines the cut surface of the penis.

Structure of the penis

The **corpora cavernosa** are paired cylindrical bodies consisting of cavernous **erectile tissue**. They are enclosed in a dense sheath of white fibrous tissue—the **tunica albuginea**. Medially the tunicae albugineae fuse to form an incomplete median **septum**, through which the cavernous tissue of the two corpora are continuous. A **deep artery** of the penis lies near the centre of each corpus cavernosum. When these arteries are dilated, the cavernous spaces are filled with blood under pressure, turning the corpora cavernosa into a rigid structure.

DISSECTION 9.6 Penis-2

Objective

I. To examine the cut section of the penis.

Instructions

1. Make a transverse section through the body of the penis, but leave the two parts connected by the skin of the urethral surface. Examine the cut surface.

2. Identify the two corpora cavernosa, the corpus spongiosum, the tunica albuginea of the corpus cavernosum and spongiosum, the urethra, and the deep artery of the penis.

The **corpus spongiosum** has a finer mesh of erectile tissue and a more delicate fibrous capsule (the tunica albuginea). Thus, when the cavernous tissue is filled with blood, it does not prevent passage of fluid in the urethra. The **arteries of the bulb** [Figs. 9.8, 9.9] traverse the corpus spongiosum, inferior to the urethra. Thus each part of the penis has a separate blood supply.

See Clinical Applications 9.1 and 9.2 for the clinical implications of the anatomy in this chapter.

CLINICAL APPLICATION 9.1 Hydrocele

A 40-day-old infant is brought to the paediatric surgery department with history of a painless, right-sided swelling in the scrotum that diminishes gradually when the child lies down. There is no history of trauma. On examination, the swelling is non-tender to touch and transilluminant (allows passage of light through it). The swelling surrounds the right testis and epididymis. A diagnosis of hydrocele is made.

Study question 1: what is a hydrocele? (Answer: a hydrocele is an abnormal collection of fluid between the parietal and visceral layers of the tunica vaginalis.)

Study question 2: what is a congenital hydrocele? (Answer: under normal circumstances, most of the processus vaginalis obliterates and the cavity of the tunica vaginalis is detached from the peritoneal cavity. If the processus vaginalis remains patent after birth, fluid from the peritoneal cavity fills the tunica vaginalis and forms a swelling around the testes. This is a congenital hydrocele.) A hydrocele can also be associated with inflammation of the testes and epididymis (epididymo-orchitis) or testicular tumours.

Study question 3: what is a haematocele? (Answer: a haematocele is a swelling around the testes due to haemorrhage into the tunica vaginalis, usually following trauma.)

CLINICAL APPLICATION 9.2 Vasectomy

A 48-year-old man opted to undergo male steriliza-tion, so that he and his wife would not have any more children. Male sterilization or vasectomy involves tying and cutting the vas deferens on both sides, as it lies in the spermatic cord. Under local anaesthesia, a skin incision is made on the front of the scrotum, above the epididymis, to access the structures in the spermatic cord. Review the coverings and contents of the spermatic cord.

Study question 1: what is the characteristic feature of the vas deferens which will enable the surgeon to dif-ferentiate it from the other structures? (Answer: the vas deferens is firm and cord-like, and easily differentiated from the other structures by its feel.)

Study question 2: what is the blood supply to the vas deferens? Name the other important artery that lies in the spermatic cord and has to be preserved during the procedure. (Answer: the vas deferens is supplied by the artery to the vas. Care should be taken not to ligate the testicular artery, as it lies in the spermatic cord.)

Note: Potency, the ability of the male to have sexual intercourse, is based on hormones secreted by the testis and is not affected by vasectomy.

CHAPTER 10
The lower back

Prior to studying the abdominal cavity, it is essential to study the thoracolumbar fascia of the back. This fascia extends from the sacrum to the neck. It binds the long extensor muscle of the vertebral column—the **erector spinae**—to the posterolateral surfaces of the vertebral bodies.

In the lumbar region, the fascia is very strong. Laterally, it gives origin to the internal oblique and transversus abdominis muscles [Fig. 10.1]. Medially, it splits into three layers—a posterior, middle, and anterior layer. The anterior and middle layers enclose the quadratus lumborum [Chapter 13].

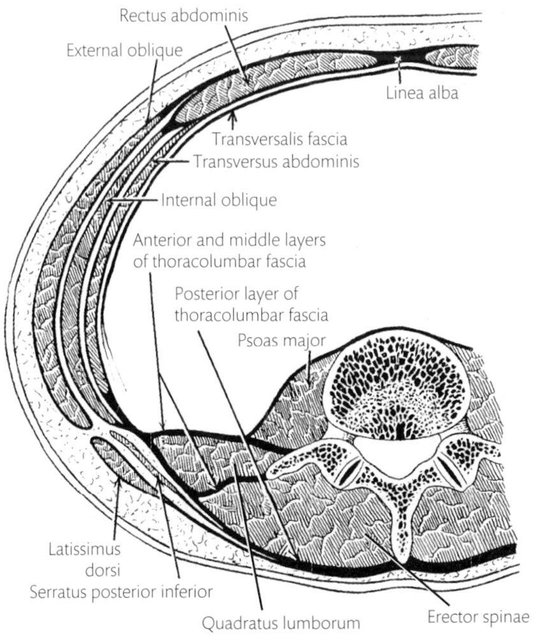

Dissection 10.1 exposes the posterior layer of the thoracolumbar fascia.

Thoracolumbar fascia

The **posterior layer** of the lumbar part of the thoracolumbar fascia passes behind the erector spinae muscle and is attached to the tips of the spines of the lumbar vertebrae. It is this layer which extends superiorly into the thoracic and cervical regions and inferiorly into the sacral region. In the

Fig. 10.1 A horizontal section through the abdominal wall at the level of the second lumbar vertebra, to show the thoracolumbar fascia.

Labels: Rectus abdominis; External oblique; Linea alba; Transversalis fascia; Transversus abdominis; Internal oblique; Anterior and middle layers of thoracolumbar fascia; Posterior layer of thoracolumbar fascia; Psoas major; Latissimus dorsi; Serratus posterior inferior; Quadratus lumborum; Erector spinae

---

DISSECTION 10.1 Exposure of the posterior layer of the thoracolumbar fascia

Objective

I. To clean the posterior surface of the posterior layer of the thoracolumbar fascia.

Instructions

1. With the body in the prone position, follow the inferior part of the latissimus dorsi to the iliac crest and expose the free posterior border of the external oblique muscle [see Fig. 4.4, Vol. 1].

2. Note the interval between the external oblique, latissimus dorsi, and iliac crest—the **lumbar triangle**—immediately superior to the iliac crest.

3. Reflect the remaining fibres of the latissimus dorsi inferiorly and those of the external oblique anteriorly. This exposes the posterior part of the internal oblique and the thoracolumbar fascia to which it is attached.

thoracic region, the thoracolumbar fascia forms a thin, transparent lamina, attached medially to the spines of the thoracic vertebrae and laterally to the angles of the ribs. It lies deep to the trapezius, rhomboids, and serratus posterior superior. In the sacral region, it stretches from the sacral spines to the ilium and sacrotuberous ligaments and fuses with the periosteum on the back of the sacrum and coccyx, inferior to the attachment of the erector spinae.

The **middle layer** of the lumbar part of the thoracolumbar fascia passes medially between the erector spinae and the quadratus lumborum to the tips of the lumbar transverse processes. The **anterior layer** passes in front of the quadratus lumborum and is attached to the anterior surfaces of the lumbar transverse processes. Thus the anterior and middle layers enclose the **quadratus lumborum**. This muscle is attached to the anterior surfaces of the lumbar transverse processes and extends from the twelfth rib superiorly to the iliolumbar ligament and iliac crest [see Fig. 8.7] inferiorly. The middle and anterior layers end superiorly by being attached to the twelfth rib, and inferiorly by being attached to the iliolumbar ligament and the adjacent iliac crest—the same structures as the quadratus lumborum.

The **anterior layer** of the thoracolumbar fascia is thin but strong. It is thickened between the transverse process of the first lumbar vertebra and the tip of the twelfth rib, to form the **lateral arcuate ligament**. This ligament gives origin to some fibres of the diaphragm. The subcostal vessels and nerve pass into the posterior abdominal wall posterior to the ligament.

Dissection 10.2 gives instructions for dissection of the thoracolumbar fascia.

DISSECTION 10.2 Thoracolumbar fascia

Objective

I. To study the three layers of the thoracolumbar fascia.

Instructions

1. Remove the remains of the latissimus dorsi. Detach the serratus posterior inferior from the posterior layer of the thoracolumbar fascia to expose the posterior layer.

2. Cut vertically through the posterior layer, from the last rib to the iliac crest. Make transverse cuts through the fascia at the upper and lower ends. Reflect the layer and expose the erector spinae.

3. Pull the erector spinae medially and follow the middle layer of the thoracolumbar fascia anterior to it. When the attachments of this layer have been defined medially, cut through it along its superior, medial, and inferior attachments. Reflect the middle layer laterally.

4. Push the quadratus lumborum medially and run your finger over the posterior surface of the anterior layer. It is better to leave this layer intact at this stage and see these structures from in front later. However, this layer may also be cut to expose the lower part of the kidney and the subcostal, iliohypogastric, and ilioinguinal nerves passing posterior to it.

CHAPTER 11
The abdominal cavity

Introduction

The abdominal cavity is enclosed by the abdominal walls and is completely filled by the abdominal viscera. The abdominal viscera include the stomach and intestines, their associated glands and ducts (liver and pancreas), blood and lymph vessels, the spleen, the kidneys, and the suprarenal glands. The kidneys, the ureters, and the suprarenal glands lie on the posterior abdominal wall, posterior to the fascia lining the abdominal cavity. The other structures lie anterior to this fascia and are surrounded to a greater or lesser extent by the peritoneal cavity.

The **peritoneum** is a tough layer of elastic areolar tissue lined with simple squamous epithelium. It lines the largest of the serous sacs of the body—the peritoneal cavity. It is similar to the pleura and pericardium in consisting of **parietal** and **visceral layers** which enclose the peritoneal cavity, and are separated from each other by a thin film of peritoneal fluid. This fluid lubricates the smooth peritoneal surfaces and facilitates movement of those parts of the abdominal viscera which are ensheathed by the visceral layer.

The **parietal peritoneum** is a simple layer on the internal surface of the abdominal walls. The **visceral peritoneum** is more complex in arrangement. It surrounds many segments of the intricately folded and tightly packed gut tube, the liver, and the spleen. The organs surrounded by the visceral peritoneum are referred to as **intraperitoneal**. The visceral peritoneum also forms mesenteries (sometimes called ligaments) which connect intraperitoneal organs to the body wall. Note that all intraperitoneal structures will have a mesentery connecting them to the body wall and that the mesentery is the only route whereby blood vessels, nerves, and lymphatics can reach the organ from the body wall [Fig. 11.1].

The **peritoneal cavity** is the slit-like interval between the parietal and visceral layers of the peritoneum and between the visceral peritoneum of adjacent intraperitoneal organs. Since these structures fill the abdomen, the peritoneal cavity is narrow and contains a very small volume of fluid. The peritoneal cavity may be distended as far as the abdominal walls allow by the introduction of fluid or air.

In the embryo, all parts of the gut tube have a mesentery, i.e. they are '**intraperitoneal**'. During development, certain parts of this tube— the duodenum and its glandular outgrowth (the pancreas), the ascending colon, and the descending colon—become applied to, and fused with, the peritoneum of the posterior abdominal wall. The mesentery disappears and the parietal peritoneum

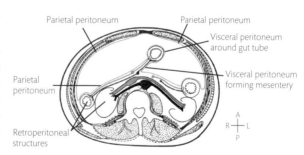

Fig. 11.1 A diagram to show the arrangement of the parietal peritoneum lining the abdominal cavity and the visceral peritoneum on the gut tube and mesentery. Note the structures which lie behind the peritoneum—the retroperitoneal structures.

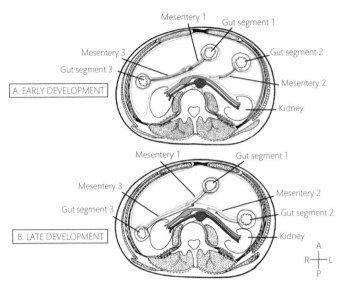

Fig. 11.2 (A) Schematic diagram showing three segments of the gut tube suspended in the peritoneal cavity by mesenteries during early development. (B) In late development, gut segments 2 and 3 and their mesenteries have adhered to the posterior abdominal wall and lie posterior to the parietal peritoneum, anterior to the kidney and other structures associated with the urogenital apparatus. Gut segment 1 remains intraperitoneal and is suspended by its mesentery. A=Anterior, P=posterior, R=right, L=left.

of the posterior abdominal wall comes to run directly over these structures [Fig. 11.2]. These structures are now '**retroperitoneal**'. As a result, the blood and lymph vessels and the nerves which originally ran in these mesenteries now lie on the posterior abdominal wall.

The paired viscera—the suprarenal glands, kidneys, and gonads—and their vessels lie on the posterior abdominal wall behind the parietal peritoneum. The retroperitoneal parts of the gut tube (duodenum, ascending colon, descending colon, pancreas) lie anterior to the paired viscera.

See Dissection 11.1 for directions on how to open the peritoneal cavity.

DISSECTION 11.1 Preliminary survey of the peritoneal cavity

Objective

I. To explore the contents of the peritoneal cavity.

Instructions

1. Open into the peritoneal cavity, taking care to avoid cutting any structure within the peritoneum.

2. Take time to explore the peritoneal cavity without damage to the peritoneum or the structures covered by it.

Posterior to the peritoneal cavity, there are three distinct layers of structures, each with its own blood and lymph vessels and nerves. From behind forwards, these are:

1. The **posterior abdominal wall**, consisting of the vertebral column and the muscles attached to it [see Fig. 10.1]. It contains the lumbar vessels and nerves. (The posterior abdominal wall is described in Chapter 13.)

2. On the posterior abdominal wall, but deep to its fascial lining, lie the **kidneys, ureters, suprarenal glands**, and great vessels—the **abdominal aorta** and **inferior vena cava**. The aorta and inferior vena cava lie on the anterior surface of the vertebral column [see Figs. 11.13, 11.59]. The kidneys, suprarenals, and their ducts lie on either side of the vertebral column. The gonads are displaced downwards from this layer, but their blood and lymph vessels and nerves still traverse it, as do the paired suprarenal and renal vessels.

3. The unpaired gut tube lies in a plane anterior to the kidney, suprarenal, and great vessels.

   (i) The retroperitoneal parts of the gut tube (**duodenum**, **ascending** and **descending colon**, and glands and blood vessels associated with them) lie posteriorly, immediately anterior to the plane of the kidney.

   (ii) The intraperitoneal parts of the gut tube which remain free—the stomach, jejunum, ileum, and transverse and sigmoid colon—lie most anteriorly. They do so by retaining the mesenteries which attach them to the posterior abdominal wall (**dorsal mesenteries**). They are supplied by unpaired visceral vessels. These are the most mobile parts of the intra-abdominal gut tube and are surrounded by the visceral peritoneum. The peritoneum surrounding the gut passes to the posterior abdominal wall from a narrow strip on the gut tube. It forms a double-layered fold of peritoneum. This double fold of peritoneum is called the **mesentery**, or ligament. Between the two layers of the fold is a variable amount of extraperitoneal fatty areolar tissue in which blood vessels, lymph vessels, and nerves run to and from the gut tube. Where the layers meet the posterior abdominal wall, they become continuous with the parietal peritoneum, and the areolar tissue between them is continuous with the extraperitoneal tissue of the abdominal walls.

In addition to the dorsal mesentery which all parts of the free gut tube have, the stomach and proximal 2–3 cm of the duodenum also have a **ventral mesentery**. The ventral mesentery attaches this part of the gut tube to the anterior abdominal wall. During development, the liver develops in this ventral mesentery and divides it into two parts. One part—the **lesser omentum**—connects the stomach and proximal duodenum to the liver. The other part—the **falciform ligament**—connects the liver to the anterior abdominal wall. The falciform ligament is the only attachment of the abdominal viscera to the anterior abdominal wall.

When the anterior abdominal wall is removed, the only parts of the viscera immediately visible are the liver, the free gut tube (stomach, jejunum, ileum, transverse colon, and sigmoid colon), and the ascending and descending parts of the colon [Fig. 11.3].

The **cavity of the lesser pelvis** extends postero-inferiorly from the abdominal cavity [Figs. 11.4, 11.5]. It lies below the linea terminalis of the bony pelvis. The pelvic cavity is bounded antero-inferiorly by the pubic symphysis, and posteriorly and superiorly by the curved sacrum and coccyx. The inferior limit of the lesser pelvis is the diamond-shaped **perineum**. A fibromuscular diaphragm—the pelvic diaphragm—stretches between the pubic symphysis and the coccyx and separates the pelvic cavity from the perineum [Fig. 11.5]. The peritoneal cavity extends

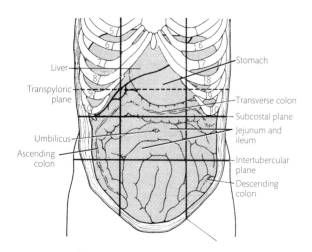

Fig. 11.3 The abdominal viscera after removal of the anterior abdominal wall and the greater omentum. Note that the eighth costal cartilage reaches the sternum in this case.

into the superior part of the pelvis above the urinary bladder and the uterus and anterior to the rectum [see Figs. 17.5, 17.6]. In the male, the peritoneal cavity is a closed sac. In the female, the uterine tubes open into it. A direct communication thus exists in the female between the pelvic cavity and the exterior through the uterus and the vagina.

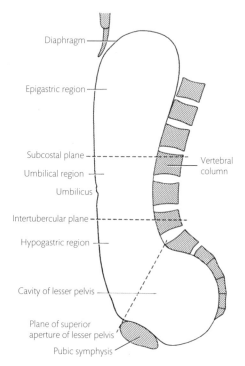

Fig. 11.4 An outline of the abdominal and pelvic cavities as seen in the median section.

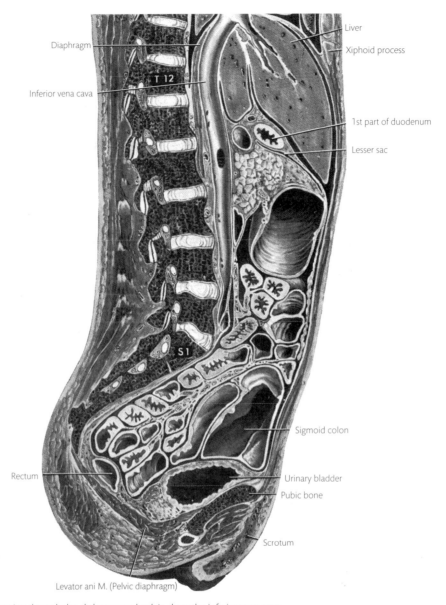

Diaphragm

Inferior vena cava

T 12

S 1

Liver

Xiphoid process

1st part of duodenum

Lesser sac

Sigmoid colon

Rectum

Urinary bladder

Pubic bone

Scrotum

Levator ani M. (Pelvic diaphragm)

Fig. 11.5 A sagittal section through the abdomen and pelvis along the inferior vena cava.

Shape of the abdominal cavity

In transverse section, the abdominal cavity is kidney-shaped because the vertebral column protrudes into it posteriorly. There is a deep paravertebral groove on each side of the vertebral column, which is separated from its thoracic counterpart by the diaphragm. Each groove lodges a kidney, a suprarenal gland, the ascending colon on the right, and the descending colon on the left [Figs. 11.6, 11.7]. Because of the curvatures of the vertebral column, the upper lumbar vertebrae lie further posteriorly than the lower. The anteroposterior extent of the abdominal cavity is therefore much greater in the superior part than in the inferior part, though it is reduced in the uppermost part where the diaphragm arches forwards, above the first lumbar vertebra [Fig. 11.4]. In the supine position, the anterior abdominal wall may be less than 5 cm from the great vessels on the anterior surface of the lower lumbar vertebral column. Similarly, the **paravertebral grooves** slope posterosuperiorly from the iliac fossa. ➔ Consequently, free fluid in the peritoneal cavity gravitates to the upper abdomen when a patient lies flat on his back [Figs. 11.4, 11.6, 11.7].

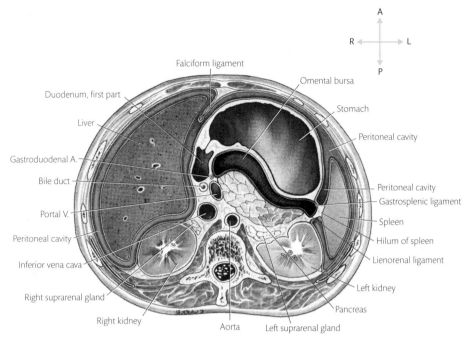

Fig. 11.6 A horizontal section through the abdomen at the level of the pylorus. Blue = peritoneal cavity. Red = lesser sac. A = anterior; P = posterior; R = right; L = left.

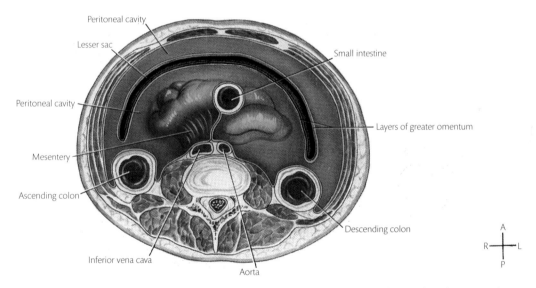

Fig. 11.7 A diagrammatic horizontal section through the abdomen at the level of the fourth lumbar vertebra. The peritoneal cavity is shown distended. Blue = peritoneal cavity. Red = lesser sac of the peritoneal cavity. A = anterior; P = posterior; R = right; L = left.

Boundaries of the abdominal cavity

The roof of the abdominal cavity is the diaphragm. The diaphragm also forms the upper parts of the lateral and posterior walls [Figs. 11.4, 11.5]. The anterior wall and a small part of each lateral wall between the ribs and the hip bone are formed by muscles and their aponeuroses. The lowest part of each lateral wall is formed by the ilium covered

internally by the iliacus muscle [see Fig. 8.3; Fig. 11.13]. The posterior wall is formed in the upper part by the vertebral column, the muscles attached to it (diaphragm, psoas, and quadratus lumborum), and the thoracolumbar fascia [see Fig. 11.13]. Below, the posterior wall is formed by the posterior part of the ilium with the iliacus muscle covering it. The posterior wall meets the anterior abdominal wall at the inguinal ligament [see Fig. 8.11].

Divisions of the peritoneal cavity—the greater sac and lesser sac

Removing the anterior abdominal wall exposes the greater part of the peritoneal cavity—the greater sac. In addition to the part exposed, there is a smaller extension of this cavity behind the stomach not visible at this stage. It is the **lesser sac**, or **omental bursa**, which lies between the stomach and the posterior abdominal wall [Figs. 11.6, 11.7]. Study the series of drawings in Fig. 11.8 to understand the development of the lesser sac. The lesser sac develops as an extension of the peritoneal cavity into the right side of the dorsal mesentery of the stomach. This extension in the double-layered dorsal mesentery creates a sac which expands beyond the limits of the stomach to the left and inferiorly [Fig. 11.8]. Superiorly, the wall of the sac extends to the left up to the diaphragm [Fig. 11.9]. To the left, the spleen develops within the two layers of the dorsal mesentery [Fig. 11.8D]. The peritoneal fold extending from the spleen to the stomach forms the **gastrosplenic ligament**. The fold extending from the spleen to the posterior abdominal wall in the region of the kidney is the **lieno-renal ligament** [Fig. 11.6]. Superior to the spleen, the dorsal mesentery passes directly from the fundus

(superior part) of the stomach to the diaphragm as the **gastrophrenic ligament**. These ligaments are simply parts of the dorsal mesentery of the stomach. They are not specially strengthened, despite the name ligament.

Part of the dorsal mesentery of the stomach is carried inferiorly by the expanding lesser sac. It forms a flattened bag of peritoneum—the **greater omentum**. In the adult, the greater omentum hangs down like an apron between the anterior abdominal wall and the anterior surface of the abdominal viscera (mainly the small and large intestines), inferior to the stomach [Figs. 11.7, 11.8C, 11.8D]. Early in development, the greater omentum contains part of the cavity of the lesser sac, but, as development proceeds, the walls fuse and convert it into a simple flap of peritoneum which often contains a considerable quantity of extraperitoneal tissue and fat. The greater omentum overlies the transverse part of the large intestine—the **transverse colon**. The transverse colon, together with its mesentery—the transverse mesocolon—fuses with the posterior surface of the greater omentum [Fig. 11.9]. The compound flap thus formed partially divides the peritoneal cavity into an antero-superior, or **supracolic**, and a postero-inferior, or **infracolic**, **compartment** [Fig. 11.9].

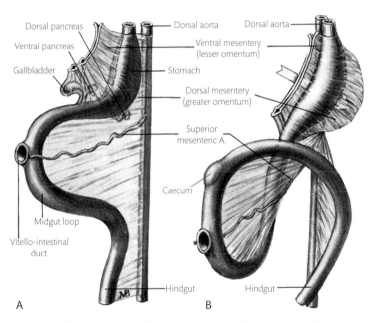

Dorsal pancreas
Ventral pancreas
Gallbladder
Dorsal aorta
Ventral mesentery (lesser omentum)
Stomach
Dorsal mesentery (greater omentum)
Dorsal aorta
Superior mesenteric A.
Caecum
Midgut loop
Vitello-intestinal duct
Hindgut
Hindgut

A   B

Fig. 11.8 A diagram to show the stages in the development of the abdominal part of the gut tube and its mesenteries. (A) Before rotation of the midgut. (B) Rotation of the midgut loop and the ballooning of the dorsal mesentery of the stomach to the left by extension of the lesser sac (indicated by the arrow) into that mesentery. (C) Return of the midgut loop into the abdomen and further growth of the lesser sac. (D) Formation of the greater omentum and the ligaments of the spleen from the dorsal mesentery of the stomach. The duodenum and ascending and descending colons are fused to the posterior abdominal wall and lose their mesentery. The other parts of the gut tube remain free and retain their mesentery.

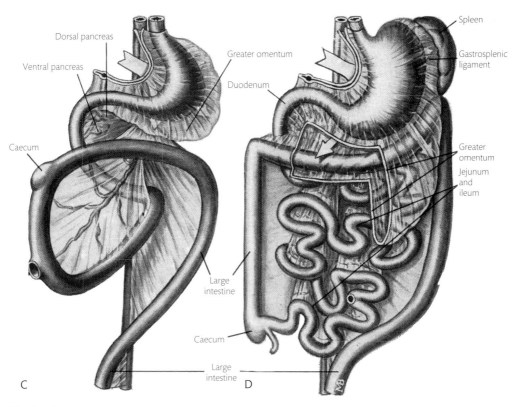

Dorsal pancreas

Ventral pancreas

Greater omentum

Duodenum

Caecum

Large intestine

Caecum

Large intestine

C

Spleen

Gastrosplenic ligament

Greater omentum

Jejunum and ileum

Large intestine

D

Fig. 11.8 (Continued)

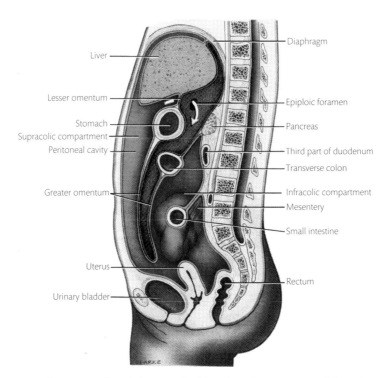

Liver

Lesser omentum

Stomach

Supracolic compartment

Peritoneal cavity

Greater omentum

Uterus

Urinary bladder

Diaphragm

Epiploic foramen

Pancreas

Third part of duodenum

Transverse colon

Infracolic compartment

Mesentery

Small intestine

Rectum

Fig. 11.9 A diagrammatic median section of the abdomen and pelvis to show the arrangement of the peritoneum. Normally, the abdominal viscera completely fill the abdominal cavity, and the peritoneal cavity is reduced to a slit. In the diagram, the cavity has been distended to make it obvious. Blue = general peritoneal cavity or greater sac. Red = lesser sac. The arrow traverses the epiploic foramen.

General arrangement of the abdominal viscera

Dissection 11.2 explores the peritoneal cavity.

DISSECTION 11.2 Exploration of the peritoneal cavity

Objectives

I. To identify and study the location of the stomach, liver, gallbladder, lesser omentum, epiploic foramen, greater omentum, and falciform ligament in the supracolic compartment.   II. To identify and study the location of the duodenum, jejunum, ileum, mesentery, caecum, vermiform appendix, ascending, transverse, descending, and sigmoid colon, transverse mesocolon, and sigmoid mesocolon in the infracolic compartment.

Instructions

The following brief description gives only the general arrangement of the abdominal viscera which may be examined without dissection. It is important to confirm the location of the abdominal organs without damage to the structures which will be dissected later. The positions given for the various structures are approximate because the abdominal viscera move with respiration and alter their position with the age and bodily habitus of the individual. The relative position of organs is also changed by distension and movement of the hollow viscera, particularly those which are free to move on a mesentery.

1. Identify the greater omentum and note its continuity with the stomach. Identify the transverse colon fused with the posterior surface of the greater omentum, a short distance inferior to the stomach.

2. The **supracolic compartment** of the peritoneal cavity lies superior to the greater omentum and transverse mesocolon. It contains the liver, stomach, spleen, and superior part of the duodenum. It lies anterior to the pancreas, duodenum, kidneys, and suprarenal glands.

3. The **liver** fills the greater part of the right hypochondrium, and is mainly under cover of the ribs and diaphragm. Most of the liver surface is covered with the peritoneum, and it is divided into a large **right** and small **left** lobes by the **falciform ligament**.

4. Examine the falciform ligament. It is attached to the anterior surface of the liver, a little to the right of the median plane. It extends to the supraumbilical part of the anterior abdominal wall.

5. The sharp **inferior margin** of the right lobe lies approximately along the right costal margin. Close to the tip of the ninth right costal cartilage, the rounded fundus of the **gallbladder** protrudes below the inferior margin of the liver. The right lobe then appears from behind the costal cartilages and almost immediately joins the left lobe between the right and left costal margins. The inferior margin of the left lobe continues in the same direction up to the eighth left costal cartilage. Here it turns more sharply upwards to meet the superior surface of the liver, posterior to the fifth left costochondral junction [Fig. 11.3].

6. The superior surface of the **right lobe** fits into the right dome of the diaphragm. It reaches the level of the upper border of the fifth rib in the right midclavicular plane. Posteriorly, it lies on the posterior part of the diaphragm, the right suprarenal gland, and the superior part of the right kidney.

7. The **stomach** lies obliquely across the supracolic compartment from upper left to lower right in a J- or C-shaped curve. The greater part is hidden by the liver, diaphragm, and ribs, but part of its anterior surface is in contact with the anterior abdominal wall, inferior to the left lobe of the liver [Fig. 11.3]. Pass a hand upwards over the anterior surface of the stomach and identify its superior rounded **fundus** and the **oesophagus** entering the right border inferior to the fundus and posterior to the liver. Lift up the inferior margin of the liver and trace the right concave border of the stomach—the **lesser curvature**—downwards. The lesser curvature runs from the entry of the oesophagus into the stomach, to a thickening—the **pyloric sphincter**—in the wall of the stomach where it meets the duodenum. Note a sharp angulation of the lesser curvature (**incisura angularis**) which marks the junction of the body of the stomach with the pyloric part [Fig. 11.10].

8. Identify the thin sheet of the peritoneum (the **lesser omentum**) which passes from the lesser curvature of the stomach to the liver. It is short where the abdominal oesophagus abuts on the liver but lengthens towards the pylorus. The lesser omentum ends in a thickened free edge on the right side. This thick margin contains the **portal vein**, the **proper hepatic artery**, and the **bile duct**, all of which run from the superior part of the duodenum to the liver [Fig. 11.11]. The small area on the liver to which the edge of the lesser omentum is attached superiorly is the **porta hepatis**.

9. Pass a finger to the left, posterior to the free edge of the lesser omentum. The finger passes through the **epiploic foramen** into the **lesser sac**, posterior to the lesser omentum and stomach. If the finger is directed upwards in the foramen, it enters a narrow extension of the lesser sac—the **superior recess** between the liver and the diaphragm [see Fig. 11.13]. A finger in the thorax pushed inferiorly between the descending aorta and the diaphragm lies posterior to the finger in the superior recess but is separated from it by the diaphragm.

10. Trace the left convex border of the stomach from the fundus to the pylorus. The fold of peritoneum which passes from this curvature is the **dorsal mesentery of the stomach**. Superiorly, it passes to the diaphragm (**gastrophrenic ligament**). Inferior to this, it extends to the spleen (**gastrosplenic ligament**). Inferiorly it forms the **greater omentum**. This greater omentum ends where the first part of the duodenum becomes adherent to the posterior abdominal wall.

11. Pull the upper part of the greater curvature of the stomach to the right and expose the **spleen** deep in the left hypochondrium. It lies posterior to the stomach and anterior to the upper part of the left kidney. Posterolaterally, the spleen lies against the diaphragm which separates it from the pleural cavity. Confirm this with a finger in the left pleural cavity. Note that the long axis of the spleen lies parallel to the tenth rib, and that the spleen lies between the ninth and eleventh ribs, posterior to the mid-axillary line. The gastrosplenic and lienorenal ligaments are attached to a narrow strip on the medial aspect of the spleen. This is the **hilus** of the spleen. Other than the hilus, the spleen is completely covered by the peritoneum [Fig. 11.6].

12. Follow the **first part of the duodenum** posterosuperiorly to the right till it turns abruptly downwards. It continues vertically as the **second part**, which is adherent to the posterior abdominal wall. It passes posterior to the attachment of the mesentery of the transverse colon [Fig. 11.12] and connects the parts of the intestine in the supracolic and infracolic compartments. The head of the pancreas lies medial to this part of the duodenum.

13. **Infracolic compartment**: turn the greater omentum up and find the **transverse colon** adherent to its posterior surface. The colon can be differentiated from the small intestine by: (i) its position; (ii) the sacculation of its wall; (iii) the thickened bands of longitudinal muscle on the wall—**taeniae coli**; and (iv) the small projecting sacs of peritoneum filled with fat—**appendices epiploicae** [Fig. 11.12]. Trace the transverse colon and its mesentery—the **transverse mesocolon**—in both directions. The transverse mesocolon is mainly fused to the greater omentum and is attached to the front of the pancreas and the second part of the duodenum [Fig. 11.13].

14. The transverse colon is continuous through the right and left **colic flexures** with the **ascending** and **descending colon** [Fig. 11.12]. The ascending and descending colon are adherent to the posterior abdominal wall in the right and left paravertebral gutters, respectively. The part of these gutters lateral to the colon are the **paracolic gutters**. They form a route of communication between the infracolic and supracolic compartments.

15. The **right colic flexure** lies anterior to the inferior part of the right kidney, close to the inferior margin of the liver. The **left colic flexure** lies at a much higher level [see Fig. 11.23] in contact with the anterior (colic) surface of the spleen.

16. The **caecum** is a blind-ended sac in the right iliac fossa. It is continuous superiorly with the ascending colon and medially with the terminal ileum and **vermiform appendix** [Fig. 11.14]. The taeniae coli pass over the surface of the caecum and converge on the base of the vermiform appendix. A blind extension of the peritoneal cavity passes upwards,

posterior to the caecum. This is the **retrocaecal recess** [Fig. 11.15]. Attempt to explore it.

17. At the left iliac fossa, the descending colon becomes continuous with the **sigmoid colon**. The sigmoid colon loops postero-inferiorly into the lesser pelvis to continue as the **rectum** on the pelvic surface of the third piece of the sacrum. Here the taeniae coli of the sigmoid colon spread out into the more uniform longitudinal muscle layer of the rectum. The short **mesentery of the sigmoid colon** is attached across the margin of the superior aperture of the lesser pelvis [Figs. 11.12, 11.13] and on the pelvic surface of the sacrum.

18. The inferior half of the duodenum, jejunum, and ileum constitute the infracolic part of the **small intestine**. They are centrally placed within a boundary formed by the caecum and colon [Fig. 11.12]. Between the caecum on the right and the sigmoid colon on the left, the boundary is incomplete and coils of small intestine lie in the lesser pelvis. The infracolic part of the **duodenum** completes this C-shaped structure. It consists of the lower half of the **second** part, the **third** part which crosses the vertebral column immediately anterior to the inferior vena cava and aorta on the third lumbar vertebra, and the short **fourth part** which joins the jejunum on the left side of the second lumbar vertebra [Fig. 11.12].

19. The jejunum and ileum lie in the free edge of the **mesentery**. The root of the mesentery runs obliquely from the duodenojejunal junction to the ileocaecal junction. It partly divides the infracolic part of the peritoneal cavity into right superior and left inferior regions. The left inferior region is continuous with the pelvic peritoneal cavity. Both regions are filled with coils of the small intestine. The vermiform appendix lies at the right extremity of the left inferior region [Figs. 11.12, 11.13].

20. Pick up the mesentery. Note the short attachment to the posterior abdominal wall and the long, complexly folded free margin containing the jejunum and ileum. The **jejunum** and **ileum** cannot be differentiated from each other clearly. The wall of the jejunum is thicker than the wall of the ileum. There is usually less fat in the mesentery of the jejunum so that the vessels and the spaces between them are more clearly visible than in the ileal mesentery. The jejunum is approximately two-fifths of the 6 m this part of the intestine is said to measure.

21. A number of variable **accessory peritoneal folds** are found in relation to the duodenum and caecum [Figs. 11.14, 11.15]. Each of these produces a peritoneal recess. These folds and recesses should be noted where present.

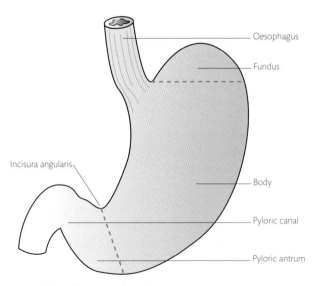

Fig. 11.10 A diagram of the anterior surface of the stomach to show its parts.

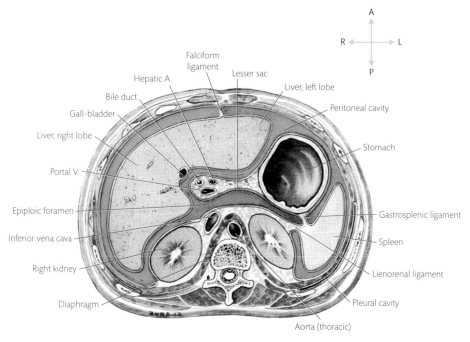

Fig. 11.11 A horizontal section through the abdomen at the level of the epiploic foramen. Blue = peritoneal cavity. Red = lesser sac. A = anterior; P = posterior; R = right; L = left.

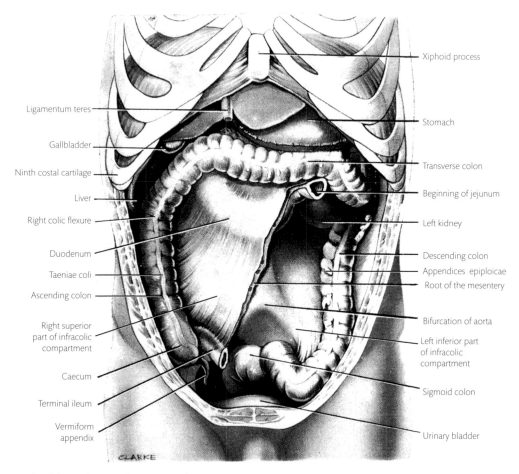

Fig. 11.12 The abdominal viscera after removal of the jejunum, ileum, and greater omentum.

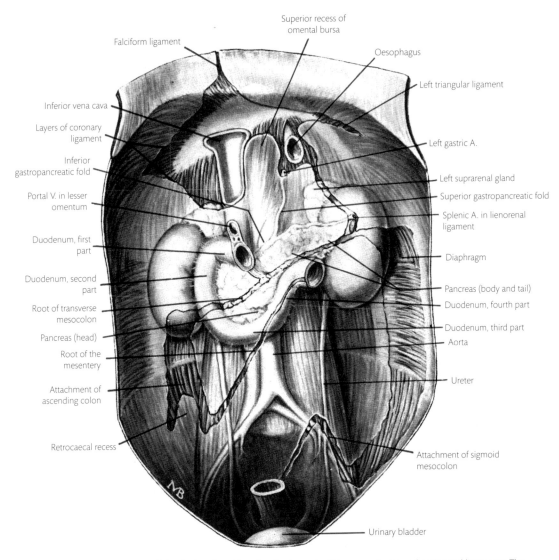

Superior recess of
omental bursa

Falciform ligament

Oesophagus

Left triangular ligament

Inferior vena cava

Layers of coronary
ligament

Left gastric A.

Inferior
gastropancreatic fold

Left suprarenal gland

Superior gastropancreatic fold

Portal V. in lesser
omentum

Splenic A. in lienorenal
ligament

Duodenum, first
part

Diaphragm

Duodenum, second
part

Pancreas (body and tail)

Root of transverse
mesocolon

Duodenum, fourth part

Duodenum, third part

Pancreas (head)

Aorta

Root of the
mesentery

Ureter

Attachment of
ascending colon

Retrocaecal recess

Attachment of sigmoid
mesocolon

Urinary bladder

Fig. 11.13 Diagram of the posterior abdominal wall to show the attachments of the mesenteries and peritoneal ligaments. The oesophagus, duodenum, and rectum are the only parts of the gut tube left *in situ*.

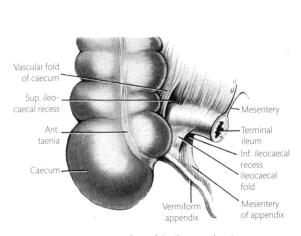

Vascular fold
of caecum

Sup. ileo-
caecal recess

Ant.
taenia

Caecum

Mesentery

Terminal
ileum

Inf. ileocaecal
recess

Ileocaecal
fold

Vermiform
appendix

Mesentery
of appendix

Fig. 11.14 The anterior surface of the ileocaecal region.

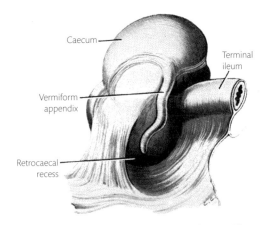

Caecum

Terminal
ileum

Vermiform
appendix

Retrocaecal
recess

Fig. 11.15 The inferior surface of the ileocaecal region. The caecum has been turned forwards to show the retrocaecal recess in which the vermiform appendix commonly lies.

Embryological basis for the adult position of the intestine

The apparently complex arrangement of the intestine described above is readily appreciated from its development [Fig. 11.8]. The **midgut** extends from the second part of the duodenum to the right two-thirds of the transverse colon. It is initially a simple loop protruding through the umbilical orifice [Fig. 11.8A]. The fixed ends of the loop are the terminal part of the duodenum and the left end of the transverse colon. This loop rotates on itself 180° anti-clockwise (as seen from the anterior surface). When the midgut loop returns to the abdomen from its position in the root of the umbilical cord, a further 90° rotation takes place in the same direction. The ends of the loop take up new positions—the duodenal end inferior to, and to the right of, the descending colon (hindgut) and its mesentery [Fig. 11.8C]. The rotation also gives the duodenum its final C shape. The small intestine falls into the central region. The caecum and other midgut parts of the colon lie anterior to the second part of the duodenum, superior to, and to the right of, the small intestine [Fig. 11.8C]. The centrally placed small intestine increases in length and displaces the surrounding parts of the large intestine outwards—the caecum and ascending colon to the right, the hindgut [Fig. 11.8D] or descending colon to the left, and the transverse colon (which lies anterior to the small intestine) upwards and forwards against the greater omentum. The mesenteries of all three parts of the colon fuse with the peritoneum adjacent to which they are applied. The mesentery of the ascending and descending colon fuses with the posterior abdominal wall. The mesentery of the transverse colon—the transverse mesocolon—fuses with the greater omentum. The ileum and jejunum retain their portion of the midgut mesentery between their fixed ends.

Peritoneal recesses

Some peritoneal folds may create recesses within the peritoneal cavity. Peritoneal recesses are often seen in relation to the duodenojejunal and ileocaecal junctions. ➲ They are of clinical importance as a loop of small intestine may become lodged and obstructed in the recess to form an internal hernia. Vascular content of the peritoneal fold may be important in surgical intervention of the hernia.

The **superior** and **inferior duodenal recesses**, when present, are to the left of the fourth part of the duodenum, behind the **superior** and **inferior duodenal folds** of the peritoneum. The inferior mesenteric vein lies behind the superior duodenal fold. The opening of the superior recess faces down; and that of the inferior recess faces up.

The **superior** and **inferior ileocaecal recesses** lie behind the **fold of the caecum** and the **ileocaecal fold** [Fig. 11.14]. The fold of the caecum contains the anterior caecal artery. The **retrocaecal recess** lies behind the caecum and may contain the vermiform appendix [Fig. 11.15].

Ligaments of the liver

Falciform ligament

The **falciform ligament** is the ventral part of the ventral mesentery (the lesser omentum is the dorsal part). It is a double fold of peritoneum attached anteriorly to the supraumbilical part of the anterior abdominal wall close to the median plane, and the diaphragm [Figs. 11.11, 11.12]. Posteriorly, the upper part of the falciform ligament passes to the right and is attached to the anterior surface of the liver. The lower part is free and this free border contains the **round ligament of the liver** passing from the umbilicus to the liver. The round ligament of the liver is the obliterated left umbilical vein. Trace the falciform ligament superiorly. On the liver, the right and left layers of peritoneum diverge to cover the right and left lobes of the liver.

Coronary ligament and right and left triangular ligaments

The peritoneum on the right and left lobes of the liver are reflected separately from the superior surface of the liver to the diaphragm [see Fig. 11.54]. On the right lobe, the peritoneum continues with the superior layer of the **coronary ligament**. Follow this fold to the right. It ends in a sharp margin—the **right triangular ligament**—where it meets the inferior layer of the coronary ligament. The left layer of the falciform ligament passes to the left as the anterior layer of the **left triangular ligament**. This ends in a sharp left margin where it becomes continuous with the posterior layer [see Fig. 11.55] of the left triangular ligament. (The inferior layer of the coronary ligament may be felt by pressing the fingers upwards, posterior to the right lobe of the liver and anterior to the right kidney. It forms the inferior margin of the **bare area** of the liver and will be seen when the liver is removed.)

Objectives

I. To identify the blood vessels at the greater curvature of the stomach.   II. To explore the lesser sac.

Instructions

1. Identify the arterial arcade (gastro-epiploic arteries) in the greater omentum, 2–3 cm from the greater curvature of the stomach.

2. Cut through the anterior layers of the greater omentum, 2–3 cm inferior to the arteries, to open the lower part of the lesser sac sufficiently to admit a hand. Explore the bursa.

Round ligament of the liver

The **round ligament of the liver** lies in the free margin of the falciform ligament and passes into a fissure on the postero-inferior (visceral) surface of the liver. (A more complete description of the ligaments of the liver is given later in the chapter, when the liver has been removed.)

Using the instructions given in Dissection 11.3 explore the lesser sac.

Lesser sac (omental bursa)

The lesser sac, or omental bursa, is an extension of the peritoneal cavity behind the stomach. It communicates with the general peritoneal cavity through the **epiploic foramen** at the right extremity of the lesser sac. The anterior margin of the epiploic foramen is formed by the portal vein, the proper hepatic artery, and the bile duct as they lie in the **free edge of the lesser omentum**. Posterior to the foramen is the inferior vena cava [Fig. 11.11]. Superiorly, the portal vein enters the liver and the inferior vena cava grooves it. Between these two veins is a narrow strip of the liver—the caudate process of the liver—which forms the superior limit of the epiploic foramen [see Fig. 11.54]. The inferior boundary of the foramen is formed by the first part of the duodenum, with the portal vein and bile duct passing posteriorly on it.

The lesser sac has a vestibule, a body, and superior, inferior, and splenic recesses. The epiploic foramen leads into the vestibule of the lesser sac. The **superior recess** of the lesser sac passes superiorly from the vestibule, on the left of the inferior vena

cava. It is posterior to the caudate lobe of the liver [see Fig. 11.54]. To the left, the vestibule opens into the main body of the bursa between the two **gastropancreatic folds**. The gastropancreatic folds are peritoneal folds produced by the left gastric artery and the common hepatic artery as they pass to the oesophageal and pyloric ends of the lesser curvature of the stomach [Fig. 11.13].

The **body** of the lesser sac lies posterior to the lesser omentum and stomach and separates the stomach from the structures on the posterior abdominal wall. (The structures posterior to the stomach are known as the 'stomach bed'.) The body of the lesser sac extends for a variable distance into the greater omentum as the **inferior recess** [Figs. 11.7, 11.8C, 11.8D, 11.9]. On the left, the bursa extends to the hilus of the spleen between the gastrosplenic and lienorenal ligaments as the **splenic recess** [Fig. 11.6].

The lesser sac gives added freedom of movement to the stomach, allowing it to expand after a meal and to slide freely on the surrounding tissues during contraction.

Dissection 11.4 examines the lesser omentum.

Lesser omentum

This double layer of peritoneum extends from the abdominal oesophagus, the lesser curvature of the stomach, and the first 2 cm of the duodenum to the liver [Fig. 11.16]. It lies posterior to the left lobe of the liver and anterior to the omental bursa. The omental bursa separates the lesser omentum from the pancreas, coeliac trunk (a branch of the aorta), and diaphragm.

Objective

I. To examine the lesser omentum.

Instructions

1. Pull the liver superiorly and tilt its inferior margin upwards to expose the lesser omentum. If this manoeuvre gives insufficient exposure, remove the left lobe of the liver by cutting through it to the left of the falciform ligament and the fissure for the round ligament (ligamentum teres); and the attachment of the lesser omentum.

On the liver, it is attached in the depths of the fissure for the ligamentum venosum [see Fig. 11.54] and around the margin of the porta hepatis. Between the duodenum and the porta hepatis is the free margin of the lesser omentum. At the free margin, the two layers enclose the **portal vein**, the **proper hepatic artery**, **bile duct**, sympathetic **nerves** on the artery, parasympathetic nerves from the anterior gastric nerves (vagus) to the gallbladder, and **lymph vessels** and nodes which drain the liver and the adjacent part of the stomach. Close to the lesser curvature of the stomach, the right and left **gastric vessels** lie between the layers of the lesser omentum. Elsewhere, the layers of the omentum enclose only extraperitoneal tissue [Figs. 11.16, 11.17].

Dissection 11.5 gives detailed instructions on how to identify and trace the structures in the lesser omentum.

Lienorenal and gastrosplenic ligaments

The thick lienorenal ligament runs from the posterior abdominal wall to the spleen. It contains the **tail of the pancreas** and the **splenic vessels**. The thin gastrosplenic ligament runs between the stomach and spleen. It contains the **short gastric** and **left gastro-epiploic arteries** (branches of the splenic artery) and the corresponding veins. **Lymph vessels** and nodes are also present in both ligaments. They drain the territories supplied by the arteries.

Dissection 11.6 gives detailed instructions on how to identify and trace the blood vessels in the greater omentum and the gastrosplenic ligament.

Dissection 11.7 gives instructions on how to dissect the stomach bed and the coeliac trunk.

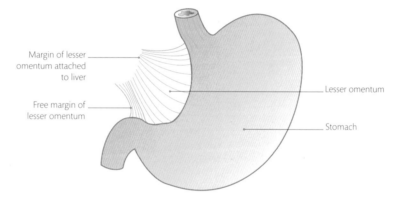

Fig. 11.16 The stomach, the first part of the duodenum, and the lesser omentum, showing the free margin of the lesser omentum and the margin attached to the liver.

Margin of lesser omentum attached to liver

Free margin of lesser omentum

Lesser omentum

Stomach

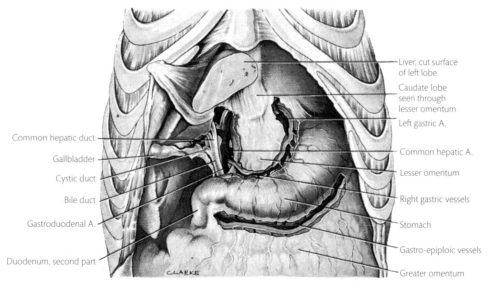

Common hepatic duct
Gallbladder
Cystic duct
Bile duct
Gastroduodenal A.
Duodenum, second part
CLARKE

Liver, cut surface of left lobe
Caudate lobe seen through lesser omentum
Left gastric A.
Common hepatic A.
Lesser omentum
Right gastric vessels
Stomach
Gastro-epiploic vessels
Greater omentum

Fig. 11.17 The interior of the abdomen after the removal of part of the left lobe of the liver. The vessels in the greater and lesser omentum are shown.

Objectives

I. To explore the contents of the lesser omentum. II. To identify and trace the left gastric vessels and their branches, the anterior vagal trunk, the right gastric vessels, the proper hepatic artery, and the portal vein.

Instructions

1. Remove the anterior layer of peritoneum from the lesser omentum, close to the lesser curvature of the stomach.

2. Find the **left gastric vessels** and follow them towards the oesophagus till they curve posteriorly round the superior surface of the lesser sac. Trace the **oesophageal branch** from it to the oesophagus.

3. Find the anterior vagal trunk on the anterior surface of the oesophagus. Trace its branches on to the stomach.

4. Trace the **right gastric artery** to the **proper hepatic artery**, and the **right gastric vein** to the portal vein. Expose the proper hepatic artery and its branches up to the porta hepatis.

5. Trace the **cystic duct** from the neck of the gallbladder to where it meets the common hepatic duct to form the bile duct. Follow the **common hepatic duct** and its tributaries (right and left hepatic ducts) to the porta hepatis and the bile duct till it passes posterior to the duodenum. Displace the proper hepatic artery and bile duct to expose the portal vein posterior to them.

6. Remove the remainder of the lesser omentum, leaving the vessels intact. Examine the abdominal wall posterior to the lesser omentum and lesser sac.

Objectives

I. To examine the lienorenal and gastrosplenic ligaments. II. To identify and trace the blood vessels in the gastrosplenic ligament and the greater curvature of the stomach.

Instructions

1. Identify the lienorenal ligament by placing one hand between the diaphragm and the spleen and the other in the lesser sac. Between the two hands is the thick lienorenal ligament which contains the **tail of the pancreas** and the **splenic vessels**.

2. Note the thin gastrosplenic ligament anterior to the hand in the lesser sac.

3. Identify and follow the short gastric and left gastro-epiploic vessels in the gastrosplenic ligament to the hilus of the spleen.

4. Confirm the attachment of the gastrosplenic ligament to the hilus of the spleen.

5. Follow the left gastro-epiploic artery through the greater omentum, parallel to the greater curvature of the stomach.

Coeliac trunk or coeliac artery

The coeliac trunk is the first unpaired branch from the abdominal aorta to the gut tube. It passes forwards for approximately 1 cm from the uppermost part of the abdominal aorta and divides into three branches: the common hepatic, splenic, and left gastric arteries [Figs. 11.18, 11.19, 11.20]. Together these arteries supply the gut tube from the lower part of the oesophagus to the descending part of the duodenum, the liver, pancreas, and spleen. The coeliac trunk is surrounded by a dense plexus of autonomic and sensory nerve fibres which are distributed with its branches.

Left gastric vessels

The left gastric artery is a small branch of the coeliac trunk which ascends on the posterior part of the diaphragm towards the oesophagus. At the cardiac end of the oesophagus, it arches forwards, raising the superior gastropancreatic fold, turns downwards and runs inferiorly along the lesser curvature of the stomach. It ends by anastomosing with the

DISSECTION 11.7 Stomach bed and coeliac trunk

Objectives

I. To remove the peritoneum from the stomach bed.   II. To identify the coeliac trunk, coeliac ganglion, left suprarenal vessels, and inferior phrenic arteries.

Instructions

1. Complete the cleaning of the gastro-epiploic vessels in the greater omentum. Follow them as far as possible in both directions. A plexus of sympathetic nerve fibres and an occasional lymph node may be found with them.

2. Cut through the stomach, the right gastric, and right gastro-epiploic vessels immediately to the left of the pylorus. Turn these structures to the left to expose the lesser sac. Remove the peritoneum from the left and posterior walls of the bursa as far inferiorly as the attachment of the greater omentum. Note the **lymph nodes (pancreaticosplenic)** on the superior border of the pancreas as it is uncovered.

3. Identify the coeliac trunk [Fig. 11.18] and remove the dense autonomic plexus from its branches. Expose the superior part of the left kidney and suprarenal gland, the three **suprarenal arteries** and the single **suprarenal vein**, and the **inferior phrenic artery** on the left crus of the diaphragm.

4. Identify the **coeliac ganglia**, one on each side of the coeliac trunk, and trace the **splanchnic nerves** superiorly from them.

5. Remove the peritoneum from the posterior surface of the stomach and trace the posterior vagal trunk and its gastric branches.

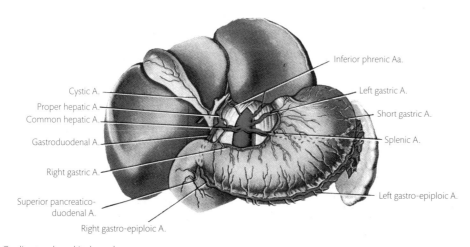

Fig. 11.18 Coeliac trunk and its branches.

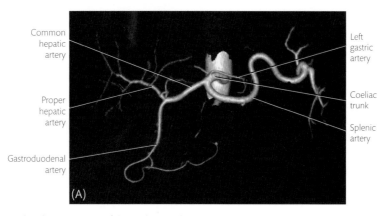

Fig. 11.19 (A) Volume-rendered 3D CT image of the coeliac trunk.

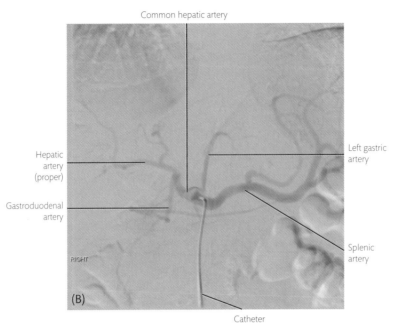

Common hepatic artery

Left gastric artery

Hepatic artery (proper)

Gastroduodenal artery

Splenic artery

RIGHT

(B)

Catheter

Fig. 11.19 (Continued) (B) Digital subtraction angiogram of the coeliac trunk. The tip of the catheter is placed in the coeliac trunk. Contrast injected into it opacifies its branches.

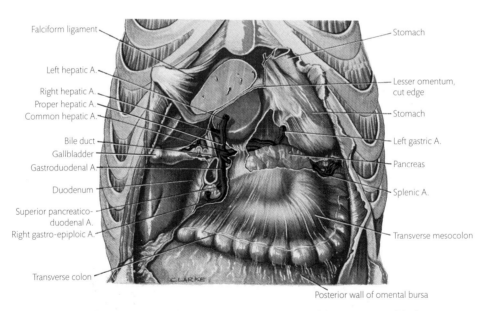

Falciform ligament

Stomach

Left hepatic A.

Right hepatic A.
Proper hepatic A.
Common hepatic A.

Lesser omentum, cut edge

Stomach

Bile duct
Gallbladder
Gastroduodenal A.

Left gastric A.

Pancreas

Duodenum

Splenic A.

Superior pancreatico-duodenal A.
Right gastro-epiploic A.

Transverse mesocolon

Transverse colon

C. CLARKE

Posterior wall of omental bursa

Fig. 11.20 The posterior wall of the omental bursa. The first part of the duodenum and the greater part of the lesser omentum are divided and the stomach turned upwards.

right gastric artery. The left gastric artery gives rise to ascending **oesophageal branches** which anastomose with oesophageal branches of the aorta in the thorax. **Gastric branches** pass to both anterior and posterior surfaces of the stomach, adjacent to the lesser curvature [Figs. 11.17, 11.18, 11.19].

The left gastric artery is accompanied by the **left gastric vein** and by branches of the va-

gal trunks to the coeliac ganglia. The left gastric vein first runs with the left gastric artery to the coeliac trunk, and then with the common hepatic artery to end in the portal vein. The tributaries of the vein correspond to the branches of the artery [Fig. 11.21]. The tributaries from the **oesophagus** are important because they anastomose with thoracic oesophageal veins which

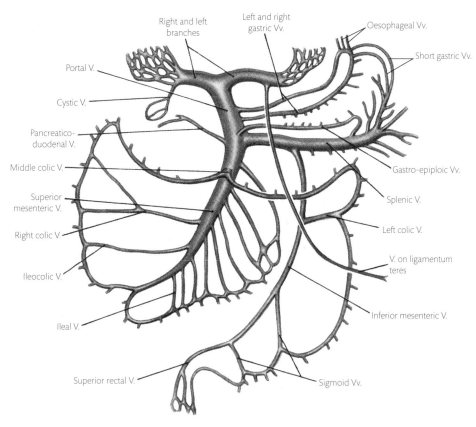

Right and left
branches

Left and right
gastric Vv.

Oesophageal Vv.

Short gastric Vv.

Portal V.

Cystic V.

Pancreatico-
duodenal V.

Middle colic V.

Superior
mesenteric V.

Right colic V.

Ileocolic V.

Ileal V.

Superior rectal V.

Gastro-epiploic Vv.

Splenic V.

Left colic V.

V. on ligamentum
teres

Inferior mesenteric V.

Sigmoid Vv.

Fig. 11.21 The portal venous system.

drain to the azygos system. ➲ This communica-tion between tributaries of the portal vein and the systemic circulation forms an alternative route for portal venous blood to reach the heart when its flow is obstructed in liver disease. In such a disease state, submucous veins in the lower oesophagus may be greatly distended and could be a source of severe haemorrhage [see Fig. 11.45].

Splenic vessels

The splenic artery is the largest branch of the coeliac trunk. It runs a sinuous course to the left along the superior border of the pancreas, poste-rior to the omental bursa and anterior to the left kidney. It enters the lienorenal ligament with the tail of the pancreas and then enters the hilum of the spleen [Figs. 11.18, 11.22, 11.23]. The splenic artery gives rise to: (1) small branches to the body and tail of the **pancreas**; (2) five or six branch-es to the **spleen**; (3) five or six slender **short gastric arteries** to the fundus of the stomach through the gastrosplenic ligament; and (4) the **left gastro-epiploic artery** which runs through the gastrosplenic ligament to the greater omen-

tum. The left gastro-epiploic artery runs towards the right, parallel to, and a short distance from, the greater curvature of the stomach. It anastomoses with the right gastro-epiploic artery, supplies both surfaces of the stomach adjacent to the greater

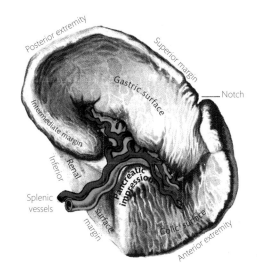

Posterior extremity

Superior margin

Gastric surface

Notch

Intermediate margin

Inferior

Renal
surface

Pancreatic
impression

Splenic
vessels

Colic surface

margin

Anterior extremity

Fig. 11.22 The visceral surface of the spleen.

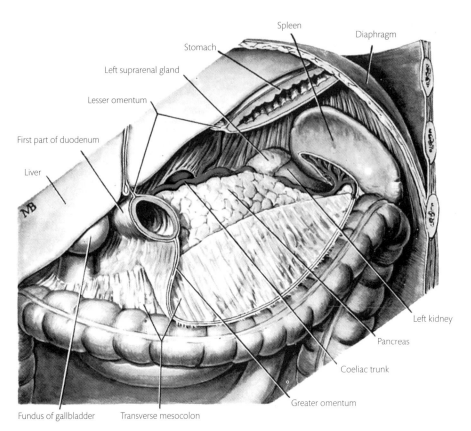

Spleen

Diaphragm

Stomach

Left suprarenal gland

Lesser omentum

First part of duodenum

Liver

Left kidney

Pancreas

Coeliac trunk

Greater omentum

Fundus of gallbladder   Transverse mesocolon

Fig. 11.23 Structures posterior to the stomach (stomach bed).

curvature, and sends small twigs into the greater omentum [Fig. 11.18].

The corresponding **veins** drain into the splenic vein. The splenic vein lies inferior to the splenic artery and runs to the right, posterior to the pancreas [Figs. 11.20, 11.21]. It unites with the superior mesenteric vein to form the portal vein.

Common hepatic artery and corresponding veins

The common hepatic artery passes to the right along the superior border of the pancreas up to the first part of the duodenum. Here it divides into the proper hepatic artery and the gastroduodenal artery.

The **proper hepatic artery** turns forwards on the duodenum, gives off the right gastric artery, and ascends in the free margin of the lesser omentum to the porta hepatis [Figs. 11.18, 11.19]. In the free margin of the lesser omentum, the proper hepatic artery lies anterior to the portal vein and to the left of the bile duct [Fig. 11.11]. Inferior to the porta hepatis, it divides into the right and left hepatic arteries which enter the corresponding lobes

of the liver. In the lesser omentum, the proper hepatic artery may give the **supraduodenal** artery to the superior part of the duodenum. The right hepatic artery gives the **cystic artery** which runs along the cystic duct to supply the gallbladder [Fig. 11.18]. The right gastric branch of the proper hepatic artery passes to the left on the duodenum, pylorus, and the lesser curvature of the stomach. It supplies these structures and anastomoses with the left gastric artery [Figs. 11.17, 11.18].

The **gastroduodenal** branch of the common hepatic artery descends posterior to the first part of the duodenum and divides into the superior pancreaticoduodenal artery and the right gastro-epiploic artery [Figs. 11.18, 11.19].

The **superior pancreaticoduodenal artery** divides into two branches which form arcades on the anterior and posterior surfaces of the head of the pancreas. Each arcade sends branches to the duodenum and the pancreas. These arcades anastomose with the inferior pancreaticoduodenal branches of the superior mesenteric artery.

The **right gastro-epiploic artery** runs to the left between the layers of the greater omentum. It anastomoses with the left gastro-epiploic artery and sends branches to the superior part of the duodenum, the right part of the stomach, and the greater omentum [Figs. 11.17, 11.18].

Variations in the arrangements of the branches of the common hepatic artery are frequent. Occasionally, the entire artery may arise from the superior mesenteric artery through enlargement of the pancreaticoduodenal arcade.

Veins draining the area supplied by the common hepatic artery enter the portal vein or one of its tributaries. The **cystic vein** enters the right branch of the portal vein [Figs. 11.17, 11.21]. The pancreaticoduodenal vein enters the portal vein. The **right gastro-epiploic vein** usually enters the superior mesenteric vein. The **right gastric vein** enters the portal vein and is united to the right gastro-epiploic vein by the **prepyloric vein**. The prepyloric vein crosses the front of the pylorus and is a landmark for the surgeon.

Spleen

The spleen lies deep in the left hypochondrium, wedged obliquely between the diaphragm, stomach, and left kidney [Fig. 11.22]. It is the largest single mass of **lymphoid tissue** in the body. It has a superolateral **diaphragmatic surface** and an inferomedial **visceral surface**, a **superior** and an **inferior margin** or border, and an **anterior** and a **posterior extremity**. The spleen is covered by peritoneum, except at the long, linear **hilus** on its concave visceral surface. The gastrosplenic and lienorenal ligaments are attached at the hilus of the spleen. Multiple branches of the splenic artery and tributaries of the splenic vein pierce the surface of the spleen at the hilus. The tip of the **tail of the pancreas** may reach it through the lienorenal ligament [Fig. 11.23].

The visceral surface is marked by the impression of the left kidney, the left colic flexure, and the stomach. The left colic flexure is applied to the **anterior extremity** of the visceral surface. The **renal surface** is in contact with the lateral part of the upper half of the left kidney. It faces inferomedially and meets the diaphragmatic surface at the blunt **inferior margin**, and the gastric surface at a low ridge (the intermediate margin) close to the hilus. The gastric surface lies adjacent to the superior border [Fig. 11.22].

The convex, posterolateral **diaphragmatic surface** lies against the diaphragm, parallel to the ninth to eleventh left ribs. It is separated from the ribs by the diaphragm, pleural cavity, and lung. This surface meets the gastric surface at the relatively sharp **superior margin**. The superior margin is notched near its anterior end. The **notches** may be palpated through the anterior abdominal wall when a grossly enlarged spleen projects below the left costal margin.

The spleen develops in the dorsal mesogastrium as a number of separate masses, each with its own blood supply. These masses fuse together but retain their separate circulations, with little or no anastomosis. ➜ Thus blockage of a branch of the splenic artery leads to death (infarction) of a segment of the spleen. Accessory splenic nodules may be found in the gastrosplenic ligament.

Abdominal part of the oesophagus

The oesophagus pierces the right crus of the diaphragm, posterior to the central tendon, 2–3 cm to the left of the median plane. It is accompanied by the anterior and posterior vagal trunks, the oesophageal branches of the left gastric artery, and the corresponding veins. It grooves the left lobe of the liver and almost immediately enters the stomach, in line with the lesser curvature. The oesophagus makes an acute angle—the **cardiac notch**—with the fundus of the stomach [Figs. 11.10, 11.24].

Replace the stomach and the left lobe of the liver if it has been removed. Review the shape and position of the stomach.

Stomach

The stomach is the most distensible part of the gut tube and lies between the oesophagus and small intestine. It is arbitrarily divided into a **fundus**, **body**, and **pylorus** [Fig. 11.10].

It has two surfaces—an anterior and a posterior surface—and two openings, or orifices—the cardiac orifice and the pyloric orifice. The **cardiac**, or oesophageal **orifice** lies approximately 10 cm posterior to the seventh left costal cartilage, 2–3 cm from the median plane. It lies between the liver anteriorly and the diaphragm posteriorly.

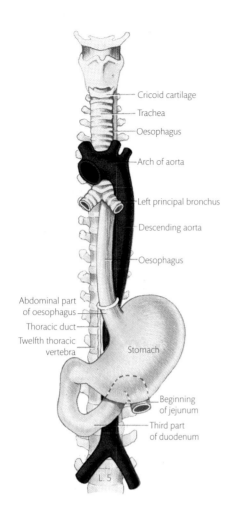

Cricoid cartilage

Trachea

Oesophagus

Arch of aorta

Left principal bronchus

Descending aorta

Oesophagus

Abdominal part of oesophagus

Thoracic duct

Twelfth thoracic vertebra

Stomach

Beginning of jejunum

Third part of duodenum

L. 5

Fig. 11.24 Schematic drawing of the oesophagus, stomach, and duodenum with adjacent structures.

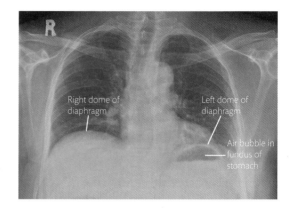

Fig. 11.25 Fundic air bubble below the left dome of the diaphragm.

The fundus of the stomach extends to the left from the cardiac orifice. It is separated from the cardiac orifice by the cardiac notch, and from the body of the stomach below by an imaginary horizontal line drawn through the cardiac opening. The fundus abuts on the left dome of the diaphragm under cover of the rib cage. It reaches the level of the fifth rib in the left mid-clavicular line. Here it is inferior and slightly posterior to the apex of the heart. In the erect posture, it is filled with a bubble of swallowed air [Fig. 11.25]. (This air moves into the pyloric portion, anterior to the vertebral column, in the supine position.)

The body of the stomach passes downwards and to the right across the supracolic compartment of the peritoneal cavity. It continues distally with the **pyloric part** of the stomach. The **incisura angularis** is a sharp angle on the lesser curvature of the stomach. An imaginary line drawn from the incisura angularis to the greater curvature separates the body from the pyloric part. The **pyloric part** of the stomach consists of a proximal dilated portion—the **pyloric antrum**—and a narrow, cylindrical portion—the **pyloric canal**. The two are separated from each other by a shallow groove—the **sulcus intermedius**. The pyloric canal is 2–3 cm long and terminates distally at the **pyloric orifice** [Fig. 11.10]. The pylorus is that portion of the stomach which is thickened by an increase in the amount of circular muscle to form the **pyloric sphincter** [Fig. 11.26]. The pylorus is highly mobile. It lies 2–3 cm to the right of the median plane but is further displaced to the right when the stomach is full. In its higher positions, the pylorus is posterior to the quadrate lobe of the liver and is separated from the pancreas by the lesser sac. The pyloric part of the stomach, along with the superior part of the duodenum, is bent across the prominent vertebral column [Figs. 11.6, 11.27].

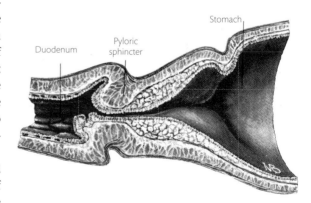

Stomach

Pyloric sphincter

Duodenum

Fig. 11.26 A longitudinal section through the gastroduodenal junction to show the thickness of the muscle forming the pyloric sphincter.

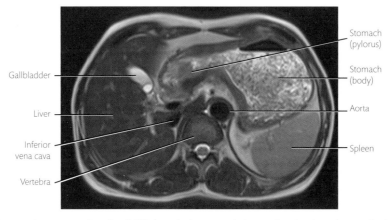

Fig. 11.27 T2W axial magnetic resonance imaging (MRI) through the upper abdomen showing the pylorus arched over the vertebral column.

The cardiac orifice and fundus are relatively fixed but move with respiration. The shape and position of the remainder of the stomach vary considerably from individual to individual, and in the same individual with age, degree of distension, position of the trunk, and state of contraction of the gastric muscle. These differences are partly due to the freedom of movement of the stomach. In thick-set individuals and children, the stomach tends to lie almost transversely across the abdomen, but in most people it is J-shaped. When J-shaped, the pyloric part lies horizontally or ascends to the superior part of the duodenum, and the lowest part of the greater curvature may even extend into the greater pelvis in the erect posture. Thus the structures in contact with the most mobile parts of the stomach are variable. Usually the anterior wall of the stomach near the lesser omentum is overlapped by the left lobe of the liver. Inferiorly, the anterior wall of the stomach is in contact with the peritoneum on the rectus sheath. Further to the left, the superior part of the stomach lies behind the anterior part of the diaphragm and rib cage [Figs. 11.3, 11.12].

The posterior wall of the stomach lies on the stomach bed but is separated from it by the omental bursa. Superiorly, the stomach bed consists of the spleen, the upper pole of the left kidney, the left suprarenal gland, and the diaphragm. Inferiorly is the upper part of the pancreas, the splenic vessels, and the mesentery of the transverse colon extending inferiorly from the pancreas [Fig. 11.23]. In the low type of a J-shaped stomach, the transverse colon and coils of the small intestine may lie posterior to its inferior part [see Fig. 11.38].

Vagal trunks

On the lower part of the thoracic oesophagus, the nerves of the oesophageal plexus unite to form the anterior and posterior vagal trunks. Each vagal trunk contains parasympathetic preganglionic fibres from both vagus nerves. The vagal trunks enter the abdomen on the oesophagus.

The **anterior gastric** nerves arise from the anterior vagal trunk. They supply the stomach and send nerve fibres to the duodenum, pancreas, and liver. The **posterior vagal trunk** sends posterior gastric nerves to the stomach. Both vagal trunks, especially the posterior, send **coeliac branches** to the coeliac plexus with the left gastric vessels.

Parasympathetic nerve fibres reach the stomach through the anterior and posterior **vagal trunks** and their branches. The **sympathetic** nerve fibres reach the stomach through the **coeliac plexus** on the branches of the coeliac trunk [Figs. 11.28, 11.29].

Vessels of the stomach

The rich arterial supply to the stomach is derived from all three branches of the coeliac trunk. The right and left gastric arteries anastomose on the lesser curvature. The right and left gastroepiploic arteries anastomose near the inferior part of the greater curvature. The superior part of the greater curvature is supplied by the short gastric arteries. Branches of all these arteries pass to both walls of the stomach at right angles to its

159

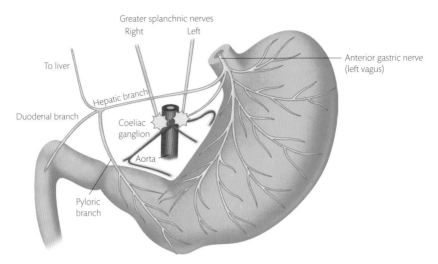

Fig. 11.28 Nerve supply to the anterior surface of the stomach. Based on a drawing by the late Dr Harsha of CMC Vellore. Reproduced with kind permission of CMC Vellore and Mrs Harsha.

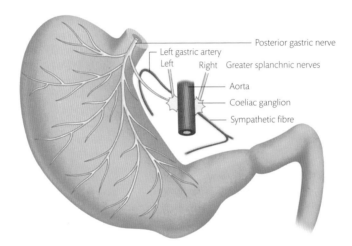

Fig. 11.29 Nerve supply to the posterior surface of the stomach. Based on a drawing by the late Dr Harsha of CMC Vellore. Reproduced with kind permission of CMC Vellore and Mrs Harsha.

long axis. The anastomosis is sufficient to permit the tying of one or more of the major arteries without ill effects [Fig. 11.18]. The **veins** draining the stomach drain with the corresponding arteries into the portal vein.

Lymph vessels run with the blood vessels to small nodes lying beside them, and through them to the **coeliac nodes** along the coeliac trunk [Fig. 11.30].

Cut open the stomach as directed in Dissection 11.8 and study the internal aspect.

Internal surface of the stomach

The internal surface of the stomach is covered by mucous membrane. It is thrown into longitudinal folds when the stomach is contracted, but is flat-

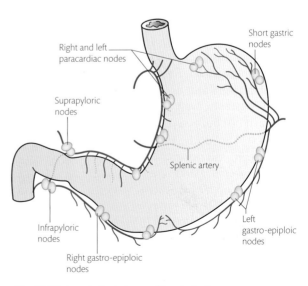

Fig. 11.30 Lymphatic drainage of the stomach.

DISSECTION 11.8 Stomach–internal aspect

Objective

I. To study the internal aspect of the stomach.

Instructions

1. Open the stomach along the greater curvature and examine the mucous membrane of the stomach with a hand lens.

tened out as it distends [Fig. 11.31A]. Groups of gastric glands open into **pits** on the surface of the stomach. Fig. 11.31B is a view of the interior of a stomach as seen through the endoscope.

Dissection 11.9 describes the dissection of the pylorus, mesentery, and superior mesenteric vessels.

The mesentery

The mesentery is a fold of peritoneum which attaches the entire jejunum and ileum (about 6 m of small intestine) to an oblique line across the posterior abdominal wall. The attachment of the mesentery to the posterior abdominal wall

is the **root of the mesentery**. The root of the mesentery extends from the duodenojejunal flexure to the ileocaecal junction and is 15 cm long. The superior mesenteric vessels run in the root of the mesentery. It crosses the anterior surface of the third part of the duodenum, aorta, inferior vena cava, right testicular or ovarian vessels, right ureter, and the right psoas muscle [Figs. 11.12, 11.13]. At the free edge of the mesentery, the two layers of peritoneum separate from each other to enclose the jejunum and ileum. Between the two layers of peritoneum, the mesentery contains the jejunal and ileal blood vessels, large **lymph vessels** known as **lacteals**, the plexus of autonomic nerves, and extraperitoneal fatty tissue.

Superior mesenteric artery

The superior mesenteric artery is the second unpaired branch of the aorta to the gut tube [Fig. 11.32]. It arises at the level of the first lumbar vertebra, 0.5 cm inferior to the coeliac trunk, posterior to the body of the pancreas and the splenic vein. It descends anterior to the left renal vein, the uncinate process of the pancreas, and the third part of the duodenum and enters the root of the mesentery. It runs in the root of the mesentery to the right iliac fossa. Here it gives branches

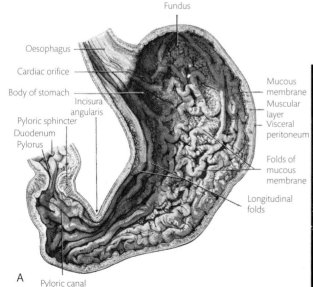

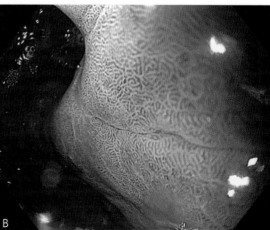

Fig. 11.31 (A) The interior of the empty contracted stomach. (B) Endoscopic view of the pyloric antrum. Image courtesy of Department of Clinical Gastroenterology, Christian Medical College, Vellore, India.

Objectives

I. To study the pylorus.   II. To identify the root of the mesentery.   III. To identify and trace the superior mesenteric vessels and the branches of the artery.

Instructions

1. Cut longitudinally through the wall of the first part of the duodenum close to the pylorus and examine the duodenal aspect of the pylorus.

2. Extend the cut through the pyloric wall to show the pyloric sphincter. The muscles of the **pyloric sphincter** push the mucous membrane of the pylorus inwards and narrow the aperture so that it appears as a small opening in the centre of a rounded knob when viewed from the duodenal side.

3. Expose the mesentery of the small intestine in the infracolic compartment by turning the transverse colon and its mesentery upwards.

4. Trace the oblique attachment of the mesentery of the small intestine from the upper left to the lower right quadrant of the posterior abdominal wall [Fig. 11.12].

5. Turn the small intestine to the left and cut through the right layer of the mesentery along the line of its attachment to the posterior abdominal wall. Strip this layer from the rest of the mesentery. Remove the fat from the **superior mesenteric vessels** in the root of the mesentery. Remove the fat from the jejunal and ileal vessels in the mesentery. Note the numerous lymph nodes and the complex mass of nerve fibres (**superior mesenteric plexus**) surrounding the vessels.

6. Trace the superior mesenteric vessels proximally and distally. Trace the branches to: (i) the caecum; (ii) the ascending colon; (iii) the transverse colon; and (iv) the duodenum and pancreas.

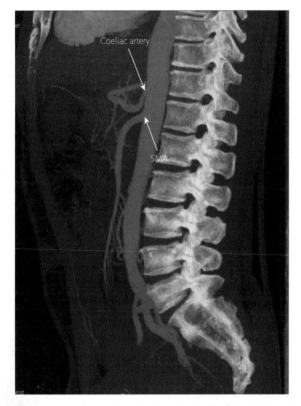

Fig. 11.32 Maximum-intensity projection image of the abdomen and pelvis, showing the aorta and the origin of the coeliac and superior mesenteric (SMA) arteries.

to the ileum and ends by anastomosing with a branch of the ileocolic artery [Figs. 11.33, 11.34].

Branches of the superior mesenteric artery

The superior mesenteric artery supplies the intestine from the middle of the second part of the duodenum to the right two-thirds of the transverse colon. The branches of the superior mesenteric artery anastomose freely with each other and with branches of the arteries supplying adjacent parts of the gut tube.

From the right side of the superior mesenteric artery arise the middle colic, the inferior pancreaticoduodenal, right colic, and ileocolic arteries. The **middle colic artery** [Fig. 11.33] arises at the lower border of the pancreas. It turns forwards into the transverse mesocolon and divides into right and left branches. These branches then form part of the **marginal artery**. The marginal artery extends along the ascending, transverse, and descending parts of the colon and receives the branches of the other colic arteries. Branches from the marginal artery pass to the colon. The middle colic artery normally supplies most of the transverse colon.

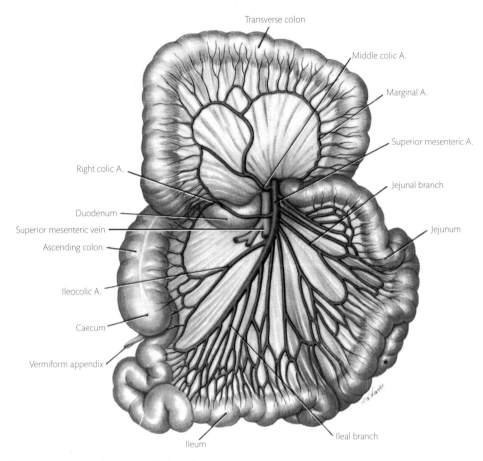

Transverse colon

Middle colic A.

Marginal A.

Superior mesenteric A.

Jejunal branch

Jejunum

Right colic A.

Duodenum

Superior mesenteric vein

Ascending colon

Ileocolic A.

Caecum

Vermiform appendix

Ileum

Ileal branch

Fig. 11.33 The superior mesenteric artery and its branches.

The **inferior pancreaticoduodenal artery** arises from the superior mesenteric artery on the duodenum and passes upwards and to the right. It forms anterior and posterior arcades, with similar arcades of the superior pancreaticoduodenal artery (a branch of the gastroduodenal artery) [Fig. 11.34]. Together, the pancreaticoduodenal arteries supply the duodenum and the head and uncinate process of the pancreas.

The **right colic artery** passes to the right across the structures of the posterior abdominal wall to join the marginal artery near the superior end of the ascending colon. It may be replaced by an enlarged ascending branch of the ileocolic artery [Fig. 11.33].

The **ileocolic artery** is a separate branch of the superior mesenteric artery, but may arise with the right colic artery. It passes downwards and to the right and divides into two branches. The ascending branch of the ileocolic artery forms the beginning of the marginal artery. A descending branch of the ileocolic artery

supplies the proximal part of the ascending colon, the caecum, the vermiform appendix, and the terminal part of the ileum. The ileocolic artery ends by anastomosing with the last ileal branch of the superior mesenteric artery. The branch to the appendix—the **appendicular artery**—enters the lowest part of the mesentery, passes posterior to the terminal ileum, and enters the mesentery of the vermiform appendix to supply the appendix [Fig. 11.14].

From the left side of the superior mesenteric artery arise 15–18 **jejunal** and **ileal branches** which enter the mesentery. They branch within the mesentery, and the branches anastomose with each other to form an arterial **arcade**. Further branches arise from the arcade to form a second, a third, or even a fourth arcade. There are usually one or two arcades in the mesentery of the jejunum and up to four arcades in the mesentery of the ileum. The last arcade sends branches known as vasa recta to each side of the small intestine. These vasa recta anastomose in the wall of the jejunum and ileum [Fig. 11.33].

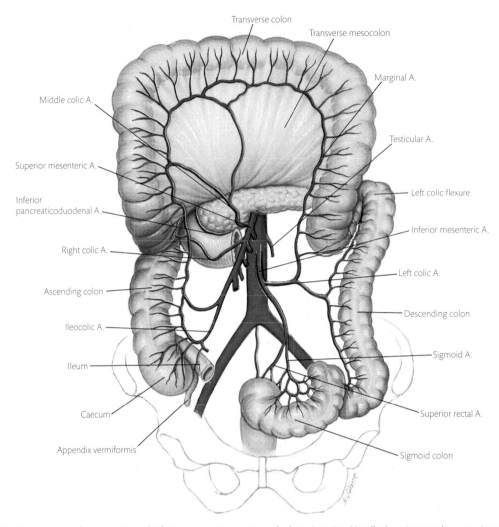

Fig. 11.34 The branches of the superior and inferior mesenteric arteries to the large intestine. Usually there is more than one sigmoid artery.

Superior mesenteric vein

This large vein lies immediately to the right of the superior mesenteric artery. Superiorly, it deviates to the right behind the pancreas and joins the splenic vein to form the portal vein. It drains blood from the territory supplied by the superior mesenteric artery. In addition, it also receives the right gastro-epiploic and pancreaticoduodenal veins and occasionally the inferior mesenteric vein [Figs. 11.21, 11.33, 11.35].

Lymph nodes of the mesentery

These numerous nodes lie between the layers of the mesentery and gradually increase in size towards the root. The lymph vessels of the small intestine are known as **lacteals** because of the milky white fat emulsion they contain. They converge on, and drain through, a series of lymph nodes, which finally unite at the root of the mesentery in the intestinal lymph trunk. The intestinal lymph trunk empties into the cisterna chyli [see Fig. 4.55; see also Fig. 13.2].

Dissect the inferior mesenteric artery and its branches by following the instructions given in Dissection 11.10.

Inferior mesenteric artery

This is the third unpaired branch of the aorta to the gut tube. It supplies the intestine from the left one-third of the transverse colon to the anal canal. The inferior mesenteric artery arises posterior to the third part of the duodenum. It descends on the left of the aorta, posterior to the peritoneum,

DISSECTION 11.10 Inferior mesenteric artery

Objective

I. To expose the inferior mesenteric artery.

Instructions

1. Turn the small intestine and its mesentery to the right.

2. Remove the peritoneum and fat on the posterior abdominal wall between the mesentery and the descending colon. Take care not to damage the left gonadal vein which lies in the extraperitoneal tissue of this region.

3. Identify the inferior mesenteric vessels, the autonomic nerves, and the lymph nodes associated with them [Fig. 11.35].

surrounded by the inferior mesenteric plexus of nerves. On the middle of the left common iliac artery, it ends by dividing into the sigmoid and superior rectal arteries [Fig. 11.35].

Branches of the inferior mesenteric artery

The branches of the inferior mesenteric artery cross the posterior abdominal wall, anterior to the plane of the kidney, ureter, and gonadal vessels.

The **left colic artery** arises a short distance below the duodenum. It passes to the left and divides into ascending and descending branches which form part of the marginal artery. The ascending branch crosses the lower pole of the left kidney and unites with the middle colic part of the marginal artery. It supplies the left colic flexure and left part of the transverse colon. The descending branch supplies the descending colon and anastomoses with the sigmoid arteries [Fig. 11.35].

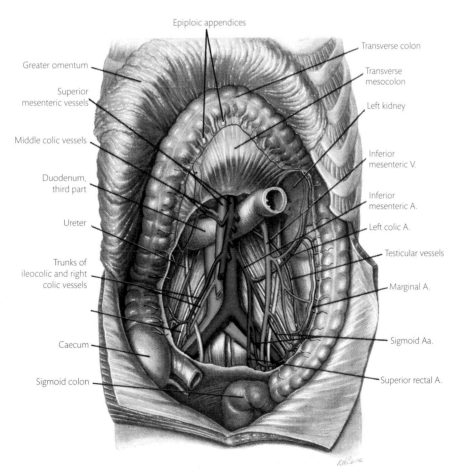

Fig. 11.35 Structures on the posterior wall of the infracolic compartment of the abdomen. The greater omentum and transverse colon are turned upwards, and the jejunum, ileum, mesentery, and peritoneum covering the posterior wall are removed.

Two or more **sigmoid arteries** pass inferiorly and to the left. They anastomose with each other and continue the marginal artery to supply the descending colon in the left iliac fossa and the sigmoid colon. The lowest sigmoid artery anastomoses with the superior rectal branch of the inferior mesenteric artery.

The **superior rectal artery** is a terminal branch of the inferior mesenteric artery and will be followed in the lesser pelvis [Fig. 11.34].

Inferior mesenteric vein

The inferior mesenteric vein is the continuation of the superior rectal vein. It ascends lateral to the inferior mesenteric artery and receives tributaries corresponding to the branches of the inferior mesenteric artery. The vein passes lateral to the duodenojejunal flexure and anterior to the left renal vein, to join the splenic vein posterior to the pancreas. It may deviate to the right and enter the superior mesenteric vein or the junction of the superior mesenteric vein and splenic vein [Fig. 11.35].

Arterial anastomoses along the gastrointestinal tract

The coeliac trunk and the superior and inferior mesenteric arteries are unpaired branches of the aorta which supply the gut tube, spleen, pancreas,

and liver. They give rise to branches which anastomose freely with each other and with the arteries supplying adjacent parts of the gut tube. The **left gastric** from the coeliac trunk anastomoses with the **oesophageal branches of the thoracic aorta**. The two **pancreaticoduodenal arteries** form a link between the coeliac trunk and the superior mesenteric artery. The jejunal and ileal branches of the superior mesenteric artery are united in the arcades. The colic branches of the superior mesenteric artery are linked with each other and with the colic branches of the inferior mesenteric artery through the marginal artery. ➲ Thus blockage of a single vessel, or even of a group of vessels, is not followed by ischaemic necrosis of any part of the intestine.

➲ If a loop of intestine is compressed at the neck of a hernial sac or twisted upon itself, as in a volvulus, blood vessels on its surface are obstructed. Death of the intestine with rupture of its wall will follow, unless the condition is treated rapidly.

Dissection 11.11 explores the small intestine—the jejenum and ileum.

Jejunum and ileum

The jejunum and ileum together measure about 6 m. They extend from the duodenojejunal junction in the left upper quadrant to the ileocaecal junction in the lower right quadrant of the abdomen. These segments of the small intestine are intraperitoneal and

---

DISSECTION 11.11 Small intestine—the jejunum and ileum

Objective

I. To study the jejunum and ileum.

Instructions

1. Examine the jejunum and ileum. Note the greater diameter and thickness of the jejunum, the lesser amount of fat in its mesentery, and the fact that the lumen is usually empty.

2. Tie two ligatures round the jejunum close to the duodenojejunal flexure; and another pair of ligatures around the ileum close to the caecum. Cut through the small intestine between each pair of ligatures and remove it by dividing the mesentery close to the

intestine. Wash out this part of the intestine with water. Remove a few inches of the jejunum and open it longitudinally. On the mucosal surface, note the mucosal folds which remain, even when the wall of the jejunum is stretched. Identify the villi with a hand lens.

3. Open the entire length of the remainder of the intestine by a longitudinal cut and note the gradual change in structure of the mucous membrane along its length. The **circular folds** become progressively smaller and less numerous from the duodenum to the terminal ileum where they are missing. The **villi** are larger and more numerous in the jejunum than in the ileum. The ileum contains aggregated lymph follicles [Figs. 11.36, 11.37].

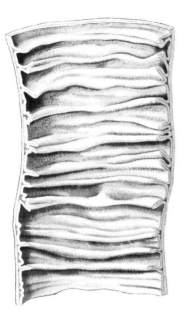

Fig. 11.36 Interior of the jejunum showing numerous mucosal circular folds.

lie in the infracolic compartment surrounded by the colon. The jejunum is wider and more thick-walled than the ileum. The mesentery of the jejunum has less fat and fewer arterial arcades. The junction of the jejunum and ileum is not clearly marked.

As in all hollow organs, the internal surface of the small intestine is lined by mucous membrane. In the jejunum and ileum, the entire thickness of the mucosa is thrown into permanent **circular folds** [Figs. 11.36, 11.37, 11.38]. The internal surface of the small intestine is covered with minute leaf- or finger-shaped projections, or **villi**, which are 0.5 mm or less in length. These are visible with a hand lens and give the mucous membrane a velvety appearance [Fig. 11.38]. The mucous membrane also contains aggregations of lymph tissue. Some lymph aggregates form **solitary lymph follicles**, 1–2 mm in diameter. Larger aggregates of **lymph follicles** are also found, especially on the antimesenteric wall of the ileum [Fig. 11.37].

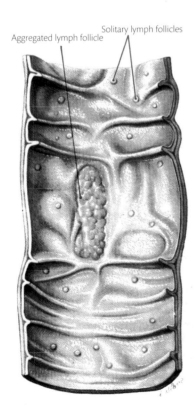

Aggregated lymph follicle

Solitary lymph follicles

Fig. 11.37 Interior of the ileum. Note the small, sparse circular folds and the solitary and aggregated lymph follicles.

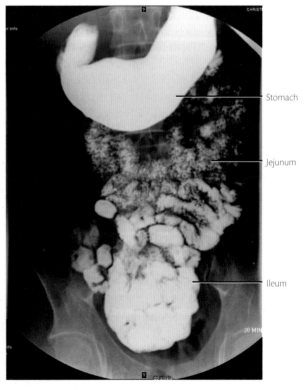

Stomach

Jejunum

Ileum

Fig. 11.38 Spot anteroposterior image from a barium meal follow-through. Note the feathery appearance of the jejunum, due to numerous circular folds of the mucosa, and the more featureless ileum.

The large intestine

The large intestine extends from the caecum in the right iliac fossa to the anus. It consists of the caecum, ascending colon, transverse colon, descending colon, sigmoid colon, rectum, and anal canal [Figs. 11.12, 11.35]. It is much shorter (1.5 m) than the small intestine and decreases in diameter from the caecum to the descending colon. All parts of it are capable of considerable distension.

Caecum

This blind end of the large intestine lies in the right iliac fossa. It is approximately 5–7 cm in length and width. The terminal ileum opens into the caecum on the left side. Superiorly, the caecum is continuous with the ascending colon [Figs. 11.14, 11.35, 11.39]. The vermiform appendix opens into the posteromedial part of the caecum. Posteriorly are the muscles, vessels, and nerves of the posterior abdominal wall—the right iliacus and psoas muscles, the right genitofemoral, femoral, and lateral femoral cutaneous nerves, and the right testicular or ovarian vessels. The vessels and nerves are anterior to the muscles. The caecum frequently overlaps the right external iliac artery and, being relatively mobile, may lie in the lesser pelvis. The caecum is almost completely covered by peritoneum [Fig. 11.15] but is frequently attached by the peritoneum to the right iliac fossa laterally and medially. Such attachment produces a wide peritoneal recess behind the caecum which may extend up posterior to the inferior part of the ascending colon. This is the **retrocaecal recess**. The vermiform appendix frequently lies in this recess. Rarely, the caecum may lie at the level of the right colic flexure, in which case the ascending colon is absent. The outer layer of smooth muscle of the wall of the caecum forms three bands on the external surface. These are the three **taeniae coli** [Fig. 11.39].

Vermiform appendix

This part of the large intestine is a narrow blind tube of very variable length. It is approximately 5–15 cm long and 5 mm in diameter. It is sus-

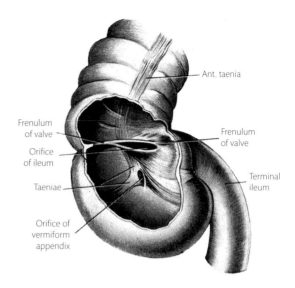

Fig. 11.39 A dried distended caecum opened to show the ileocaecal orifice and valve.

pended by a small extension of the mesentery—the mesentery of the appendix—which descends posterior to the terminal ileum [Fig. 11.14]. The base of the appendix is attached to the posteromedial surface of the caecum, 2–3 cm inferolateral to the ileocaecal junction. The tip of the appendix is very variable in position. Frequently, it lies in the retrocaecal recess but may extend into the lesser pelvis [Figs. 11.14, 11.40, 11.41]. In the pelvis, it may lie close to the right ovary, right uterine tube, and right ureter [see Fig. 15.2B].

The appendix has the same peritoneal and muscle coats as the small intestine. At the base, the longitudinal muscle is continuous with the three **taeniae coli** of the caecum [Fig. 11.39]. The mucous membrane of the appendix contains an abundance of **lymph follicles**.

Vessels and nerves

The caecum and appendix are supplied by branches of the **ileocolic artery**. The appendicular artery arises from the ileocolic artery and passes in its mesentery, posterior to the terminal ileum. **Lymph vessels** pass to nodes in the mesentery of the appendix, and to others scattered along the ileocolic artery. Nerves from the **superior mesenteric plexus** reach the caecum and appendix on the ileocolic artery.

Follow the instructions given in Dissection 11.12 to study the caecum.

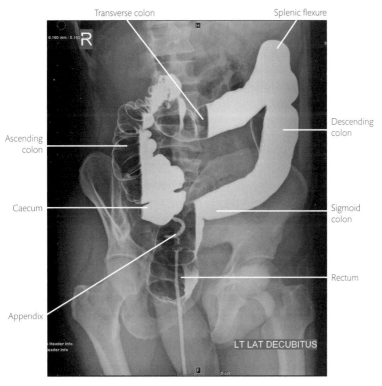

Transverse colon

Splenic flexure

Descending colon

Ascending colon

Sigmoid colon

Caecum

Rectum

Appendix

LT LAT DECUBITUS

Fig. 11.40 A radiograph of the partly emptied colon outlined by barium introduced as an enema. The narrow, irregular parts of the lumen are produced by contraction of the muscles of the colon.

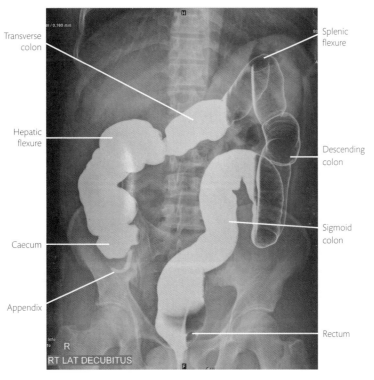

Transverse colon

Splenic flexure

Hepatic flexure

Descending colon

Sigmoid colon

Caecum

Appendix

Rectum

RT LAT DECUBITUS

Fig. 11.41 Spot anteroposterior image from a barium enema, with the patient in the right lateral decubitus position.

Ileocaecal orifice

Normally, the ileum enters the caecum obliquely through a horizontal slit. At the point of entry the mucosa is partly invaginated into the caecum to form folds (the **ileocaecal valve**) above and below the opening. Medially and laterally, these folds meet to form ridges—the **frenula of the valve** [Fig. 11.39].

Ascending colon

The ascending colon is 12–20 cm long. It begins in the right iliac fossa as an upward continuation from the caecum. It ascends on the right iliacus, the iliac crest, and the quadratus lumborum in the right paravertebral gutter [Figs. 11.13, 11.42]. It is anterior to the right **lateral cutaneous nerve of the thigh** and the **ilio-inguinal** and **iliohypogastric nerves**. It ends in the right colic flexure by turning sharply to the left to continue with the transverse colon. The right colic flexure lies on the lower part of the right kidney and posterior to the liver [see Fig. 11.64].

The peritoneum covers the front and sides of the ascending colon and holds it against the posterior abdominal wall. Anterior to the ascending colon is

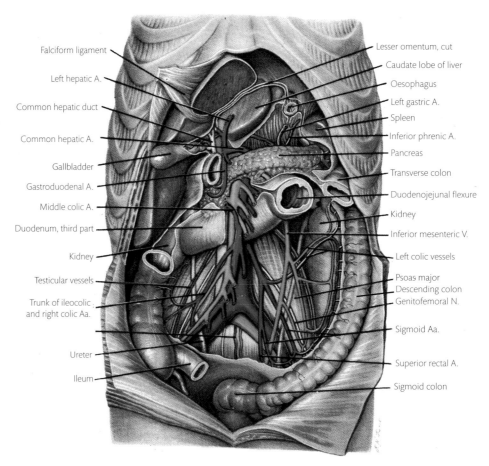

Fig. 11.42 Structures on the posterior abdominal wall.

Falciform ligament
Left hepatic A.
Common hepatic duct
Common hepatic A.
Gallbladder
Gastroduodenal A.
Middle colic A.
Duodenum, third part
Kidney
Testicular vessels
Trunk of ileocolic and right colic Aa.
Ureter
Ileum

Lesser omentum, cut
Caudate lobe of liver
Oesophagus
Left gastric A.
Spleen
Inferior phrenic A.
Pancreas
Transverse colon
Duodenojejunal flexure
Kidney
Inferior mesenteric V.
Left colic vessels
Psoas major
Descending colon
Genitofemoral N.
Sigmoid Aa.
Superior rectal A.
Sigmoid colon

the anterior abdominal wall, but the greater omentum and small intestine may intervene [Fig. 11.12].

Vessels and nerves

The ascending colon and right colic flexure are supplied by the **ileocolic** and **right colic** branches of the superior mesenteric artery and nerves from the **superior mesenteric plexus**. **Lymph vessels** end in nodes on the medial side of the colon and along its vessels.

Transverse colon

The transverse colon is usually the longest (40–50 cm) and most mobile part of the colon [Figs. 11.23, 11.35, 11.40, 11.41]. It begins anterior to the right kidney and the second part of the duodenum, posterior to the liver and the fundus of the gallbladder. It then descends anterior to the coils of the small intestine and ascends on the left to the **left colic flexure** [see Fig. 11.64]. Here it is anterior to the lateral margin of the **left kidney**, immediately inferior to the **spleen**, and posterior to the left margin of the greater omentum. The left colic flexure lies at a higher level than the right flexure and is more acute and further lateral [Fig. 11.23]. It is attached to the diaphragm by a short fold of peritoneum—the **phrenicocolic ligament**. Between the right and left colic flexures the transverse colon forms a dependent loop. The lowest part of the loop may reach well below the umbilicus in the erect position but is usually superior to it in the recumbent position. If the small intestines are distended, the transverse colon may be pushed superiorly, anterior to the liver [Fig. 11.12]. ➔ If distended with gas in this location, it may mask the normal liver dullness and mimic the presence of gas in the peritoneal cavity.

The transverse colon is suspended from the posterior abdominal wall by the **transverse mesocolon** [Figs. 11.9, 11.23, 11.35]. The root of the transverse mesocolon is attached to the posterior abdominal wall on the second part of the duodenum, the head and lower margin of the body of the pancreas, and the anterior surface of the left kidney [Fig. 11.13]. This double fold of the peritoneum is fused to the posterior surface of the greater omentum [Fig. 11.9], except at the lateral ends [Figs. 11.13, 11.23]. It contains the middle colic vessels and branches of the right and left colic vessels with their accompanying nerves and lymph vessels.

Vessels and nerves

The transverse colon is mainly supplied by the **middle colic** vessels, but its extremities and the flexures also receive blood from the **right** or **left colic arteries** [Fig. 11.33]. Nerves accompany all these arteries. Those on the right and middle colic arteries are derived from the **superior mesenteric plexus** and transmit sympathetic and vagal nerve fibres. Those on the left colic artery are derived from the **inferior mesenteric plexus** and transmit sympathetic and pelvic parasympathetic nerve fibres. **Lymph vessels** and nodes lie on the arteries. (The superior and inferior mesenteric plexuses of nerves are described later.)

Descending colon

The descending colon extends from the left colic flexure to the superior aperture of the pelvis, near the inguinal ligament. It is retroperitoneal and is attached to the posterior abdominal wall in the left paravertebral gutter and iliac fossa. At first, it lies anterior to the lateral surface of the left kidney and medial to the diaphragm. It then descends on the left transversus abdominis and quadratus lumborum to the iliac crest, anterior to the same nerves as the ascending colon—the left iliohypogastric, ilio-inguinal, and lateral cutaneous nerve of the thigh. It continues in the left iliac fossa on the iliacus [Fig. 11.35]. At the inguinal ligament, it turns medially and lies on the left femoral nerve, left psoas, left gonadal vessels, and left genitofemoral nerve. It continues as the sigmoid colon, anterior to the external iliac vessels [Figs. 11.40, 11.41, 11.42].

➔ The pressure of the lowest part of the descending colon on the testicular and external iliac veins may account for the greater frequency of varicose veins in the left spermatic cord and left lower limb.

Vessels and nerves

The blood supply to the descending colon is by the **left colic** and **upper sigmoid** branches of the inferior mesenteric vessels [Fig. 11.34]. These are accompanied by nerves from the **inferior mesenteric plexus** and the corresponding lymph vessels and nodes [see Figs. 11.59, 13.2].

Dissection 11.13 describes how to mobilize the descending colon to study the posterior relations of the same.

Sigmoid colon

This part of the colon varies in length from 15 to 80 cm. It extends from the end of the descending colon to the pelvic surface of the third sacral vertebra where it continues as the rectum [Figs. 11.34, 11.35]. The sigmoid colon is attached to the posterior abdominal wall and the posterosuperior wall of the pelvis by a double fold of peritoneum—the **sigmoid mesocolon**. Usually the sigmoid colon lies free in the lesser pelvis inferior to the small intestine. When long, depending on the length of its mesentery, it may extend into any part of the abdomen.

The root of the **sigmoid mesocolon** has a ʌ-shaped attachment to the posterior wall of the abdomen and lesser pelvis. It begins at the end of the descending colon and ascends on the surface of the external iliac vessels to the middle of the common iliac artery. Here it turns sharply downwards and to the right across the rim of the lesser pelvis to the third piece of the sacrum [Fig. 11.13]. Just lateral to the apex of the ʌ, a pocket-like extension of the peritoneal cavity passes upwards, posterior to the root of the mesocolon, in front of the left ureter. This is the **intersigmoid peritoneal recess**. The **inferior mesenteric artery** divides near the apex of the ʌ into two branches. The superior rectal artery enters the right limb of the sigmoid mesocolon, and the sigmoid arteries enter the left limb [Fig. 11.34]. Rarely, the sigmoid mesocolon begins at the iliac crest and runs directly to the third piece of the sacrum. In this case, the sigmoid colon could be said to start at the iliac crest where the blood supply by the sigmoid arteries begins.

Taeniae coli

Taeniae coli are three ribbon-like thickenings of the longitudinal muscle of the caecum and colon. They start at the root of the vermiform appendix and are present on the caecum, and ascending, transverse, descending, and sigmoid colon. They end in the terminal part of the sigmoid colon by spreading out to become continuous with the longitudinal muscle of the rectum. These thickenings are uniformly spaced around the circumference of the colon. In the ascending and descending colon, the taeniae are anterior, posteromedial, and posterolateral in position. In the transverse colon, the taeniae are anterior, posterior, and superior. Between the taeniae coli, the wall of the colon and caecum bulges outwards, forming three rows of puckered pouches called **sacculations** [Fig. 11.34].

Lymph nodes of the large intestine

Small nodes lie near the marginal artery and along the arteries passing to it. From these nodes, the lymph drains to nodes on the branches of the superior mesenteric artery and then enters the **intestinal lymph trunk**. Lymph draining with the inferior mesenteric artery enters the **lumbar lymph nodes** beside the aorta. All the lymph from the large intestine finally reaches the cisterna chyli [see Fig. 13.2].

Dissection 11.14 describes the dissection of the large intestine.

Peritoneum of the large intestine

The peritoneum forms an incomplete covering for the ascending colon, descending colon, and upper part of the **rectum** as these parts are applied to the posterior abdominal and pelvic walls. The transverse colon is intraperitoneal and is attached to the posterior abdominal wall by the transverse mesocolon. The inferior third of the rectum has no contact with the peritoneum. There are small projecting fat-filled pouches of peritoneum on the surface of the colon. These are the **appendices epiploicae**. They are numerous on the sigmoid and transverse colon but are absent from the caecum, appendix, and rectum [Fig. 11.35].

DISSECTION 11.14 Large intestine

Objective

I. To examine the external and internal aspects of the large intestine.

Instructions

1. Cut through the colon between ligatures at the junction of the descending and sigmoid parts. Remove the caecum and colon in one piece, dividing the peritoneum and blood vessels close to them.

2. Examine the external surface of the colon.

3. Wash out the colon and open it longitudinally. Examine its internal surface.

4. Cut a transverse section through the vermiform appendix and examine the cut surface with a hand lens.

DISSECTION 11.15 External surface of the duodenum and pancreas

Objective

I. To expose the external surface of the duodenum and pancreas.

Instructions

1. Expose the anterior surface of the pancreas and define the limits of the gland.

2. Trace the duodenum from the pylorus to the duodenojejunal flexure.

When not distended, the **mucous layer** of the colon forms a number of crescentic folds on the internal aspect. Many small **solitary lymph follicles** bulge the mucous membrane, but neither villi nor aggregated lymph follicles are present.

Dissection 11.15 exposes the anterior surface of the duodenum and pancreas.

Duodenum

The duodenum is the widest and most fixed part of the small intestine. It is approximately 25 cm long and is bent in a C-shaped curve. The concavity of the curve faces to the left and upwards and is filled by the head of the pancreas. The duodenum connects the parts of the gut tube that lie in the supracolic and infracolic compartments as it passes posterior to the attachment of the transverse mesocolon. The duodenum lies across the vertebral column and extends into the paravertebral gutters [Figs. 11.13, 11.42].

The **first** (superior) **part** of the duodenum passes upwards, backwards, and to the right from the pylorus. It lies superior to the pancreas. The portal vein, inferior vena cava, gastroduodenal artery, and bile duct lie posterior to the first part of the duodenum. The quadrate lobe of the liver and the neck of the gallbladder lie anterior to it. The first part is approximately 5 cm long but appears much shorter in an anteroposterior radiograph because of its oblique direction [Figs. 11.13, 11.42]. In radiographs, it forms the **duodenal cap**. The first half of the first part of the duodenum has the greater and lesser omentum attached to it and is free to move with the stomach. The second half has no mesentery.

Posterior to the neck of the gallbladder, the first part of the duodenum turns sharply downwards to form the **second** (descending) **part**. The second part is 8 cm long and is completely retroperitoneal. It lies anterior to the medial part of the right kidney and right psoas major (anterior to the renal vessels and ureter) down to the level of the third lumbar vertebra [see Fig. 11.64]. In the supracolic compartment, the second part is posterior to the liver and **gallbladder**. Then it passes posterior to the beginning of the transverse mesocolon to enter the infracolic compartment. In the infracolic compartment, it lies behind the jejunum [Fig. 11.42]. Medially, it is applied to the head of the pancreas. Two-thirds of the way along its length, the **bile** and **main pancreatic ducts** pierce the wall of the second part of the duodenum to enter its posteromedial aspect [see Fig. 11.48].

The **third** (horizontal) **part** of the duodenum is also retroperitoneal. It is nearly 10 cm long and passes horizontally to the left, inferior to the pancreas. It lies anterior to the right psoas muscle, right ureter, right testicular or ovarian artery, vertebral column, inferior vena cava, and aorta at the origin of the inferior mesenteric artery. The anterior surface is covered with peritoneum, except where the root of the mesentery and the superior mesenteric vessels cross it [Fig. 11.35].

The short **fourth** (ascending) **part** of the duodenum passes upwards on the left psoas muscle to

DISSECTION 11.16 Duodenum

Objective

I. To study the external and internal features of the duodenum.

Instructions

1. Divide the peritoneum along the right side of the second part of the duodenum. Separate this part of the duodenum from the deeper structures and turn it to the left.

2. Identify the aorta and vertebral bodies thus exposed.

3. Replace the duodenum and remove the peritoneum and fat surrounding the fourth part. Identify the **inferior mesenteric vein** lateral to the fourth part, the superior mesenteric vessels medial to it, and part of the left renal vein superior to it.

4. A slender fibromuscular band may be seen passing from the superior surface of the duodenojejunal flexure to the right crus of the diaphragm. This is the **suspensory muscle of the duodenum**.

5. Open the entire length of the duodenum by cutting along its convex side. Clean the interior to expose the mucosal surface.

6. Identify a longitudinal fold on the posteromedial wall of the second part of the duodenum. Identify an elevation—the **greater duodenal papilla**—at the proximal end of this fold. This elevation is often covered by a circular fold of mucosa [Fig. 11.43]. The **bile** and **pancreatic ducts** open by a common orifice on the greater duodenal papilla. (The position of the opening of the ducts will be confirmed when the ducts are traced to the duodenum.)

7. The **lesser duodenal papilla** lies superior and anterior to the greater duodenal papilla. The accessory pancreatic duct enters the second part of the duodenum at the lesser duodenal papilla. This papilla is smaller and more difficult to find than the greater duodenal papilla.

the left of the aorta and the head of the pancreas. It lies anterior to the left sympathetic trunk and the testicular or ovarian artery [Figs. 11.13, 11.35]. It bends anteriorly at the **duodenojejunal flexure**, 2–3 cm to the left of the median plane at the level of the second lumbar vertebra. A double fold of peritoneum suspends the duodenojejunal flexure from the posterior abdominal wall. A small slip of muscle—the **suspensory ligament of the duodenum**—may be present in this peritoneal fold.

The position of the duodenum is variable. The first half of the superior part is very mobile. The horizontal part may pass to the duodenojejunal flexure without a recognizable ascending part, and the entire duodenum may lie at a higher or lower level.

Vessels and nerves

The superior part of the duodenum receives small arteries from the **proper hepatic** (through the supraduodenal branch), **right gastric**, **right gastro-epiploic**, and **gastroduodenal arteries**. The remainder of the duodenum is supplied by the superior and inferior **pancreaticoduodenal arteries**. These arteries form arcades anterior and posterior to the head of the pancreas. Occasionally, this anastomosis may replace the hepatic artery.

The **lymph vessels** drain to nodes that lie between the duodenum and pancreas. These nodes drain to nodes on the coeliac trunk or superior mesenteric artery. Nerves reach the duodenum from the **coeliac** and **superior mesenteric plexus** on the corresponding arteries.

Using instructions given in Dissection 11.16 study the surface features, relations and internal surface of the duodenum.

Internal surface of the duodenum

The **mucous layer** is similar to that of the jejunum, but the **villi** are short and broad. **Circular folds** begin approximately 2 cm from the pylorus [Figs. 11.43A, 11.43B]. They are small and irregular but become large and numerous further distally. Two elevations—the greater and lesser duodenal papillae—are seen on the posteromedial wall of the second part of the duodenum. The **bile** and **pancreatic ducts** open by a common orifice on the greater duodenal papilla. The accessory pancreatic duct, when present, opens on the lesser duodenal papilla. A small longitudinal fold of mucosa extends down from the greater duodenal papilla [Fig. 11.43A].

Dissect the splenic vein and the terminal parts of the superior and inferior mesenteric veins following the instructions given in Dissection 11.17.

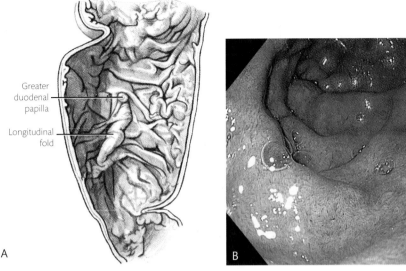

A

B

Fig. 11.43 (A) The internal surface of the posterior wall of the descending part of the duodenum. The greater duodenal papilla lies at the upper end of the longitudinal fold and is hooded by a circular fold. (B) Endoscopic view of the duodenum. Image courtesy of Department of Clinical Gastroenterology, Christian Medical College, Vellore, India.

175

In figure:
Greater duodenal papilla
Longitudinal fold

DISSECTION 11.17 Splenic vein and terminal parts of the superior and inferior mesenteric veins

Objective

I. To identify and trace the splenic vein, the terminations of the superior and inferior mesenteric veins, and the beginning of the portal vein.

Instructions

1. Lift the tail of the pancreas from the spleen, and the body of the pancreas from the posterior abdominal wall.

2. Identify the **splenic vein** on the posterior surface of the pancreas, and follow it to its junction with the superior mesenteric vein. The splenic and superior mesenteric veins unite to form the **portal vein**.

3. Trace the **inferior mesenteric vein**. It usually enters the splenic vein but may enter the beginning of the portal vein or the superior mesenteric vein.

4. Follow the superior mesenteric vessels upwards, anterior to the uncinate process of the pancreas and posterior to the junction of the body and head of the pancreas.

5. Follow the portal vein downwards to the junction of the splenic and superior mesenteric veins.

Portal vein

The portal vein drains the abdominal and pelvic parts of the alimentary canal (except for the lowest part of the rectum and anal canal), the spleen, the pancreas, and the gallbladder. It enters the liver through the porta hepatis, from which it gets its name. At the porta hepatis, the portal vein divides into right and left branches which empty the portal venous blood into the liver sinusoids (large-diameter capillaries). Venous systems uniting two groups of capillaries elsewhere in the body are called **portal venous systems** after this vein [Fig. 11.44].

The portal vein begins posterior to the junction of the body and head of the pancreas by the union of the **splenic** and **superior mesenteric veins**. As it ascends posterior to the first part of the duodenum, it receives a **pancreaticoduodenal vein** and, more superiorly, the right and left **gastric veins**. It ascends in the free edge of the lesser omentum and ends by dividing into the right and left branches which enter the porta hepatis. The **right branch** of the portal vein receives the **cystic vein** from the gallbladder and enters the right lobe of the liver. The **left branch** passes to the left, gives branches to the caudate and quadrate lobes, unites with the **ligamentum teres** and **ligamentum venosum**, and enters the left lobe of the liver. Small **para-umbilical veins** pass

The abdominal cavity

176

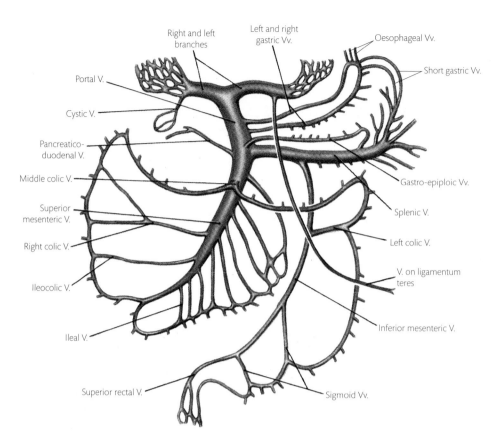

Fig. 11.44 A diagram of the portal venous system.

from the umbilicus and reach the left branch of the portal vein along the ligamentum teres [Fig. 11.44].

The inferior vena cava lies posterior to the entire length of the portal vein but is separated from it superiorly by the epiploic foramen. The **bile duct** and first the gastroduodenal artery and then the proper hepatic artery are anterior to the portal vein [see Fig. 11.47].

The portal vein and the hepatic artery empty blood into the sinusoids of the liver. The portal vein transports the products of carbohydrate and protein digestion from the intestine and the products of red cell destruction from the spleen. (Fats are mostly transported through the lacteals to the thoracic duct.) The tributaries and branches of the portal vein contain up to one-third of the total volume of blood in the body.

Sites of porto-systemic anastomosis

The portal vein communicates with the systemic circulation at certain sites where venous blood can drain into both the portal system and the systemic (or caval) system. These sites of **porto-systemic**

anastomosis are clinically important [Fig. 11.45]. Porto-systemic anastomosis occurs at the following sites: (1) At the lower end of the oesophagus, where the **oesophageal veins** drain upwards through the azygos vein into the superior vena cava, and down through the left gastric vein to the portal vein. (2) At the umbilicus, where venous blood drains through the lateral thoracic and superficial epigastric veins to the axillary and femoral veins, and through the **para-umbilical veins** to the portal vein. (3) In the rectum, where venous blood drains through the inferior and middle rectal veins to the internal iliac veins and the inferior vena cava, and through the **superior rectal vein** to the portal vein. Less importantly, porto-systemic anastomosis occurs (4) at the bare area of the liver, where there may be anastomosis between veins draining into the right branch of the portal vein and the lumbar or azygos veins, and (5) in the region of the right and left colic flexures, where colic veins may communicate with retroperitoneal veins.

These sites of porto-systemic anastomosis are clinically important. ➲ If the portal vein is obstructed and blood cannot flow through the

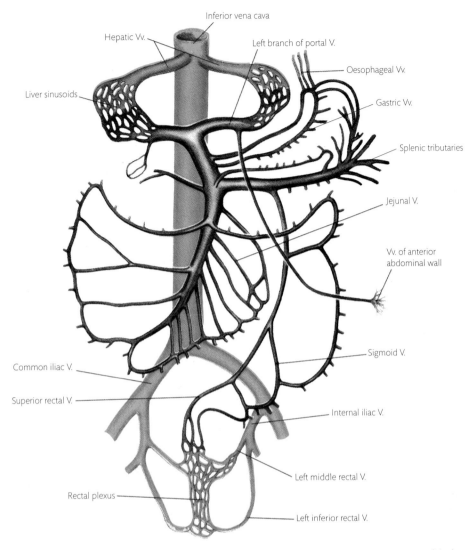

Inferior vena cava

Hepatic Vv.

Left branch of portal V.

Oesophageal Vv.

Liver sinusoids

Gastric Vv.

Splenic tributaries

Jejunal V.

Vv. of anterior
abdominal wall

Common iliac V.

Superior rectal V.

Sigmoid V.

Internal iliac V.

Left middle rectal V.

Rectal plexus

Left inferior rectal V.

Fig. 11.45 A diagram of the portal venous system (grey) to show its anastomoses with the systemic venous system (blue).

liver, the anastomosis may enlarge to transport the portal venous blood to the heart through the superior and inferior venae cavae. The back pressure in the tributaries of the portal vein may cause distension and bleeding from the submucous venous plexus in the lower oesophagus and rectum.

Splenic vein

Five or six veins draining the spleen emerge from the hilus of the spleen and unite to form the splenic vein. The splenic vein runs first in the lienorenal ligament, then on the left kidney, left psoas mus-

cle, left crus of the diaphragm, and the aorta. It lies on the posterior surface of the pancreas. It ends by uniting with the superior mesenteric vein to form the portal vein, anterior to the inferior vena cava [Figs. 11.20, 11.44].

Tributaries

The tributaries of the splenic vein correspond to the branches of the splenic artery. They are the veins draining the spleen, the short gastric veins, the left gastro-epiploic veins, and the veins draining the pancreas. In addition, the inferior mesenteric vein usually joins the splenic vein.

Dissection 11.18 traces the bile duct and the pancreatic duct to the duodenum.

Objective

I. To trace the bile duct and the terminal part of the pancreatic duct into the duodenum.

Instructions

1. Free the third part of the duodenum and the uncinate process of the pancreas from the posterior abdominal wall. Turn the descending part of the duodenum and the head of the pancreas to the left.

2. Look for the posterior part of the pancreaticoduodenal vessels and the bile duct on the head of the pancreas. The **bile duct** lies in a groove on the posterior surface of the head, with the vein on its left side passing to the portal vein.

3. Trace the bile duct inferiorly from the lesser omentum, and find its union with the pancreatic duct close to the duodenum.

4. Expose the structures posterior to the pancreas.

Ducts of the liver

The liver develops from a hollow branching outgrowth of that part of the primitive gut tube which forms the duodenum. The proximal part of the outgrowth forms the system of bile ducts leading to the duodenum. Bile is secreted into bile canaliculi which lead into progressively larger ducts. These ducts finally unite to form the right and left **hepatic ducts**. The two hepatic ducts join to form the **common hepatic duct**. The **cystic duct** from the gallbladder joins the common hepatic duct to form the **bile duct** [Fig. 11.46]. Bile produced in the liver either flows directly to the duodenum or into the gallbladder when the sphincter on the duodenal opening of the bile duct is closed. Bile is concentrated in the gallbladder.

Bile duct

This duct is approximately 10 cm long and 0.5 cm wide. It begins by the union of the common hepatic and cystic ducts. It lies to the right of the proper hepatic artery and anterior to the portal vein. It descends first in the free edge of the lesser omentum, and then posterior to the first part of the duodenum where it lies to the right of the gastroduodenal artery [Fig. 11.47]. It then deviates slightly to

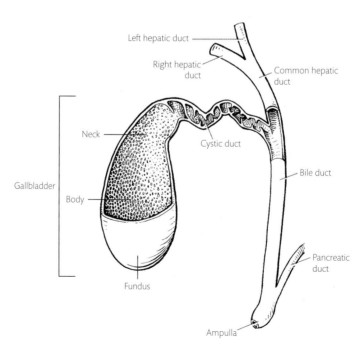

Fig. 11.46 Gallbladder and extrahepatic parts of the biliary system.

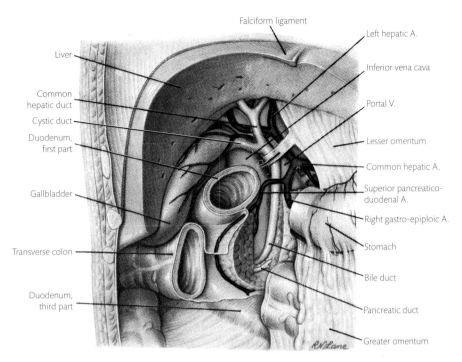

Fig. 11.47 A diagram to show the extrahepatic biliary system. The arrow indicates the epiploic foramen.

the right in a groove on the posterior surface of the head of the pancreas. It enters the posteromedial wall of the second part of the duodenum, a little inferior to its middle [Fig. 11.48].

The duct passes obliquely through the duodenal wall, expanding to form the **ampulla** [Fig. 11.48].

The ampulla bulges the mucous membrane of the duodenum inwards as the **greater duodenal papilla** where the duct pierces it. The terminal part of the **pancreatic duct** runs with the bile duct for a short distance and joins it either before or during its passage through the duodenal wall.

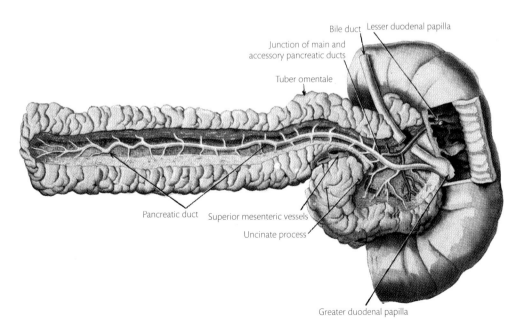

Fig. 11.48 Duct system of the pancreas, viewed from the posterior side.

DISSECTION 11.19 Blood vessels and ducts of the pancreas

Objectives

I. To complete the exposure of the splenic and superior mesenteric vessels, and the portal vein.   II. To identify the pancreatic branches of the splenic vessels.   III. To dissect the duct system of the pancreas.

Instructions

1. Turn the tail and body of the pancreas to the right, stripping the splenic artery and vein from its posterior surface. Identify the vessels passing to the pancreas from the splenic vessels.

2. Detach the superior mesenteric vessels, portal vein, and gastroduodenal artery from the pancreas, identifying and then dividing their glandular branches or tributaries. Divide the bile duct near the first part of the duodenum, and remove the duodenum and pancreas in one piece.

3. On the posterior surface of the pancreas, make two cuts into the gland, parallel and close to the superior and inferior margins of the body. Pick away the lobules of the gland between the cuts to expose the greyish-white duct. Trace the duct in both directions [Fig. 11.48], taking care to expose the accessory pancreatic duct and its tributaries in the head of the pancreas. Follow both ducts to the duodenum and identify their openings on the inner surface of the duodenum.

Here a **sphincter** of smooth muscle controls the discharge of bile and pancreatic secretions into the duodenum. The strongest part of the sphincter surrounds the bile duct alone and lies proximal to the ampulla and the junction with the pancreatic duct. When this sphincter contracts, bile passes along the cystic duct to the gallbladder but does not enter the pancreatic duct. The remainder of the bile duct contains very little muscle.

The point of union of the common hepatic and cystic ducts is very variable but is usually close to the porta hepatis. The arrangement of the bile and pancreatic ducts is also variable.

The main parts of the splenic, superior and inferior mesenteric veins have been exposed in Dissection 11.17. Dissection 11.19 further explores the blood vessels and ducts of the pancreas.

Pancreas

The pancreas is an elongated gland which lies across the upper part of the posterior abdominal wall and extends from the duodenum to the spleen. It lies at the junction of the supracolic and infracolic compartments of the peritoneal cavity [Fig. 11.13].

The expanded **head of the pancreas** lies in the concavity of the duodenum, overlapping the second and third parts. The head is anterior to the inferior vena cava [Figs. 11.13, 11.47], the bile duct, and the aorta. The bile duct grooves its superolateral part. The **uncinate process** of the pancreas extends posteriorly from the inferior part of the head and passes between the superior mesenteric vessels and the aorta [Fig. 11.42]. The head is crossed anteriorly by the transverse colon or its mesentery, and the first 2–3 cm of the duodenum. The head of the pancreas joins the body, anterior to the formation of the portal vein.

The **body** of the pancreas passes to the left across the aorta and the superior mesenteric artery, the left crus of the diaphragm, left psoas major, left renal vessels, and the left kidney [Figs. 11.6, 11.23, 11.34, 11.42]. It is posterior to the lesser sac and stomach. A small projection from the superior part of the pancreas—the **tuber omentale**—is in contact with the lesser omentum, immediately inferior to the coeliac trunk. The splenic artery runs a sinuous course along the upper margin of the body. The splenic vein lies on its posterior surface and is joined by the inferior and superior mesenteric veins. The blunt end of the body—the **tail**—lies in the lienorenal ligament and may touch the hilus of the spleen [Fig. 11.22].

Vessels and nerves

The **pancreaticoduodenal arteries** and **veins** supply the head. The splenic **vessels** supply the remainder of the pancreas. Sympathetic and parasympathetic nerve fibres reach the gland along the arteries from the coeliac and superior mesenteric plexuses. **Lymph nodes** lie along the superior border of the pancreas (pancreaticosplenic nodes) and on the pancreaticoduodenal arteries.

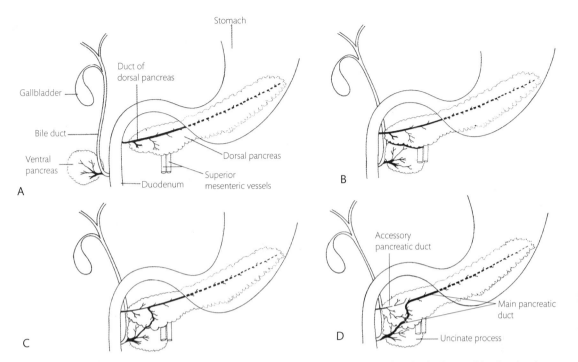

Fig. 11.49 (A, B, C, D) A diagram to show the formation of the adult pancreas and pancreatic ducts by the fusion of the dorsal and ventral pancreatic buds in the embryo.

Ducts of the pancreas

Developmentally, the pancreas arises as two separate hollow branching outgrowths from the duodenum. The smaller outgrowth—the ventral pancreatic bud—arises in common with the hepatic outgrowth. The dorsal pancreatic bud arises more proximally. The dorsal pancreas forms part of the head, the body, and the tail of the pancreas. The ventral pancreas forms the posterior part of the head and uncinate process. The ventral pancreas moves into a position dorsal to the dorsal pancreas. The two rudiments fuse, and their ducts communicate in the substance of the gland.

The duodenal end of the **main pancreatic duct** is derived from the duct of the ventral pancreas. The remainder of the main pancreatic duct is derived from the duct of the dorsal pancreas. The accessory duct is derived from the duodenal end of the dorsal pancreatic duct. It usually communicates with the main pancreatic duct and opens into the duodenum, 2–3 cm proximally [Fig. 11.49].

The main pancreatic duct begins in the tail of the pancreas, runs through the body slightly superior to the centre, and receives small tributaries throughout its course. At the head, it bends infe-

riorly, usually communicates with the accessory duct, and then drains the uncinate process and the posterior part of the lower part of the head. It joins the bile duct as it pierces the duodenal wall at the greater duodenal papilla [Figs. 11.48, 11.50].

The **accessory pancreatic duct** receives tributaries from the upper part of the head and from its lower anterior part. Normally, the accessory duct connects with the main duct. The accessory pancreatic duct may be entirely separate or simply a tributary of the main duct without a separate entry to the duodenum. This is a matter of some clinical importance when the main duct is obstructed at the **hepatopancreatic ampulla**.

Where the pancreatic duct joins the bile duct, weak **sphincters** are found in the pancreatic duct and on the combined channel. The pancreatic sphincter prevents reflux of bile into the pancreatic duct when the common duct is closed. ➔ The greater duodenal papilla can be catheterized under direct vision using a duodenal endoscope. The bile or pancreatic duct may then be filled with X-ray-opaque material to visualize the duct system, a procedure known as endoscopic retrograde cholangiopancreatography (ERCP) [Fig. 11.50].

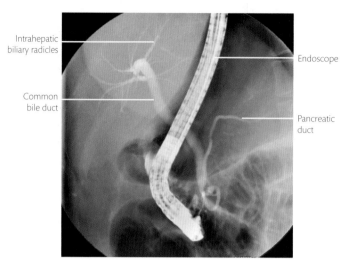

Fig. 11.50 Endoscopic retrograde cholangiopancreatography (ERCP) image in a patient who has previously undergone cholecystectomy.

Liver

The liver is the largest gland in the body. Most of it lies under cover of the ribs and costal cartilages and is in contact with the diaphragm. The diaphragm separates the liver from the pericardium and the right pleura [Figs. 11.3, 11.51].

Dissection 11.20 describes the procedure for the removal of the liver.

The liver is a soft, dark brown, highly vascular organ. It is readily torn in abdominal injuries and may be a source of severe intra-abdominal bleeding. The shape of the liver is determined by the surrounding organs. In the cadaver, it retains the shape of a blunt wedge with its rounded base

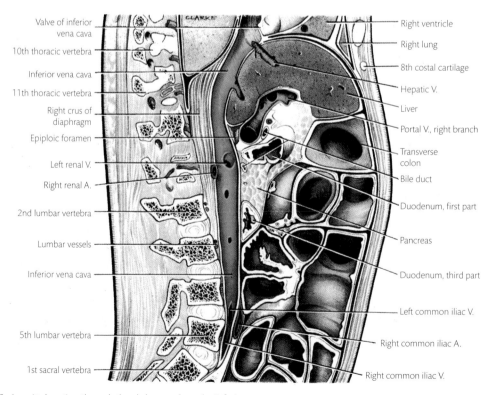

Fig. 11.51 A sagittal section through the abdomen along the inferior vena cava.

Objective

I. To cut the peritoneal reflections from the liver and the inferior vena cava and remove the liver.

Instructions

1. With one hand in the pleural cavity and the other in the peritoneal cavity, examine the position of the liver. Note that the liver extends to the level of the fifth rib in the right mid-clavicular line, filling this dome of the diaphragm and part of the left dome anterior to the stomach. The right lobe of the liver is separated from the costodiaphragmatic recess of the pleura by the diaphragm.

2. Pull the liver downwards, and divide the anterior layers of the coronary and left triangular ligaments. Avoid injury to the inferior vena cava.

3. Identify the inferior vena cava between the liver and the diaphragm, and strip the liver downwards from it. While doing so, find and divide the hepatic veins entering the inferior vena cava and divide the remaining peritoneal connections of the liver to the diaphragm. If the inferior vena cava is buried deeply in the liver, divide it and remove a segment of it with the liver.

to the right. The liver has two surfaces—a **diaphragmatic surface** and a **visceral surface** [Figs. 11.52, 11.53, 11.54]. The diaphragmatic surface is arbitrarily divided into superior, anterior, right, and posterior parts. Together, these parts form the curved surface which is in contact with the diaphragm. The visceral surface faces posteroinferiorly. It is separated from the anterior part of the diaphragmatic surface by the sharp inferior margin, and from the posterior part of the diaphragmatic surface by an indistinct posterior border. The liver is divided into four lobes—the right, left, caudate, and quadrate lobes—by fissures and the attachment of ligaments.

Fissures of the liver

There are a number of fissures on the visceral surface and the posterior part of the diaphragmatic surface [Fig. 11.54]. A deep fissure extends almost vertically across the visceral surface. The upper part of this fissure is the **fissure for the ligamentum venosum**, and the lower part is the **fissure for the ligamentum teres**. The fissure for the ligamentum venosum separates the **left lobe** of the liver from the **caudate lobe** [Fig. 11.54] and has the upper part of the lesser omentum attached in its depths. The fissure for the ligamentum teres extends vertically across the visceral surface and separates the left lobe of the liver from the **quadrate lobe** [Fig. 11.54]. Near the middle of the visceral surface is a short transverse fissure called the **porta hepatis**. This fissure extends to the right between the caudate and quadrate lobes. The inferior part of the lesser omentum extends to the right to surround the porta hepatis and form the free edge of the lesser omentum [Fig. 11.54]. The free edge of the lesser omentum encloses the branches of the hepatic artery, branches of the portal vein, and the hepatic and cystic ducts as they enter and leave the liver at the porta hepatis.

The right margin of the caudate lobe is separated from the right lobe by a sulcus containing the **inferior vena cava**. The right margin of the quadrate lobe is separated from the right lobe by the **gallbladder** in its fossa. The inferior vena cava does not form a complete right margin for the caudate lobe. Inferiorly, a small strip of the caudate lobe—the **caudate process**—extends to the right

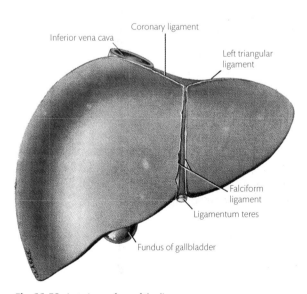

Fig. 11.52 Anterior surface of the liver.

Labels: Coronary ligament; Inferior vena cava; Left triangular ligament; Falciform ligament; Ligamentum teres; Fundus of gallbladder

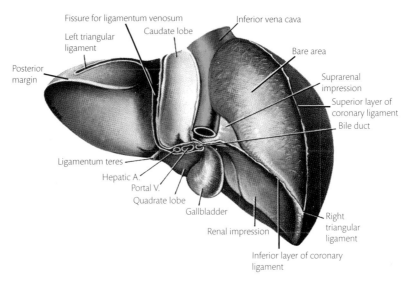

Fig. 11.53 Posterior surface of the liver.

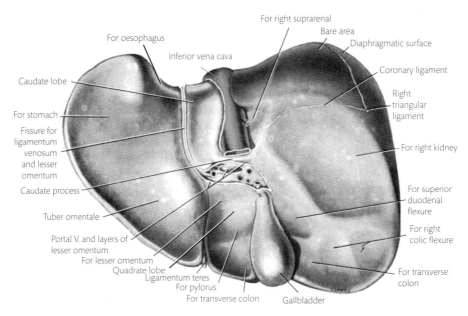

Fig. 11.54 The postero-inferior (visceral) surface of the liver.

between the inferior vena cava and the portal vein in the porta hepatis. This caudate process forms the upper wall of the **epiploic foramen** [Fig. 11.54] and unites the caudate and right lobes of the liver.

The ligamentum teres is the fibrous remnants of the (left) umbilical vein of the fetus, and the ligamentum venosum is a remnant of the ductus venosus. In the fetus, these vessels are continuous with each other through the left branch of the portal vein. The left umbilical vein carries oxygenated blood from the placenta to the left branch of

the portal vein. The ductus venosus is a channel which bypasses the liver and carries this oxygenated blood directly to the inferior vena cava.

Surfaces of the liver

Diaphragmatic surface

The diaphragmatic surface is arbitrarily divided into superior, anterior, right, and posterior parts. The right part lies between the seventh and eleventh ribs in the right mid-axillary line. The diaphragm separates the liver from the pleura down to the tenth rib and from the lung down to the eighth rib in quiet respiration.

The anterior part of the diaphragmatic surface is triangular. The **falciform ligament** is attached vertically to this surface [Fig. 11.52] and marks the division of the liver into right and left lobes anteriorly. A part of the anterior surface is in contact with the anterior abdominal wall between the right and left costal margins [Fig. 11.3].

The superior part of the diaphragmatic surface is convex. It is slightly flattened centrally, inferior to the pericardium—the **cardiac impression**. It rises almost to the level of the nipple on the right side and to the level of the fifth intercostal space in the left mid-clavicular plane [Fig. 11.3]. On the left, the superior part meets the visceral surface at a sharp posterior margin [Fig. 11.53].

The posterior part of the diaphragmatic surface is narrow in the left lobe but widens at the fissure for the ligamentum venosum. This part of the diaphragmatic surface includes the **caudate lobe**. The caudate lobe forms the anterior wall of the superior recess of the lesser sac. At the right margin of the caudate lobe, the peritoneum turns posteriorly on the inferior vena cava and extends towards the left on the diaphragm. This peritoneum thus forms the right and posterior walls of the superior recess of the lesser sac.

The **inferior vena cava** lies in a deep groove (occasionally buried in the liver), immediately to the right of the caudate lobe. The two main **hepatic veins** enter it at the upper end of the groove, and some smaller veins enter it at a lower level. The posterior part of the diaphragmatic surface to the right of the inferior vena cava is broad and not covered by peritoneum. This is the **bare area of the liver**. Direct contact between the liver and the diaphragm in the bare area permits passage of lymph vessels and small veins through the diaphragm. A slight depression immediately to the right of the lower end of the caval groove and partly in the bare area marks the position of the right suprarenal gland [Fig. 11.54].

Visceral surface

The visceral surface [Fig. 11.54] is irregular in shape and fits the upper abdominal viscera which lie postero-inferior to it. The left lobe lies in relation to the stomach and oesophagus, both of which leave an impression on it. A small part of the left lobe—the tuber omentale—is in contact with the lesser omentum, close to the porta hepatis [Figs. 11.54, 11.55].

The most obvious feature on the right lobe is the **gallbladder**. It extends from near the porta hepatis to a shallow notch on the inferior margin. It is anterior to the second part of the duodenum and the transverse colon. To the left of the gallbladder,

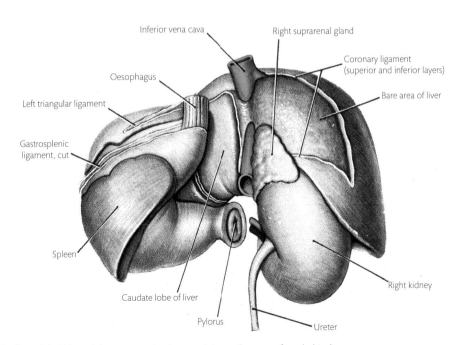

Fig. 11.55 The liver, right kidney, right suprarenal, spleen, and stomach as seen from behind.

the quadrate lobe overlies the lesser omentum, pylorus, beginning of the duodenum, and the transverse colon. To the right of the gallbladder, the visceral surface is in contact with the junction of the first and second parts of the duodenum, the upper part of the right kidney, and the right colic flexure [Figs. 11.54, 11.55].

Peritoneal covering and ligaments of the liver

The peritoneum covers the surface of the liver, except the bare area (which includes the groove for the inferior vena cava) and the fossa for the gallbladder. The peritoneal attachments of the liver are readily understood if it is realized that the liver develops in the ventral mesentery of the stomach and upper duodenum. As a result, the **ventral mesentery** is divided by the liver into two parts—a part which connects the liver to the anterior abdominal wall (the **falciform ligament**) and a part which connects the liver to the stomach and duodenum (the **lesser omentum**). Most of the ligaments described below are double folds of peritoneum enclosing connective tissue.

Falciform ligament

The falciform ligament extends from the supraumbilical part of the anterior abdominal wall to the anterior part of the diaphragmatic surface of the liver, between the right and left lobes. At the liver, the peritoneum forming the right and left layers of the falciform ligament separate and cover the right and left lobes of the liver. The inferior or free edge of the falciform ligament contains the **ligamentum teres**—the obliterated part of the left umbilical vein. At the superior part of the diaphragmatic surface, the peritoneum covering the right lobe of the liver turns up to form the superior layer of the right coronary ligament. Similarly, the peritoneum covering the left lobe turns up and continues as the anterior layer of the left triangular ligament [Figs. 11.52, 11.53].

Coronary ligament

The coronary ligament is formed by the reflection of peritoneum from the right lobe of the liver to the diaphragm. The two layers of the coronary ligament—the superior and inferior layers—form the boundaries of the bare area of the liver. Traced to the right, the two layers of the coronary ligament meet at the right triangular ligament [Figs. 11.53, 11.54].

Triangular ligaments

There are two triangular ligaments—right and left. The right triangular ligament extends between the right lobe of the liver and the diaphragm. It is continuous with the two layers of the coronary ligament. The left triangular ligament extends from the superior surface of the left lobe of the liver to the diaphragm [Figs. 11.53, 11.54, 11.55].

Lesser omentum

This double fold of peritoneum attaches the lesser curvature of the stomach and the proximal duodenum to the visceral surface of the liver. The attachment to the liver is L-shaped. The vertical limb of the 'L' lies deep in the fissure for the ligamentum venosum (between the left and caudate lobes). The horizontal limb of the 'L' surrounds the porta hepatis and the structures which lie in it—the terminal branches of the hepatic artery and portal vein, the right and left hepatic ducts, lymph vessels and nodes, and nerves [Fig. 11.54].

Ligamentum venosum

The ligamentum venosum lies in the fissure by the same name, between the caudate and left lobes of the liver. It is the obliterated part of the ductus venosus [Fig. 11.54].

Vessels and nerves of the liver

The liver receives blood through the **hepatic artery** and **portal vein**. Blood drains from the liver to the inferior vena cava through the right and left **hepatic veins** and by some smaller veins. The right and left **lobes of the liver** receive separate branches of the hepatic artery and portal vein and give rise to separate tributaries of the hepatic veins and ducts. All of the **quadrate lobe** and the left part of the **caudate lobe** are supplied and drained by the vessels of the left lobe. The right part of the caudate lobe is supplied and drained by the vessels of the right lobe [Figs. 11.44, 11.47].

The **nerves** supplying the liver are derived from the coeliac plexus and from the gastric branches of the vagal trunks. Some sensory fibres in the right phrenic nerve supply the gallbladder and its ducts.

Lymph vessels emerge either through the porta hepatis to nodes in the lesser omentum or pass from the bare area through the diaphragm to thoracic lymph nodes.

Gallbladder

The gallbladder is a piriform sac with a storage capacity of 30–60 ml. It concentrates bile produced by the liver and discharges it into the duodenum. The gallbladder lies in a shallow fossa along the right edge of the quadrate lobe of the liver. Usually it is directly in contact with the liver substance and has venous communications with it [Figs. 11.54, 11.56]. Occasionally, it may be suspended from the liver by a short mesentery or be partly buried in it.

Antero-inferiorly, the rounded **fundus of the gallbladder** protrudes below the inferior margin of the liver. It touches the anterior abdominal wall where the right linea semilunaris meets the ninth costal cartilage [Fig. 11.3]. The fundus is continuous with the **body** of the gallbladder and the body is continuous with the **neck** which is close to the right extremity of the porta hepatis [Fig. 11.46]. The fundus of the gallbladder lies anterior to the transverse colon; the body lies on the second part of the duodenum, and the neck lies anterior to the first part of the duodenum [Figs. 11.47, 11.54].

Vessels and nerves of the gallbladder

The gallbladder is supplied by the **cystic artery**, a branch of the right hepatic artery [Fig. 11.18] and drained by the **cystic vein**, a tributary of the portal vein. **Lymph vessels** from the gallbladder pass to nodes on the cystic duct and in the porta hepatis. Nerves reach it along the artery from the coeliac plexus (sympathetic), the vagus (parasympathetic), and the right phrenic nerve (sensory).

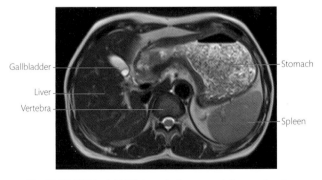

Fig. 11.56 T2W axial MRI through the upper abdomen showing the liver, gallbladder, spleen, and stomach.

Cystic duct

The cystic duct is 2 cm or more in length. It descends from the neck of the gallbladder between the layers of the lesser omentum and joins the common hepatic duct to form the bile duct [Fig. 11.46].

Dissection 11.21 describes the dissection of the structures in the porta hepatis.

Structures in the porta hepatis

Near the porta hepatis, the common hepatic duct, hepatic artery, and portal vein divide into right and left branches [Figs. 11.47, 11.54]. These pass together into the corresponding lobes of the liver. The hepatic ducts are anterior to the arteries and both are anterior to the veins. The right branch of the portal vein receives the cystic vein and enters the right lobe of the liver. The left branch of the portal vein passes between the caudate and quadrate lobes and supplies both. It unites with the ligamentum venosum and the ligamentum teres and enters the left lobe of the liver.

In Dissection 11.22 you will be instructed on how to trace the blood vessels in the liver.

Dissection 11.23 explores the interior of the gallbladder.

DISSECTION 11.21 Structures in the porta hepatis

Objective

I. To identify and trace the hepatic ducts, branches of the portal vein, and the hepatic artery in the porta hepatis.

Instructions

1. Expose the structures in the porta hepatis—the right and left hepatic ducts, the right and left branches of the portal vein, the right and left branches of the hepatic arteries—and follow them to their entry into the liver. Their arrangement is variable and may not correspond to the following description.

DISSECTION 11.22 Blood vessels in the liver

Objective

I. To trace branches of the hepatic artery and portal vein and tributaries of the hepatic vein within the substance of the liver.

Instructions

1. Trace a branch of the portal vein, hepatic artery, and hepatic duct for some distance into the liver. Note their branches to the liver tissue.

2. Trace one of the hepatic veins backwards from the inferior vena cava into the liver.

3. Inspect the cut surface of a slice of the liver with a hand lens.

DISSECTION 11.23 Interior of the gallbladder

Objective

I. To examine the interior of the gallbladder.

Instructions

1. Make a longitudinal incision through the wall of the gallbladder and cystic duct. Wash out the interior with a jet of water and examine the lining.

Internal surface of the gallbladder and cystic duct

The mucous membrane of the gallbladder is complexly folded to increase the surface area. It has a honeycomb appearance to the unaided eye. From the neck of the gallbladder, a prominent fold of mucous membrane runs spirally along the cystic duct—the **spiral fold**. It may help to maintain the patency of the cystic duct [Fig. 11.46].

Abdominal structures in contact with the diaphragm

The upper part of the posterior surface of each kidney and suprarenal gland is in contact posteriorly with each half of the diaphragm. Anterior to this, the right lobe of the liver fills the right dome. The stomach, the left lobe of the liver, and the spleen fill the left dome. Parts of the right and left lobes

of the liver lie inferior to the central tendon. The liver, stomach, and spleen are separated by the diaphragm from parts of the pleural cavities.

Replace the upper abdominal organs that have been removed, and confirm their positions relative to the pleural cavities.

The autonomic nervous system

Dissection 11.24 gives instructions on how to identify the coeliac ganglia and trace its branches.

The general arrangement of the autonomic nervous system is described in Chapter 1 and illustrated in Fig. 1.9. The autonomic nervous system in the abdomen consists of sympathetic and parasympathetic nerves which innervate the smooth muscle and glands of the abdominal viscera.

Sympathetic nervous system

This part of the abdominal autonomic nervous system consists of: (1) the lumbar portion of the sympathetic trunks and their branches and (2) the sympathetic plexuses.

Sympathetic trunk

The right and left **sympathetic trunks** lie on the anterolateral surface of the lumbar vertebra. Each trunk consists of a series of ganglia united by nerve fibres [Fig. 11.57]. Superiorly, it continues with the thoracic part of the sympathetic trunk by passing through the diaphragm. Inferiorly, it continues with the pelvic part of the sympathetic trunk

DISSECTION 11.24 Coeliac ganglia

Objective

I. To identify the coeliac ganglia and trace their branches.

Instructions

1. Find a **coeliac ganglion** on each side of the coeliac trunk. Each ganglion lies in the plexus of nerves on the aorta, anterior to the corresponding crus of the diaphragm.

2. Trace branches of the ganglia to the suprarenal glands, the coeliac trunk, and inferiorly along the aorta to form plexuses on the superior and inferior mesenteric arteries.

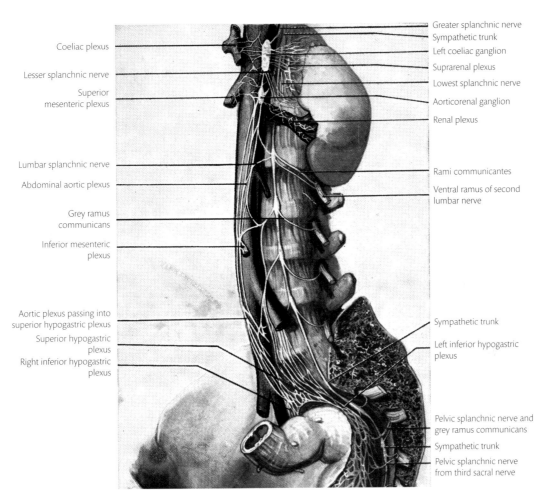

Coeliac plexus

Lesser splanchnic nerve

Superior
mesenteric plexus

Lumbar splanchnic nerve

Abdominal aortic plexus

Grey ramus
communicans

Inferior mesenteric
plexus

Aortic plexus passing into
superior hypogastric plexus

Superior hypogastric
plexus

Right inferior hypogastric
plexus

Greater splanchnic nerve

Sympathetic trunk

Left coeliac ganglion

Suprarenal plexus

Lowest splanchnic nerve

Aorticorenal ganglion

Renal plexus

Rami communicantes

Ventral ramus of second
lumbar nerve

Sympathetic trunk

Left inferior hypogastric
plexus

Pelvic splanchnic nerve and
grey ramus communicans

Sympathetic trunk

Pelvic splanchnic nerve
from third sacral nerve

Fig. 11.57 Sympathetic plexuses in the abdomen and pelvis.

by passing behind the common iliac vessels. The abdominal and pelvic viscera get their sympathetic supply through the sympathetic trunk through branches which arise in the thorax (the greater, lesser, and least splanchnic nerves [see Figs. 4.13B, 4.14B]), in the abdomen (the lumbar splanchnic nerves [Fig. 11.57]), and in the pelvis (the sacral splanchnic nerves [see Fig. 13.6]).

Bundles of **preganglionic fibres** to the sympathetic trunk arise from the thoracic and upper lumbar segments of the spinal cord and enter the sympathetic trunk through **white rami communicantes**. The preganglionic fibres to the body wall end on the cells of the ganglia at various levels. These ganglia send sympathetic nerves to the body wall through **post-ganglionic fibres** which reach the lumbar nerves through **grey rami communicantes**.

The sympathetic trunk also gives sympathetic nerves to the abdominal viscera. These are the **lumbar splanchnic nerves** which arise from

the lumbar part of the sympathetic trunk. They are preganglionic fibres which join the inferior part of the abdominal aortic plexus [Fig. 11.57].

Abdominal autonomic plexuses

A series of somewhat variable, inter-related autonomic plexuses are found in the abdomen and pelvis. These include the coeliac plexus, aorticorenal plexus, superior mesenteric plexus, abdominal aortic (intermesenteric) plexus, inferior mesenteric plexus, superior hypogastric plexuses, and inferior hypogastric plexuses (the last lies in the pelvis). In addition to the sympathetic nerves, these plexuses contain ganglia and carry preganglionic parasympathetic nerves from the vagus and pelvic splanchnic nerves [Fig. 11.57].

The **coeliac plexus** lies on the aorta and the crus of the diaphragm around the coeliac trunk. It is posterior to the lesser sac and partly overlapped by the pancreas on both sides and the inferior vena cava on the right [Figs. 11.28, 11.29, 11.57]. Embedded in the coeliac plexus on each side of the coeliac trunk are the large, nodular **coeliac ganglia**. The ganglia give rise to most of the post-ganglionic sympathetic nerve fibres in the plexus. Preganglionic fibres pass directly through the coeliac ganglion to the suprarenal glands and to the smaller ganglia on the coeliac trunk and the superior mesenteric artery.

The coeliac plexus is part of the abdominal autonomic plexuses and continues through it with the **superior mesenteric** and **renal plexuses** on the corresponding arteries. The plexuses on the renal arteries give rise to subsidiary plexuses along the gonadal arteries and the ureter.

The **abdominal aortic** or **intermesenteric plexus** consists of two or three intercommunicating strands of nerve fibres over each side of the abdominal aorta [Fig. 11.57]. They arise in the coeliac and superior mesenteric plexuses and are reinforced by lumbar splanchnic nerves from each lumbar sympathetic trunk. The lumbar splanchnic nerves descend obliquely at the sides of the aorta and unite with the lowest part of the aortic plexus. The plexus extends along the branches of the abdominal aorta below the superior mesenteric artery. Inferior to the bifurcation of the aorta, the abdominal aortic plexus continues as the superior hypogastric plexus.

The **superior hypogastric plexus** lies anterior to the aortic bifurcation and between the two common iliac arteries. It is also known as the **presacral nerve**. It lies on the front of the fifth lumbar vertebra and the left common iliac vein. On the sacral promontory, this plexus divides into the right and left

inferior hypogastric (pelvic) **plexuses** around the corresponding internal iliac arteries [Fig. 11.57].

Parasympathetic nervous system

The parasympathetic nerves to the abdomen and pelvic organs are from the vagus and the second, third, and fourth sacral nerves. Preganglionic fibres from the vagus run through the coeliac and superior mesenteric plexuses. Preganglionic fibres from the sacral nerves run through the inferior mesenteric and superior and inferior hypogastric plexuses. They synapse with parasympathetic ganglia found in or near the organ they innervate.

Start the study of the suprarenals and kidneys by exposing these glands and the blood vessels supplying them.

Using instructions given in Dissection 11.25 explore the suprarenals, kidneys, ureters, and the blood vessels supplying them.

Suprarenal glands

The suprarenal or adrenal glands consist of two parts—the cortex (developed from the coelomic epithelium) and the medulla (developed from the neural crest cells and bearing similarity to the sympathetic ganglion). Each suprarenal gland lies against the superomedial surface of the corresponding kidney, enclosed in the renal fascia. A little fatty connective tissue separates it from the kidney.

The **right gland** is pyramidal in shape. It is related to the diaphragm posteromedially, the

---

DISSECTION 11.25 Exposure of the suprarenals, kidneys, ureters, and their blood vessels

Objectives

I. To expose the suprarenals and kidneys.   II. To identify and trace the renal vessels and tributaries of the renal veins.

Instructions

1. Remove the fat and fascia from the anterior surface of the left kidney and suprarenal gland.

2. Find the left suprarenal vein and the left testicular or ovarian vein. Trace both to the left renal vein.

3. Follow the left renal vein from the left kidney to the inferior vena cava.

4. Displace the vein and expose the left renal artery. Follow its branches to the left kidney, left suprarenal gland, and ureter.

5. Follow the ureter down in the abdomen.

6. Turn the left kidney medially to expose its posterior surface and that of its vessels and the ureter. Identify the muscles, vessels, and nerves, which are posterior to them.

7. Carry out the same dissection on the right side, but note that the testicular or ovarian and suprarenal veins drain directly to the inferior vena cava.

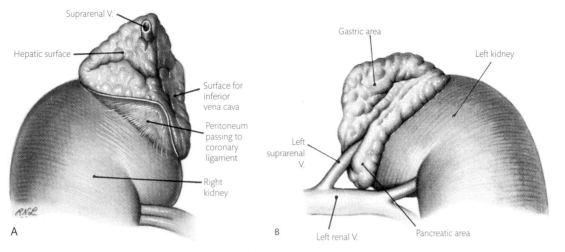

Fig. 11.58 (A) Anterior surface of the right suprarenal gland. (B) Anterior surface of the left suprarenal gland.

inferior vena cava anteromedially, the liver anteriorly, and the kidney inferolaterally. Superiorly, it lies on the bare area of the liver, but lower down it is covered by peritoneum [Fig. 11.58A].

The **left gland** is crescentic in shape. It is related to the diaphragm posteromedially, the stomach anteriorly (with the lesser sac and pancreas intervening), and the kidney inferolaterally [Fig. 11.58B].

Vessels of the suprarenal glands

The abundant blood supply to the gland is obtained through many small **arteries** which enter the surface of the adrenal cortex. These arteries arise from three different sources—the inferior suprarenal arteries arise from the renal arteries, the middle suprarenal arteries from the aorta, and the superior suprarenal arteries from the inferior phrenic arteries [Fig. 11.59]. The arteries supply the cortex of the suprarenal and pierce it to enter and supply the medulla. The **suprarenal veins** run inwards from the cortex to the medulla and emerge from the suprarenal as a single vein. The right suprarenal vein drains into the inferior vena cava, and the left into the left renal vein.

Dissection 11.26 explores the cut section of the suprarenal gland.

The kidneys

The kidneys are reddish-brown in colour and approximately 10 cm long, 5 cm wide, and 2.5 cm thick. They are ovoid in shape, but the medial margin is deeply indented and concave at its middle. On the medial margin is a wide, vertical cleft—the **hilus**—which transmits the structures entering and leaving the kidney—the ureter, renal vessels, lymphatics, and nerves. Within the kidney, and immediately lateral to the hilus, is a fat-filled space—the **sinus** of the kidney. The hilus lies approximately at the level of the first lumbar vertebra [Figs. 11.59, 11.60].

The kidneys lie in the upper part of the paravertebral gutters, posterior to the peritoneum, against the structures on the sides of the last two thoracic and first three lumbar vertebrae. They are angulated in such a way that the anterior and posterior surfaces face anterolateral and posteromedial, respectively, and the superior ends are medial to the inferior ends. In addition, the right kidney lies at a lower level than the left. (The superior end of the right kidney is at the eleventh intercostal space and that of the left kidney at the eleventh rib [Figs. 11.13, 11.60, 11.61]).

The ureter extends from the hilus of the kidney to the urinary bladder [Fig. 11.59]. The upper end of the ureter expands to form the **pelvis of the kidney** [Figs. 11.62A, 11.62B]. The pelvis passes through the hilus into the sinus of the kidney. In the sinus, two to three short, funnel-like tubes—the **major calyces**—open into the renal pelvis. The renal vessels lie anterior to the pelvis, but some of their branches and tributaries pass posterior to it. Lymph vessels and autonomic and sensory nerve fibres also pass through the hilus into the sinus of the kidney.

Each kidney is enclosed in a dense fibrous **capsule**, which is readily stripped from its surface.

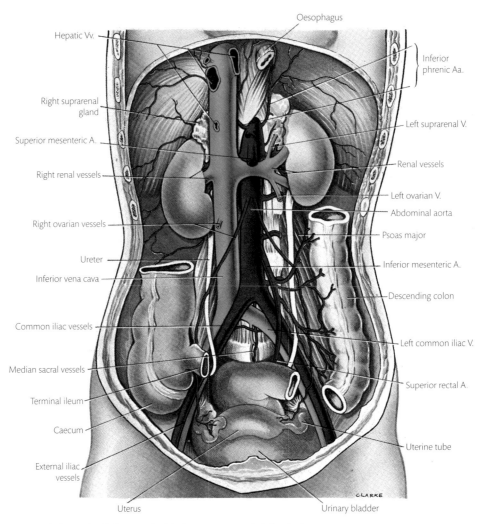

Right suprarenal gland

Superior mesenteric A.

Right renal vessels

Right ovarian vessels

Ureter

Inferior vena cava

Common iliac vessels

Median sacral vessels

Terminal ileum

Caecum

External iliac vessels

Uterus

Hepatic Vv.

Oesophagus

Inferior phrenic Aa.

Left suprarenal V.

Renal vessels

Left ovarian V.

Abdominal aorta

Psoas major

Inferior mesenteric A.

Descending colon

Left common iliac V.

Superior rectal A.

Uterine tube

Urinary bladder

CLARKE

Fig. 11.59 Posterior abdominal wall showing the inferior vena cava and abdominal aorta.

The capsule passes through the hilum to line the sinus. The fibrous capsule is surrounded by a fatty capsule—the **perirenal fat**. Around the perirenal fat is a sheath of loosely fitting fascia—the **renal fascia**. The renal fascia encloses the kidney and

DISSECTION 11.26 Suprarenal gland

Objective

I. To study the cut section of the suprarenal gland.

Instructions

1. Follow the left suprarenal vein into the gland, removing the anterior surface of the gland to expose the extent of the medulla.

2. Examine the cut surfaces with a hand lens.

suprarenal gland. It is continuous laterally with the transversalis fascia (on the inner aspect of the transversus abdominis), superiorly with the diaphragmatic fascia (on the inferior surface of the diaphragm), and medially with the fascia around the renal vessels. Inferiorly, the anterior and posterior layers of the renal fascia are only loosely united. External to the renal fascia, there may be a considerable accumulation of extraperitoneal fat—the **pararenal fat**.

The developing kidney is first formed in the pelvis and subsequently ascends to the lumbar region. During the ascent, the kidney receives its blood supply from successive sources, some of which persist beyond the developmental period as accessory renal arteries. Such accessory arteries may be found arising from the aorta and entering the lower pole of a normally placed kidney [Fig. 11.63].

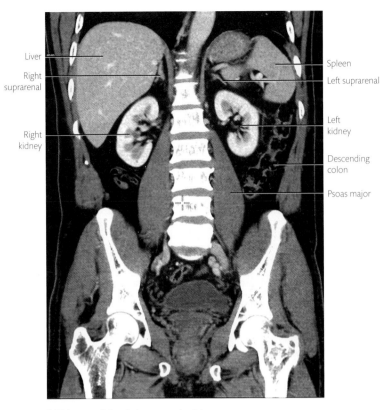

Fig. 11.60 Coronal reconstructed CT image of the abdomen and pelvis.

Liver

Right suprarenal

Right kidney

Spleen

Left suprarenal

Left kidney

Descending colon

Psoas major

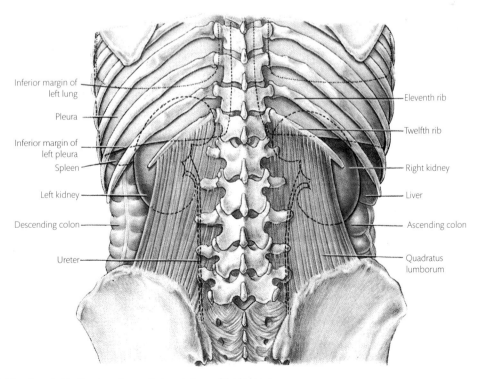

Fig. 11.61 View from behind to show the posterior relations of the kidneys.

Inferior margin of left lung

Pleura

Inferior margin of left pleura

Spleen

Left kidney

Descending colon

Ureter

Eleventh rib

Twelfth rib

Right kidney

Liver

Ascending colon

Quadratus lumborum

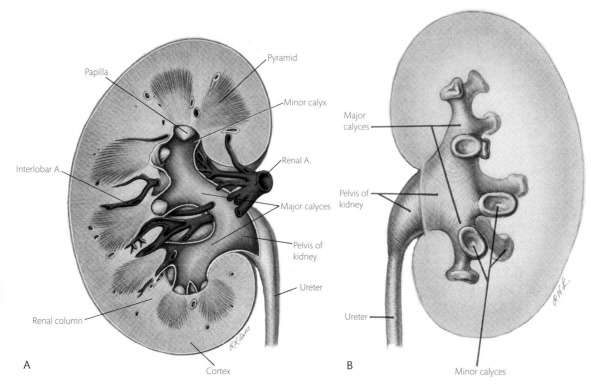

Papilla
Pyramid
Minor calyx
Interlobar A.
Renal A.
Major calyces
Major calyces
Pelvis of kidney
Pelvis of kidney
Ureter
Renal column
Minor calyces
Cortex
A
B

Fig. 11.62 (A) Coronal section of the kidney. Note the papillae projecting into the minor calyces. (B) The pelvis and calyces of the kidney from a cast. The cupped appearance of the lesser calyces is due to each having a renal papilla inserted into it.

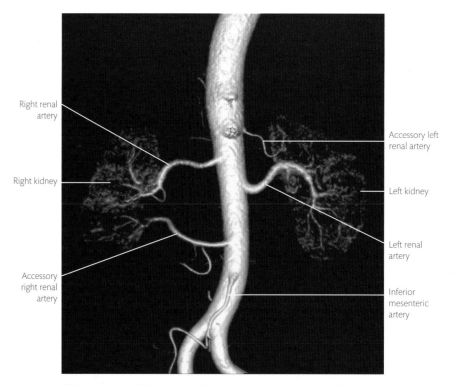

Right renal artery
Accessory left renal artery
Right kidney
Left kidney
Left renal artery
Accessory right renal artery
Inferior mesenteric artery

Fig. 11.63 Volume-rendered 3D image from a CT angiogram of the abdominal aorta. Image of the coeliac artery and the superior mesenteric artery have been removed to demonstrate the renal arteries. Note the accessory renal arteries to the right renal lower pole and to the left renal upper pole.

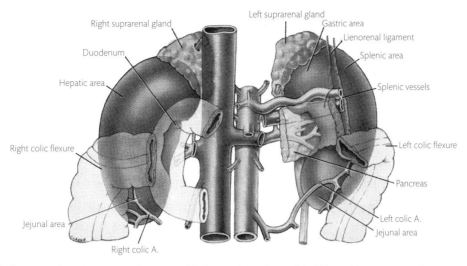

Fig. 11.64 A diagram to show the structures in contact with the anterior surfaces of the kidneys. The pancreas, colon, suprarenal glands, and duodenum are shown as though transparent.

When first formed, the rudiments of the two kidneys are close together. At this stage, the lower poles of the kidney may fuse together to form an anomalous **horseshoe kidney** in front of the aorta. The ascent of a horseshoe kidney is stopped by the inferior mesenteric artery.

Structures in contact with the kidney

Posteriorly, the upper part of both kidneys lies on the diaphragm. The lower part lies in relation to the psoas major medially and the quadratus lumborum, the anterior layer of the thoracolumbar fascia [Chapter 13], and the transversus abdominis laterally [Fig. 11.61]. The **subcostal** vessels and nerve and the **iliohypogastric** and **ilio-inguinal nerves** lie between the kidney and the anterior layer of the thoracolumbar fascia [see Fig. 13.4].

The **diaphragm** separates the upper part of each kidney from the pleura and the twelfth rib. Occasionally, there is a defect in the diaphragm in this region, and the kidney may be in contact with the pleura and the last rib [see Fig. 12.3].

The upper part of the **right kidney** is wedged between the posterior abdominal wall and the visceral surface of the liver [Figs. 11.55, 11.60]. Here the anterior surface of the right kidney is separated from the liver by the suprarenal gland and the peritoneum of the **hepatorenal recess**. Inferiorly, the right kidney is separated from the liver and gallbladder by the descending part of the duodenum medially and the right flexure of the colon inferolaterally. The lower end of the kidney lies in the infracolic compartment [Fig. 11.64].

The upper part of the **left kidney** is posterior to the suprarenal gland, the lesser sac, the attachment of the lienorenal ligament, and more laterally the spleen. Anterior to the left renal hilus lies the body of the pancreas [Fig. 11.13] with the splenic vessels and the attachment of the greater omentum and transverse mesocolon on it. Inferior to this, the left kidney lies in the infracolic compartment, with the descending colon along its lateral margin, the jejunum anterior and the duodenojejunal flexure medial to it [Fig. 11.64]. The descending colon, pancreas, splenic vessels, and the left suprarenal gland are in direct contact with the kidney without intervening peritoneum.

Dissection 11.27 explores the interior of the kidney.

The **sinus of the kidney** is a considerable space within the kidney which contains the greater part of the pelvis of the kidney, the calyces, blood and lymph vessels, and nerves of the kidney.

Structure of the kidney

On the cut surface of the kidney, note the paler **cortex** adjacent to the capsule and the darker conical **pyramids** of the **medulla**. The pyramids are capped with the cortex which extends inwards between them as the **renal columns**. The apex of each pyramid forms a small conical projection—the **renal papilla**. The renal papilla opens into the minor calyx [Figs. 11.62A, 11.62B].

DISSECTION 11.27 Interior of the kidney

Objective

I. To study the interior of the kidney.

Instructions

1. Remove the anterior wall of the renal sinus piece-meal, beginning at the hilum. Divide the vessels entering this wall of the sinus.

2. Define the calyces.

3. Expose the contents of the sinus.

4. Remove the anterior part of the kidney by making a clean coronal slice from the lateral margin through the sinus.

Vessels of the kidney

The right and left renal arteries arise from the aorta. Close to the hilus of the kidney, they divide into four or five **segmental arteries**. Most of these branches pass anterior to the pelvis of the kidney, but one or two pass posterior to it. The right and left renal veins drain the kidneys into the inferior vena cava [Fig. 11.59]. **Nerves** to the kidney are derived from the renal plexus.

Pelvis of the kidney and calyces

The calyces are short, funnel-like tubes. There are two orders of calyces—the major and minor calyces. There are approximately ten minor calyces, the ends of which form cup-shaped expansions over one or two renal papillae and receive urine from it. The minor calyces empty into two or three major calyces, which, in turn, empty into the renal pelvis [Fig. 11.62].

The renal pelvis and calyces are surrounded by fat, vessels, and nerves in the renal sinus. The pelvis emerges through the lower part of the hilus. It tapers down and joins the ureter near the inferior pole of the kidney [Fig. 11.62]. The extrarenal part of the right pelvis is related anteriorly to the second part of the duodenum and the renal vessels. The left pelvis is related to the renal vessels and pancreas [Fig. 11.64].

Abdominal part of the ureter

The ureter is a muscular tube, 25 cm long and 5 mm wide. It extends from the pelvis of the kidney to the urinary bladder in the pelvis. The first half of the ureter lies in the abdomen. It begins as a continuation of the renal pelvis and descends almost vertically in front of the tips of the lumbar transverse processes. It enters the lesser pelvis anterior to the origin of the external iliac artery [Figs. 11.59, 11.65].

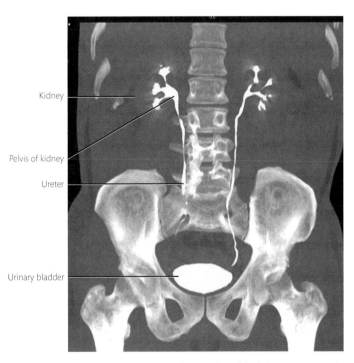

Kidney

Pelvis of kidney

Ureter

Urinary bladder

Fig. 11.65 An intravenous pyelogram showing the kidney outlines, calyces, pelvis of the kidney, ureters, and urinary bladder.

Blood supply

Small branches pass to the ureter from the renal artery, testicular or ovarian artery, aorta, and common iliac arteries. (The pelvic part of the ureter also receives branches from the internal iliac arteries and vesical or uterine arteries.) These arteries form a longitudinal anastomosis on the ureter. **Lymph vessels** drain to lumbar, common, and internal iliac nodes.

See Clinical Applications 11.1–11.5 for the practical implications of the anatomy in this chapter.

CLINICAL APPLICATION 11.1 Splenomegaly and its identification by physical examination

Splenomegaly refers to an enlargement of the spleen. Various conditions lead to splenomegaly. They are broadly classified as conditions which cause: (1) expansion of lymphoid tissue in response to infection; (2) resumption of extramedullary haematopoiesis; (3) increased reticulo-endothelial activity due to haemolysis; (4) involvement by lymphoproliferative disease; and (5) vascular congestion due to portal hypertension—increased pressure in the portal vein.

Study question 1: why would portal hypertension result in splenomegaly? (Answer: the splenic vein drains directly into the portal vein. Increased pressure in the portal vein would lead to venous congestion within the spleen, causing it to enlarge.)

Study question 2: is the spleen normally palpable? (Answer: no. The anterior pole of the spleen normally extends only up to the mid-axillary line. It would have to be enlarged 2–3 times its normal size to be palpable beyond the left costal margin.)

Study question 3: in which direction does the spleen enlarge? And why? (Answer: the spleen enlarges downwards and medially from the left costal margin towards the right iliac fossa. The phrenicocolic ligament and the left colic flexure prevent it from expanding inferiorly.)

Study question 4: what other anatomical features help to identify a palpable mass in the abdomen as the spleen? (Answer: (1) the apposition of the diaphragmatic surface of the spleen to the inferior surface of the left dome of the diaphragm makes the organ move with respiration; and (2) the superior border is often notched anteriorly. Palpating the notch on an abdominal mass helps confirm the clinical finding of an enlarged spleen.)

CLINICAL APPLICATION 11.2 Appendicitis

A 13-year-old boy presented with low-grade fever, vomiting, and acute abdominal pain which was initially periumbilical and later shifted to the right iliac fossa. On examination, palpation of the abdomen revealed maximum tenderness at McBurney's point. A diagnosis of acute appendicitis was considered.

Study question 1: where is McBurney's point? What is the significance of maximum tenderness at McBurney's point? (Answer: McBurney's point is a point at the junction of the medial two-thirds and lateral one-third of a line joining the right anterior superior iliac spine to the umbilicus. This is the point of maximum tenderness in acute appendicitis.)

Study question 2: why is there shifting of pain from the periumbilical region to the right iliac fossa? (Answer: the periumbilical pain occurs because of stimulation of sensory nerve fibres from the appendix—visceral pain. The pain shifts and localizes to the right iliac fossa as the inflammation progresses to involve the parietal peritoneum overlying the appendix—parietal pain. Visceral pain is typically dull and poorly localized. Parietal pain is sharp and well localized.)

Study question 3: what is the cause of appendicitis? (Answer: in 50–80% of individuals, appendicitis is caused by obstruction of the lumen of the appendix by faecal matter (faecolith), parasites, a tumour, or lymphoid hyperplasia. Continued secretion of mucus within an obstructed appendix results in raised intraluminal pressure, impairment of venous drainage, and mucosal ischaemia. This is often complicated by bacterial proliferation, abscess formation, or even perforation of the appendix.)

Study question 4: why is appendicitis more common in younger individuals? (Answer: histological examination of the appendix reveals the presence of abundant lymphoid tissue in the mucosa and submucosa of younger individuals. As age advances, the lymphoid tissue progressively atrophies. As such infections are more likely to cause lymphoid hyperplasia and trigger appendicitis in younger individuals.)

CLINICAL APPLICATION 11.3 Portal hypertension

A 65-year-old man with a history of chronic alcohol abuse presented to the emergency department with a sudden bout of massive blood vomiting (haematemesis). On examination, he was pale and restless, with low blood pressure and increased heart rate. The abdomen was grossly distended with fluid. Dilated veins were seen on the anterior abdominal wall. Ultrasonography showed free fluid in the peritoneal cavity, shrunken liver, dilated portal vein, and moderate splenomegaly. Endoscopy revealed bleeding oesophageal varices in the lower oesophagus. Based on the history of excessive alcohol intake and clinical findings, a diagnosis of liver cirrhosis with portal hypertension was made.

Study question 1a: why is the liver shrunken? (Answer: ethanol damages the liver, causing hepatocellular necrosis and fibrosis around the sinusoids. Ultimately, the liver becomes shrunken, fibrotic, and cirrhotic, with increased portal vascular resistance.)

Study question 1b: what do you understand by the term portal hypertension? (Answer: portal hypertension literally means increased pressure in the portal vein. Increased portal vascular resistance due to cirrhosis leads to decreased blood flow through the liver and hypertension in the portal vein. Common causes of portal hypertension are portal vein thrombosis, cirrhosis of the liver,

and hepatic vein thrombosis. The normal portal venous pressure is about 7–10 mmHg.)

Study question 2: what are the effects of portal hypertension? (Answer: portal hypertension leads to back pressure changes such as dilatation of the portal vein, splenomegaly, and enlargement of collateral vessels. The collateral channels at sites of porto-systemic anastomosis open up to form alternate routes for the portal venous blood to reach the heart. With time, these channels become dilated to accommodate the increased blood flow through them.)

Study question 3: what are oesophageal varices? (Answer: oesophageal varices are enlarged submucosal veins in the lower end of the oesophagus. They usually occur subsequent to portal vein obstruction and increased blood flow through the oesophageal veins. Rupture of oesophageal varices was the cause of massive haematemesis (vomiting of blood) in this patient.)

Study question 4: what explanation can you provide for the dilated veins on the anterior abdominal wall? (Answer: the dilated veins on the anterior abdominal wall are the result of opening up of collateral channels between the periumbilical veins (portal circulation) and the superficial veins of the anterior abdominal wall (systemic circulation).)

CLINICAL APPLICATION 11.4 Obstructive jaundice

A 48-year-old woman presented to the emergency room with recurring attacks of severe right upper abdominal pain. She also complained of generalized itching and passage of dark-coloured urine and pale-coloured stools. Examination revealed yellowish discoloration of the sclera. Ultrasonography, CT abdomen, and ERCP revealed dilated bile ducts and stones in the common bile duct (CBD). The presence of stones in the CBD causing obstruction to the flow of bile is called **choledocholithiasis**. Bile duct stones usually originate in the gallbladder.

Study question 1: what are gallstones? (Answer: gallstones are stones formed within the gallbladder. The process of gallstone formation is complex. The vast majority of gallstones are asymptomatic and produce

symptoms of colicky pain only on obstruction of the cystic duct or CBD.)

Study question 2: what are the other causes of extrahepatic biliary obstruction? (Answer: other common causes of obstruction are carcinoma of the bile duct, helminths (parasites) in the bile duct, stricture of bile ducts, carcinoma of the head of the pancreas, and periampullary carcinoma around the ampulla of Vater. All these conditions can cause obstruction to the flow of bile into the duodenum.)

Study question 3: what is Courvoisier's law? (Answer: Courvoisier's law states that in a case of obstructive jaundice, if the gallbladder is palpable, it is unlikely to be due to gallstone disease. Fig. 11.66 is an ERCP image showing gallstones in the CBD.)

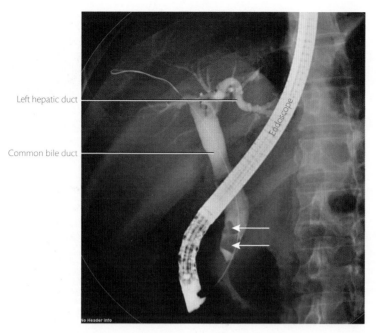

Left hepatic duct

Common bile duct

Endoscope

Fig. 11.66 Endoscopic retrograde cholangiopancreatography (ERCP) image showing calculi in the common bile duct (white arrows) (the patient had undergone a cholecystectomy earlier).

CLINICAL APPLICATION 11.5 Renal tumour

A 65-year-old man presented with haematuria (passage of blood in the urine) and dull pain in the left lumbar region. On abdominal examination, the left kidney was palpable. On scrotal examination, there was a soft swelling on the left which felt like a bag of worms. The scrotal swelling was diagnosed as a varicocele. Further investigation showed the presence of a renal malignancy. The patient underwent surgery to have the kidney removed.

Study question 1: is the kidney normally palpable? (Answer: no, a normal-sized kidney is not palpable.)

Study question 2: what anatomical features help to distinguish an enlarged left kidney from an enlarged spleen? (Answer: an enlarged kidney, but not an enlarged spleen, is bimanually palpable, i.e. palpable with both hands when the hands are placed on the anterior and posterior surfaces of the abdomen. The splenic notch is felt on palpation of an enlarged spleen.)

Study question 3: what is a varicocele? What is the likely cause for the left-sided varicocele in this patient? (Answer: dilated and tortuous veins of the pampiniform plexus constitute a varicocele. It is possible that the tumour cells from the kidney invaded and blocked the left renal vein and obstructed venous drainage of the left testis.)

Study question 4: what structures at the hilum of the kidney would have to be ligated and cut during the nephrectomy? (Answer: the renal vessels and ureter which lie at the hilus need to be ligated and cut. The renal vein is anterior to the renal artery at the hilus, and the ureter is posterior to both.)

CHAPTER 12
The diaphragm

The diaphragm is a thin, fibromuscular, dome-shaped partition between the thoracic and abdominal cavities. It is an important muscle of inspiration and its position changes constantly with respiration. When it contracts, the **dome** of the diaphragm is partially flattened; the abdominal contents are displaced downwards, and the vertical extent of the thoracic cavity is increased. When it relaxes, it rises and may go up to the level of the fourth rib, superior to the nipple, in full expiration [see Fig. 2.2; Fig. 12.1].

The fibrous, central part of the diaphragm—the **central tendon**—is slightly depressed by the heart. The more elevated right and left parts of the diaphragm form the right and left **domes** of the diaphragm. The right dome, supported by the liver, lies at a slightly higher level (a little inferior to the nipple in the male) than the left [see Fig. 4.9; Figs. 12.1, 12.2].

Dissection 12.1 gives instructions on dissecting the origin of the diaphragm.

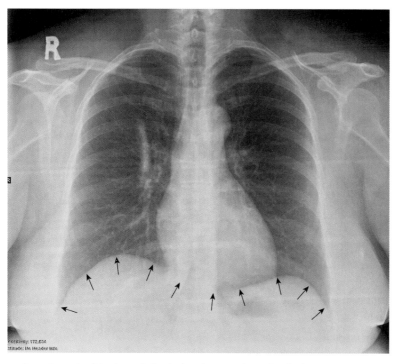

Fig. 12.1 An anteroposterior radiograph of the thorax in inspiration. Arrows point to the diaphragm.

DISSECTION 12.1 The diaphragm

Objectives

I. To expose the vertebral and costal attachments of the diaphragm.   II. To identify the intercostal vessels and nerves as they enter the abdomen.

Instructions

1. Strip the peritoneum from the **diaphragm**, and expose its crura on the anterior surfaces of the upper two or three lumbar vertebrae.

2. Find the **arcuate ligaments**. They are fibrous arches anterior to the aorta, psoas, and quadratus lumborum from which the diaphragm arises [Fig. 12.2].

3. Expose the slips of the diaphragm arising from the internal surface of the lower six costal cartilages.

4. Identify the intercostal vessels and nerves entering the abdominal wall between the costal cartilages.

5. Review the anterior attachments of the diaphragm to the xiphoid process.

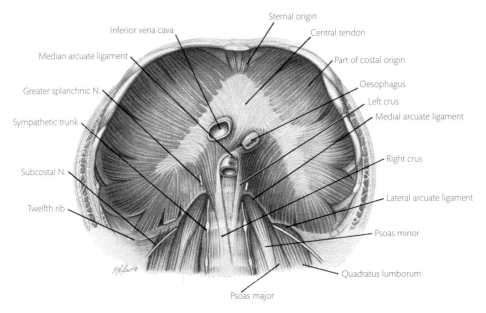

Fig. 12.2 The abdominal surface of the diaphragm.

Labels: Inferior vena cava; Sternal origin; Central tendon; Median arcuate ligament; Part of costal origin; Greater splanchnic N.; Oesophagus; Left crus; Sympathetic trunk; Medial arcuate ligament; Right crus; Subcostal N.; Lateral arcuate ligament; Twelfth rib; Psoas minor; Quadratus lumborum; Psoas major

Attachments of the diaphragm

The diaphragm arises from the margins of the inferior aperture of the thorax and passes upwards and inwards to the edges of the flat, C-shaped central tendon. The anterior fibres run horizontally backwards. The posterior fibres are almost vertical and pass upwards to the central tendon. There is a deep recess between the posterior thoracic wall and the posterior fibres of the diaphragm—the **costodiaphragmatic recess**.

The diaphragm takes origin from the sternum, the lower six costal cartilages, the upper lumbar vertebra, and the three arcuate ligaments [Fig. 12.2].

The **sternal origin** is by two small slips which arise from the xiphoid process.

The **costal origin** is by wide slips from each of the lower six costal cartilages. These slips interdigitate with slips of origin of the transversus abdominis.

The **vertebral origin** is from: (1) the crura; and (2) the arcuate ligaments.

The **right** and **left crura** are thick, fleshy muscle bundles which are attached to the anterior surfaces of the upper lumbar vertebral bodies. The left crus is attached to the upper two lumbar vertebrae, and the right crus to the upper three lumbar vertebrae. The crura are also attached to the intervening intervertebral discs and the tendinous slips that

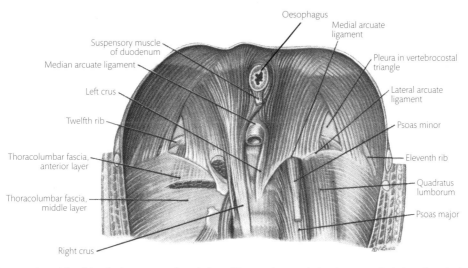

Oesophagus
Medial arcuate ligament
Suspensory muscle of duodenum
Pleura in vertebrocostal triangle
Median arcuate ligament
Lateral arcuate ligament
Left crus
Psoas minor
Twelfth rib
Eleventh rib
Thoracolumbar fascia, anterior layer
Quadratus lumborum
Thoracolumbar fascia, middle layer
Psoas major
Right crus

Fig. 12.3 The posterior origin of the diaphragm, seen from in front. The vertebrocostal triangles are particularly well marked.

bridge the lumbar vessels on the vertebral bodies. They lie on each side of the aorta. As the fibres of the right crus ascend towards the central tendon, they deviate to the left and encircle the oesophageal hiatus.

The **median arcuate ligament** is a tendinous band which unites the medial sides of the right and left crura superiorly. This ligament lies on the anterior surface of the aorta [Fig. 12.3]. The **medial arcuate ligament** is a tendinous thickening of the fascia over the psoas major. It stretches from the lateral side of each crus to the transverse process of the first (or second) lumbar vertebra.

The **lateral arcuate ligament** is a linear thickening of the anterior layer of the thoracolumbar fascia [Fig. 12.3; see also Fig. 13.4]. It extends from the medial arcuate ligament over the anterior surface of the quadratus lumborum to the twelfth rib.

Fibres from the lateral part of the lateral arcuate ligament may be missing [Fig. 12.3]. Such a deficiency is known as the **vertebrocostal triangle** and is thought to represent an incomplete closure of the embryonic **pleuroperitoneal canal**. ➲ When the vertebrocostal triangle is present, it leaves the pleura almost directly in contact with the kidney and makes a potential site for herniation of abdominal contents into the thorax.

The muscle fibres of the diaphragm converge and are inserted into the C-shaped **central tendon**. This tendon has a larger **median part** which expands anteriorly towards the xiphoid process, and **right and left horns** which curve posteriorly

into the corresponding halves of the diaphragm [Fig. 12.2].

Foramina in the diaphragm

There are three large and numerous small openings, or foramina, in the diaphragm. These foramina allow for passage of structures between the thoracic and abdominal cavities. The **inferior vena cava** pierces and fuses with the central tendon of the diaphragm, 2–3 cm to the right of the median plane, approximately at the level of the eighth thoracic vertebra. When the diaphragm contracts, it compresses the abdominal viscera, lowers the intrathoracic pressure, and pulls the inferior vena cava open. These actions facilitate blood flow from the abdomen into the thorax. Slender branches of the **right phrenic nerve** and some lymph vessels from the liver also traverse the foramen with the inferior vena cava [Fig. 12.2].

The **oesophagus** passes obliquely through an oval opening, or a hiatus, in the muscular right crus of the diaphragm, posterior to the central tendon, 2–3 cm to the left of the median plane. It lies approximately at the level of the tenth thoracic vertebra. Other structures passing through the oesophageal hiatus are the anterior and posterior **vagal trunks**, the oesophageal branches of the left gastric artery, and communications between the veins of the stomach and thoracic oesophagus [Fig. 12.2].

The **aortic hiatus** lies posterior to the median arcuate ligament of the diaphragm and anterior to the twelfth thoracic vertebra. The hiatus also transmits the **thoracic duct**, the **azygos vein**, and lymph vessels which descend to the cisterna chyli from the thorax [Fig. 12.2].

In addition to structures passing through these three apertures, a number of smaller structures pass between the thorax and the abdomen through, or around, the diaphragm. They are:

1. The **phrenic nerves**. The left nerve pierces the diaphragm lateral to the pericardium. (The right phrenic nerve enters the abdomen lateral to the inferior vena cava.)
2. The **superior epigastric vessels** enter the abdomen between the sternal and costal origins of the diaphragm.
3. The **musculophrenic vessels** enter the abdomen between the slips of origin from the seventh and eighth costal cartilages.
4. The lower five intercostal nerves enter the abdomen between the slips of origin from the lower six costal cartilages.
5. The **subcostal vessels** and **nerves** enter the abdomen posterior to the lateral arcuate ligaments.
6. The **sympathetic trunks** enter the abdomen posterior to the medial arcuate ligaments.
7. The **splanchnic nerves** pierce the right and left crura.
8. The **hemiazygos vein** pierces the left crus.

Nerves and vessels

The motor supply to the diaphragm is from the **phrenic nerves** which arise from the third, fourth, and fifth cervical ventral rami—mainly the fourth. They descend in the thorax, pierce the diaphragm, branch on the inferior surface of the diaphragm, and supply it. The sensory supply to the diaphragm is through the phrenic and lower intercostal nerves. The high level of origin of the phrenic nerves is due to the caudal movement of the diaphragm and viscera during development.

The principal arteries supplying the diaphragm are the **inferior phrenic arteries** from the abdominal aorta [see Fig. 11.59], the **musculophrenic** branch of the internal thoracic artery [see Fig. 3.11], and the **pericardiacophrenic** arteries which accompany the phrenic nerves.

See Clinical Application 12.1 for the practical implications of the anatomy in this chapter.

CLINICAL APPLICATION 12.1 Diaphragmatic hernia

Protrusion of abdominal contents into the thoracic cavity through an opening in the diaphragm is called a **diaphragmatic hernia**. Congenital diaphragmatic hernias are most commonly due to posterolateral developmental defects (Bochdalek's hernias). Other hernias, anteromedial or retrosternal hernias (of Morgagni) occur between the xiphoid and costal origins of the diaphragm.

Study question 1: left side congenital diaphragmatic hernias are more common than right. Use your knowledge of anatomy to explain why this may be so. (Answer: the presence of the liver on the right side covers the defect.)

Study question 2: what is the likely presentation of newborns with this condition? (Answer: the most prominent symptom is breathing difficulty because of compromised thoracic space and poorly developed lungs.)

Study question 3: what would a plain radiograph in this case show? (Answer: bowel loops in the thoracic cavity and hypoplastic lungs.)

Acquired herniae are seen in the middle-aged, most commonly due to weakness in the musculature around the oesophageal hiatus. Study question 4: which part of the diaphragm contains the oesophageal opening? What is the position of the oesophageal opening? (Answer: muscle fibres from the right crus of diaphragm loop around the oesophagus to the left of the midline at T. 10 vertebral level.)

Traumatic diaphragmatic injury may be suspected with penetrating lower chest wounds. Study question 5: at what level does the summit of the diaphragmatic dome lie? (Answer: the dome of the diaphragm can reach the level of the fifth rib, the right side being higher than the left. Hence penetrating wounds below the level of the nipple can injure the diaphragm.)

CHAPTER 13
The posterior abdominal wall

Blood vessels of the posterior abdominal wall

The major blood vessels of the abdomen—the abdominal aorta, the inferior vena cava, the common iliac vessels, and the initial segments of the azygos and hemiazygos veins—lie on the posterior abdominal wall.

Dissection 13.1 describes the dissection of the blood vessels of the posterior abdominal wall.

The abdominal aorta

The abdominal aorta lies in the midline and descends on the vertebral column from the aortic hiatus in the diaphragm (at the level of the T. 12 vertebra) to its bifurcation into the common iliac vessels on the fourth lumbar vertebra [Fig. 13.1A]. It is partially surrounded by sympathetic plexuses, lymph vessels, and lymph nodes.

The aorta is related posteriorly to the anterior longitudinal ligament on the lumbar vertebrae, and the left lumbar veins which pass transversely to the inferior vena cava. Superiorly, the aorta lies between the crura of the diaphragm. Inferiorly, it lies between the sympathetic trunks. The fourth part of the duodenum and coils of the jejunum are on its left side. The inferior vena cava lies on its right.

Structures that lie anterior to the aorta from above downwards, are: (1) the pancreas and splenic vein, partly separated from the aorta by the superior mesenteric artery; (2) the left renal vein between the aorta and superior mesenteric artery; (3) the third part of the duodenum; (4) the root of the mesentery; and (5) the peritoneum separating it from coils of the small intestine.

DISSECTION 13.1 Posterior abdominal wall-1

Objectives

I. To expose the aorta and inferior vena cava. II. To study the sympathetic trunk, lumbar vessels, and cisterna chyli. III. To identify and trace the branches of the abdominal aorta and tributaries of the inferior vena cava.

Instructions

1. Expose the abdominal aorta and inferior vena cava.

2. Identify the lymph nodes which lie adjacent to them.

3. Identify the sympathetic trunks which lie on each side of the aorta on the anterior surface of the psoas major muscle. The right sympathetic trunk lies posterior to the inferior vena cava. Trace the branches of the sympathetic trunks.

4. Clean the proximal parts of the lumbar arteries.

5. Between the right crus of the diaphragm and the aorta, expose the cisterna chyli and the azygos vein. Trace the cisterna chyli upwards to the thoracic duct, and trace the azygos vein inferiorly to the posterior surface of the inferior vena cava at the level of the renal veins.

6. Find and trace the testicular or ovarian vessels.

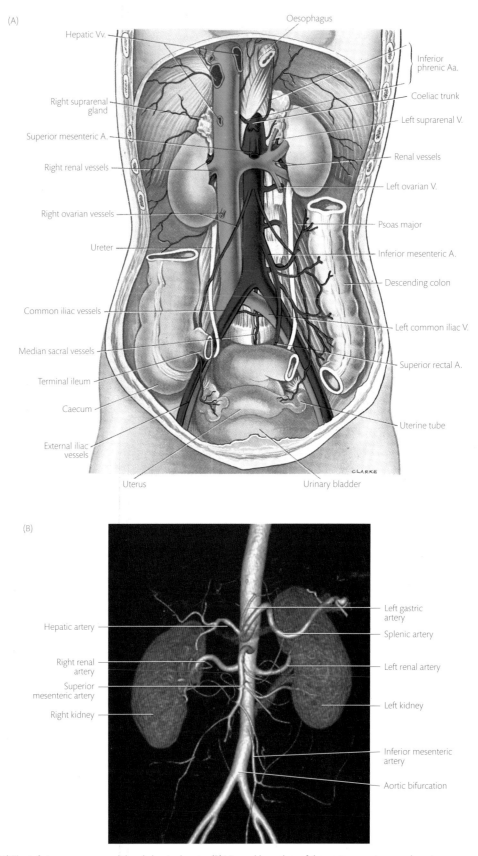

(A)

Oesophagus

Hepatic Vv.

Inferior phrenic Aa.

Right suprarenal gland

Coeliac trunk

Left suprarenal V.

Superior mesenteric A.

Renal vessels

Right renal vessels

Left ovarian V.

Right ovarian vessels

Psoas major

Ureter

Inferior mesenteric A.

Descending colon

Common iliac vessels

Left common iliac V.

Median sacral vessels

Superior rectal A.

Terminal ileum

Caecum

Uterine tube

External iliac vessels

Uterus

Urinary bladder

CLARKE

(B)

Hepatic artery

Left gastric artery

Splenic artery

Right renal artery

Left renal artery

Superior mesenteric artery

Left kidney

Right kidney

Inferior mesenteric artery

Aortic bifurcation

Fig. 13.1 (A) The inferior vena cava and the abdominal aorta. (B) Visceral branches of the aorta, seen in a renal angiogram.

In a slim person, the inferior part of the abdominal aorta is very close to the anterior abdominal wall. It may be compressed against the lumbar vertebral column by firm pressure on the anterior abdominal wall, just above the umbilicus.

Branches of the abdominal aorta

There are three sets of branches arising from the aorta. (1) Unpaired ventral branches to the gut tube and its derivatives. These are the coeliac trunk, the superior and inferior mesenteric arteries. (These arteries have been dissected and discussed already.) (2) Paired lateral branches to the structures derived from the intermediate mesoderm of the embryo—the suprarenal glands, the kidneys, and the ovaries or testes. (3) Paired posterolateral branches to the diaphragm (the inferior phrenic arteries) and to the abdominal wall (the lumbar arteries). In addition, the median sacral artery is an unpaired branch which arises from the posterior surface of the aorta at its bifurcation and continues down into the lesser pelvis [Fig. 13.1B].

Inferior phrenic arteries

The **inferior phrenic arteries** are the first paired branches of the abdominal aorta. They pass superolaterally over the crura of the diaphragm near the superior margins of the suprarenal glands. They send many small **superior suprarenal arteries** to the suprarenal gland and then ramify on the inferior surface of the diaphragm.

Middle suprarenal arteries

Small **middle suprarenal arteries** arise near the origin of the superior mesenteric artery. They pass laterally to the suprarenal glands, the right goes posterior to the inferior vena cava.

Renal arteries

Large paired renal arteries arise from the aorta at the level of the upper part of the second lumbar vertebra. They cross the corresponding crus of the diaphragm and the psoas muscle to reach the kidneys. At the hilus of the kidney, each renal artery branches to supply the kidney. In addition to the branches to the kidney, each renal artery sends small arteries to the ureter and to the suprarenal gland—the **inferior suprarenal artery**. The right renal artery passes posterior to the inferior vena cava and the right renal vein. The left renal artery is posterior to its vein [see Fig. 11.64].

An accessory renal artery is not uncommon. It usually arises from the aorta, passes anterior to the ureter (and the inferior vena cava if right-sided), and enters the antero-inferior part of the kidney [see Fig. 11.63].

Testicular and ovarian arteries

Each testicular artery is a long, slender vessel that arises from the front of the aorta, a short distance inferior to the renal arteries. It runs inferolaterally anterior to the ureter as it lies on the posterior abdominal wall and posterior to the intestines and mesenteric vessels. It runs to the corresponding deep inguinal ring and enters the inguinal canal. The **right testicular artery** lies anterior to the inferior vena cava, right psoas, right ureter, and right external iliac artery. It is posterior to the third part of the duodenum, the right colic vessels, the ileocolic vessels, the superior mesenteric vessels, and the caecum. The **left testicular artery** has most of the same structures posterior to it, except for the inferior vena cava. Anteriorly are the duodenum, the inferior mesenteric vein, the left colic and sigmoid vessels, and the inferior part of the descending colon [see Fig. 11.35].

The **ovarian arteries** are very similar to the testicular arteries in their course, except that they enter the lesser pelvis by crossing the external iliac arteries at the brim of the pelvis [Fig. 13.1A]. The left ovarian artery is posterior to the sigmoid colon and sigmoid mesocolon. The right is posterior to the terminal ileum.

Lumbar arteries

Four pairs of lumbar arteries arise from the posterior surface of the abdominal aorta, in series with the posterior intercostal arteries. They pass laterally on the surface of the upper four lumbar vertebral bodies, and then backwards, deep to the psoas muscle, with the corresponding lumbar veins and the rami communicantes of the lumbar nerves.

Common iliac arteries

See Common iliac arteries, p. 208.

The inferior vena cava

This is the widest vein of the body. It drains venous blood from the lower limbs, most of the abdominal wall, the kidneys and suprarenal glands, and most of the pelvis and perineum. Venous blood from the remaining abdominal viscera—the spleen and the gut tube and its associated glands—drains to the liver in the portal vein and reaches the inferior vena cava, only after circulating through the liver.

The inferior vena cava begins by the union of the right and left **common iliac veins** on the anterior surface of the fifth lumbar vertebra. It ends by entering the right atrium, after piercing the central tendon of the diaphragm and the pericardium [see Fig. 4.22; Fig. 13.1A]. The inferior vena cava ascends to the right of the median plane, at first with the aorta on its medial side and the right ureter laterally. The vertebral column, right psoas major, right sympathetic trunk, and right lumbar arteries lie posterior to it. The inferior vena cava then arches forwards on the right crus of the diaphragm, anterior to the right renal artery, right coeliac ganglion, and right middle suprarenal artery. It grooves the liver between the right and caudate lobes [see Fig. 11.53]. Here it is anterior to the medial part of the right suprarenal gland and the posterior part of the diaphragm [see Fig. 11.51].

Anterior to the inferior vena cava, as it ascends, are: (1) the right common iliac artery; (2) the superior mesenteric vessels in the root of the mesentery; (3) the ileocolic and right colic vessels; (4) the third part of the duodenum; (5) the right testicular or ovarian artery; (6) the head of the pancreas and the bile duct; (7) the portal vein and the first part of the duodenum; (8) the lesser omentum anterior to the epiploic foramen; and (9) the liver tissue between the right and caudate lobes.

Tributaries

- The **third** and **fourth lumbar** veins. (The first and second lumbar veins drain into the ascending lumbar vein.)
- The **right testicular** or **ovarian vein**. Each gonadal (**testicular** or **ovarian**) **vein** is formed by the union of the veins in the **pampiniform plexus**. The testicular vein begins at the deep inguinal ring; the ovarian vein begins at the superior aperture of the pelvis. The gonadal veins ascend accompanying the corresponding arteries. The left gonadal vein enters the left renal vein; the right gonadal vein enters the inferior vena cava, inferior to the renal vein. This apparent asymmetry of the gonadal and suprarenal veins is because the part of the left renal vein which receives these vessels is the remnant of the **left inferior vena cava**.

- The **renal veins**. As the inferior vena cava lies to the right of the median plane, the right renal vein is much shorter than the left. Both renal veins lie anterior to the corresponding arteries. The right renal vein passes posterior to the second part of the duodenum and may be overlapped by the right margin of the head of the pancreas. The long left vein receives the left suprarenal and testicular or ovarian veins, and usually the hemiazygos vein close to the kidney. The left renal vein passes to the right, posterior to the inferior border of the pancreas and the inferior mesenteric vein. It crosses the median plane in the angle between the aorta and the superior mesenteric artery [Fig. 13.1A].
- The **right suprarenal vein**. (The left suprarenal vein drains into the left renal vein [Fig. 13.1A].)
- The **inferior phrenic veins** though the left may pass with the left suprarenal vein to the left renal vein.
- The **right** and **left hepatic veins** drain the lobes of the liver into the inferior vena cava as it grooves the liver.
- The azygos vein arises from the posterior surface of the inferior vena cava and ascends into the thorax.
- Common iliac veins—see Common iliac veins, p. 209.

The azygos and hemiazygos veins

The azygos and hemiazygos veins usually begin in the abdomen, the hemiazygos from the posterior surface of the left renal vein and the azygos from the posterior surface of the inferior vena cava at the same level. The azygos vein ascends into the thorax through the aortic hiatus. The hemiazygos vein enters the thorax by piercing the left crus of the diaphragm. Either or both veins may arise from the union of the **subcostal** and **ascending lumbar veins** [see Fig. 4.55].

Common iliac arteries

The common iliac arteries are terminal branches of the abdominal aorta. They arise on the anterior surface of the fourth lumbar vertebra. They are surrounded by extensions of the aortic sympathetic and lymph plexuses. Each artery passes inferolaterally to the superior surface of the sacro-iliac joint where it divides into **internal** and **external** iliac arteries. Both common iliac arteries are anterior to the corresponding sympathetic trunk. The superior rectal vessels and some sigmoid arteries lie anterior to the left common iliac artery. The right common iliac artery is anterior to the beginning of the inferior vena cava and the right common iliac vein [Fig. 13.1A].

Common iliac veins

The common iliac veins begin on the medial surface of the psoas muscle by the union of the internal and external iliac veins. They end by uniting together to form the inferior vena cava, 2 cm to the right of the median plane on the fifth lumbar vertebra. Each common iliac vein receives an iliolumbar vein. The median sacral vein joins the left common iliac vein.

The right common iliac vein is posterior to the corresponding artery. The left is inferomedial to its artery and runs a longer course to reach the inferior vena cava [Fig. 13.1A].

External iliac arteries

The external iliac arteries begin immediately anterior to the sacro-iliac joints as a continuation of the common iliac arteries. They pass inferolaterally along the margins of the superior aperture of the lesser pelvis, at first medial to and then anterior to the psoas. Each external iliac artery gives off a **deep circumflex iliac artery** and an **inferior epigastric artery**, immediately superior to the inguinal ligament at the mid-inguinal point. The external iliac continues as the femoral artery by passing posterior to the inguinal ligament.

Each external iliac artery is at first anterior and then lateral to its vein. Anteriorly, it is crossed by the ureter, the vas deferens in the male or the round ligament of the uterus in the female, the genital branch of the genitofemoral nerve, and the ovarian vessels [Fig. 13.1A]. On the right, the caecum and appendix may lie anterior to it. On the left, the end of the descending colon is anterior to its distal part.

External iliac veins

Each external iliac vein ascends with its artery, passing from its medial to its posterior surface and being crossed by the same structures. Each vein receives the inferior epigastric vein and the deep circumflex iliac vein. It passes lateral to the internal iliac artery and unites with the internal iliac vein to form the common iliac vein.

The lymph nodes of the posterior abdominal wall

The lymph nodes of the posterior abdominal wall are scattered along the iliac vessels, the aorta, and the inferior vena cava [Fig. 13.2].

The **external iliac nodes** lie on the external iliac vessels. The nodes situated medially receive lymph from the lower limb and pelvic viscera. The external iliac nodes situated laterally receive lymph from the areas supplied by the inferior epigastric and deep circumflex iliac arteries. All this lymph ascends through other external iliac nodes to the **common iliac nodes**. There are two groups of common iliac nodes: a lateral group along the common iliac vessels, and a medial group in the angle between the common iliac vessels. The lateral group receives lymph from the lower limb and pelvis through the external and internal iliac nodes. The medial group receives lymph from the pelvic viscera directly and through the internal iliac and sacral nodes. The efferents of the common iliac nodes pass to the lumbar nodes.

The **lumbar nodes** are scattered along the aorta and inferior vena cava. They receive lymph directly from adjacent structures, like the posterior abdominal wall, kidneys, ureters, testes or ovaries, uterine tubes, uterus, caecum, and ascending and transverse colons. Lymph from the descending colon and pelvis reaches the lumbar lymph nodes through the inferior mesenteric nodes. Lymph from the lower limbs also reach the lumbar lymph nodes through the common iliac nodes. The efferent vessels from the lumbar nodes form the right and left **lumbar lymph trunks**, which drain to the cisterna chyli [Fig. 13.2].

Cisterna chyli

This white lymph sac is approximately 4 mm wide and 5 cm long. It is often tortuous and branched. It lies on the upper two lumbar vertebrae between the aorta and azygos vein, behind the right crus of the diaphragm. It receives the **lumbar lymph trunks** inferiorly, the **intestinal lymph trunk** (which drains the liver, stomach, and small intestine)

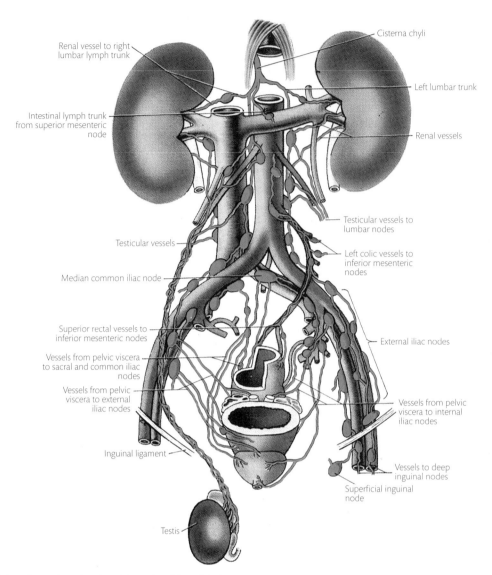

Fig. 13.2 Lymph vessels and nodes of the male pelvis and abdomen.

about the middle, and lymph vessels from the lower intercostal nodes superiorly [Fig. 13.2]. It continues as the **thoracic duct** through the aortic hiatus [see Fig. 4.55]. A similar distended lymph sac may be present on the left of the aorta.

Muscles and fasciae of the posterior abdominal wall

Three muscles on each side of the vertebral column—the quadratus lumborum, psoas, and iliacus—form the greater part of the posterior abdominal wall, and each is enclosed in fascia [Figs. 13.3, 13.4, 13.5].

Quadratus lumborum

This muscle arises from the iliolumbar ligament (which extends between the transverse process of the fifth lumbar vertebra to the iliac crest), the adjacent part of the iliac crest, and the lower two to four lumbar transverse processes. Narrowing slightly as it ascends, it gets inserted into the medial part of the anterior surface of the twelfth rib. It is also inserted into the upper lumbar transverse processes, posterior to its slips of origin. **Nerve supply**: direct branches of the upper four lumbar ventral rami. **Action**: it is a lateral flexor of the lumbar vertebral column. It aids in inspiration by holding the twelfth rib down when the diaphragm and intercostal muscles contract.

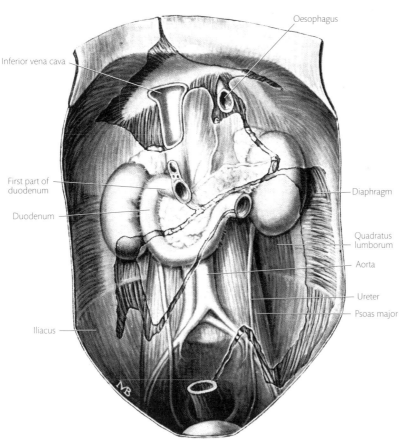

Fig. 13.3 Posterior abdominal wall with attachments of the mesenteries and peritoneal ligaments. The oesophagus, duodenum, and rectum are the only parts of the gut tube left *in situ*.

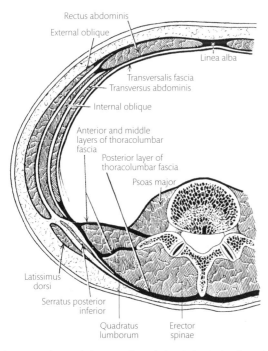

Fig. 13.4 A horizontal section through the abdominal walls at the level of the second lumbar vertebra.

The quadratus lumborum lies between the anterior and middle layers of the **thoracolumbar fascia** [Fig. 13.4]. These layers fuse at the lateral margin of the quadratus lumborum and are attached above to the twelth rib and below to the iliolumbar ligament and iliac crest, anterior and posterior to the muscle. Part of the anterior layer is thickened to form the lateral arcuate ligament, and it continues upwards to the twelfth rib, posterior to the pleura [see Figs. 8.7, 11.61, 12.3].

Psoas major

This long muscle arises from the anterior surfaces of the upper four lumbar transverse processes, medial to the quadratus lumborum; from the sides of the last thoracic and upper four lumbar intervertebral discs, adjacent margins of the vertebral bodies; and from the tendinous arches which unite these margins lateral to the lumbar arteries.

The muscle runs down along the margin of the superior aperture of the lesser pelvis and enters the thigh, posterior to the inguinal ligament. Its

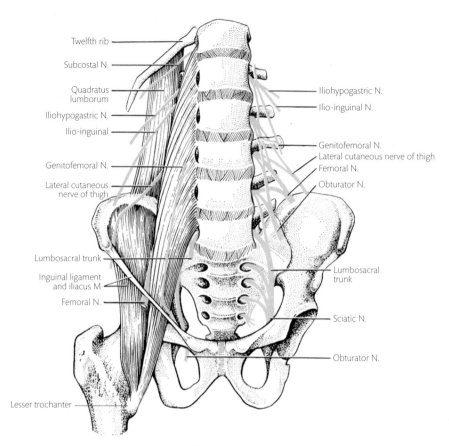

Fig. 13.5 Drawing showing lumbar plexus, sacral plexus, and iliacus, psoas, and quadratus lumborum.

tendon then passes postero-inferiorly to the lesser trochanter of the femur [Fig. 13.5]. **Nerve supply**: branches from the second to fourth lumbar ventral rami and from the femoral nerve. **Action**: see under Iliacus [see Fig. 12.2; Fig. 13.4].

Psoas minor

This small muscle is not always present. It arises with the uppermost fibres of the psoas major, descends on the anterior surface of the psoas major, forms a thin tendon, and is inserted into the thickened lower part of the fascia covering the psoas and iliacus. **Nerve supply**: the first lumbar ventral ramus. **Action**: see under Iliacus [see Fig. 12.3].

Iliacus

The iliacus arises from the upper part of the floor of the iliac fossa. It converges on to, and fuses with, the lower part of the psoas major. It is inserted with the psoas major to the lesser trochanter of the femur and an area immediately inferior to the

lesser trochanter. **Nerve supply**: the femoral nerve [Fig. 13.5; see also Fig. 17.7].

Actions of the psoas and iliacus

The psoas major and iliacus are flexors of the hip joint. As they are inserted lateral to the axis of rotation, they also rotate the thigh medially. The psoas muscles are lateral flexors of the lumbar vertebral column.

➲ An inflamed appendix can cause psoas spasm, with resulting flexion and medial rotation of the right thigh.

➲ When the neck of the femur is broken, the psoas and iliacus rotate the distal segment of the femur (and the entire limb with it) laterally, and the toes are characteristically pointed outwards.

Fascia of the psoas and iliacus

The psoas is enclosed in a sheath of fascia which fuses above with the periosteum of the vertebral column and the anterior layer of the thoracolumbar fascia. It is thickened to form the **medial arcuate**

Objectives

I. To study the muscles of the posterior abdominal wall.
II. To study the vessels and nerves of the posterior abdominal wall.

Instructions

1. Expose the muscles of the posterior abdominal wall by removing the fascia covering the quadratus lumborum, psoas, and iliacus. Avoid injury to the vessels and nerves related to the muscles (the main vessels lie anterior to the fascia; the nerves are posterior to it). Note that the vessels on the iliacus are branches of the iliolumbar artery.

2. Push the inferior vena cava laterally and expose the right sympathetic trunk. Trace both sympathetic trunks superiorly to the medial arcuate ligaments and inferiorly into the pelvis, posterior to the common iliac vessels.

3. Find and trace the branches of both sympathetic trunks to the superior hypogastric plexus.

4. Detach the psoas major from the intervertebral discs and vertebral bodies on one side. The lumbar vessels are now exposed.

5. Trace the **lumbar vessels** and the rami communicantes posteriorly, deep to the tendinous arches from which the psoas arises.

ligament. Below, the psoas fascia is fused with the arcuate line of the bony pelvis and the fascia covering the iliacus (the iliac fascia).

The **iliac fascia** is attached to the inner lip of the iliac crest, the inguinal ligament, and the transversalis fascia [see Fig. 8.11]. In the thigh, it forms the posterior wall of the femoral sheath [see Fig. 8.13]. It is often thickened by the insertion of the psoas minor into it.

Dissection 13.2 describes the dissection of the muscles, vessels, and nerves of the posterior abdominal wall.

Nerves of the posterior abdominal wall

Sympathetic trunk

The thoracic part of each sympathetic trunk becomes continuous with the lumbar part, posterior to the medial arcuate ligament. In the abdomen, the trunk lies in the groove between the anterior border of the psoas major and the vertebral bodies, anterior to the lumbar vessels. It enters the pelvis by passing posterior to the common iliac vessels [see Fig. 12.2; Fig. 13.6].

Branches

The **rami communicantes** are long. They run from the sympathetic trunks to the ventral rami of the lumbar nerves. The first two or three lumbar ventral rami are united to the sympathetic trunk by white and grey rami communicantes. The remaining lumbar and all sacral ventral rami are united to the trunk by only a grey ramus. Visceral branches (**lumbar splanchnic nerves**) arise irregularly from the trunk. They pass into the pelvis through the abdominal aortic and hypogastric plexuses [Fig. 13.6].

Subcostal nerve

The subcostal nerve is the ventral ramus of the twelfth thoracic nerve [Figs. 13.5, 13.7]. It sends a branch to the ventral ramus of the first lumbar nerve and then passes inferolaterally on the anterior surface of the quadratus lumborum. It enters the abdomen, posterior to the lateral arcuate ligament. At the lateral border of the quadratus lumborum, it pierces the transversus abdominis to run in the abdominal wall between the transversus and the internal oblique.

Use the instructions given in Dissection 13.3 to dissect the lumbar plexus.

Lumbar nerves

Five lumbar ventral rami emerge through the intervertebral foramina below the corresponding vertebrae and pass into the posterior part of the psoas major [Fig. 13.5]. Here they are connected to the sympathetic trunk by rami communicantes

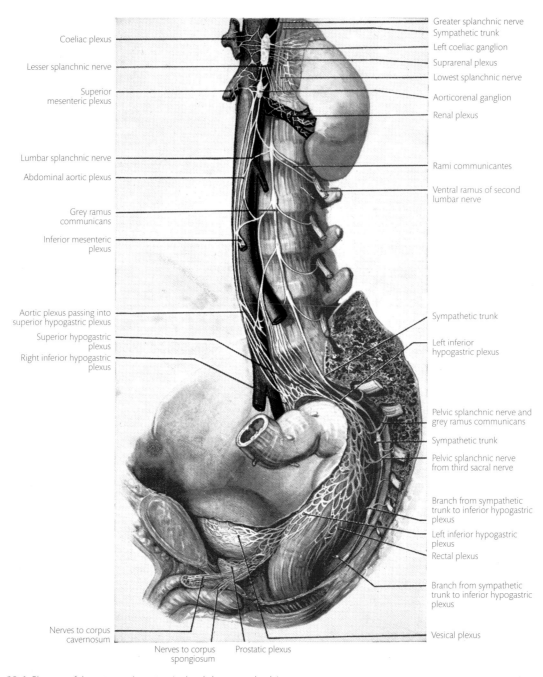

Coeliac plexus

Lesser splanchnic nerve

Superior
mesenteric plexus

Lumbar splanchnic nerve

Abdominal aortic plexus

Grey ramus
communicans

Inferior mesenteric
plexus

Aortic plexus passing into
superior hypogastric plexus

Superior hypogastric
plexus

Right inferior hypogastric
plexus

Nerves to corpus
cavernosum

Nerves to corpus
spongiosum

Prostatic plexus

Greater splanchnic nerve

Sympathetic trunk

Left coeliac ganglion

Suprarenal plexus

Lowest splanchnic nerve

Aorticorenal ganglion

Renal plexus

Rami communicantes

Ventral ramus of second
lumbar nerve

Sympathetic trunk

Left inferior
hypogastric plexus

Pelvic splanchnic nerve and
grey ramus communicans

Sympathetic trunk

Pelvic splanchnic nerve
from third sacral nerve

Branch from sympathetic
trunk to inferior hypogastric
plexus

Left inferior hypogastric
plexus

Rectal plexus

Branch from sympathetic
trunk to inferior hypogastric
plexus

Vesical plexus

Fig. 13.6 Plexuses of the autonomic system in the abdomen and pelvis.

and give branches to the intertransverse muscles, psoas, and quadratus lumborum. The ventral rami of the **fourth lumbar nerve** divides into two. The upper division joins with the first, second, and third to form the lumbar plexus. The lower division joins the fifth lumbar ventral ramus to form the **lumbosacral trunk**. The lumbosacral trunk enters the pelvis to join the sacral plexus [Fig. 13.7].

Lumbar plexus

This plexus is formed in the substance of the psoas major by the ventral rami of the first three and part of the fourth lumbar ventral rami. It receives a

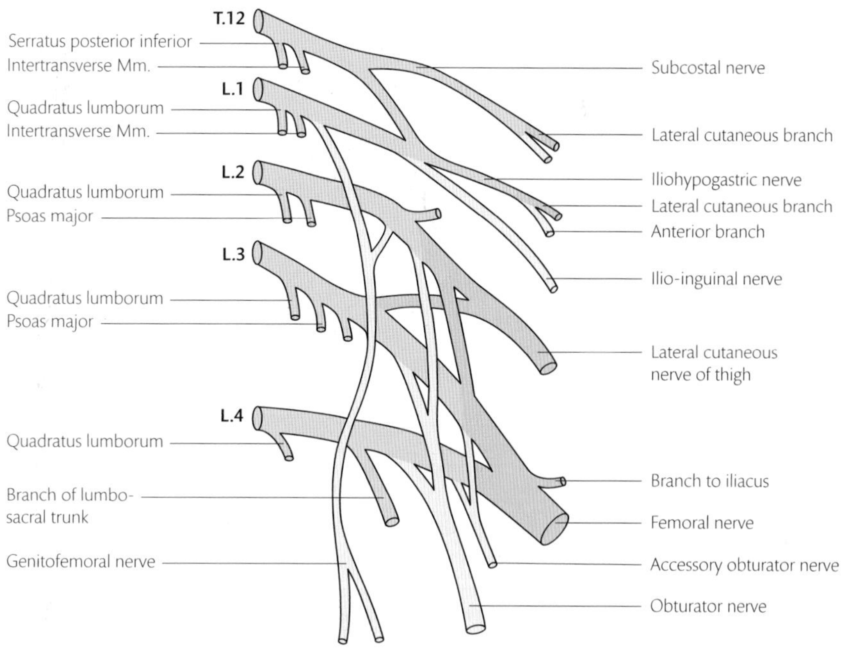
T.12
Serratus posterior inferior
Intertransverse Mm.
L.1
Quadratus lumborum
Intertransverse Mm.
L.2
Quadratus lumborum
Psoas major
L.3
Quadratus lumborum
Psoas major
L.4
Quadratus lumborum
Branch of lumbo-
sacral trunk
Genitofemoral nerve
Subcostal nerve
Lateral cutaneous branch
Iliohypogastric nerve
Lateral cutaneous branch
Anterior branch
Ilio-inguinal nerve
Lateral cutaneous
nerve of thigh
Branch to iliacus
Femoral nerve
Accessory obturator nerve
Obturator nerve

Fig. 13.7 A diagram of the lumbar plexus. Ventral rami are yellow; ventral divisions are pale yellow; dorsal divisions are orange.

DISSECTION 13.3 Lumbar plexus

Objective

I. To remove the psoas major on one side and study the formation and branches of the lumbar plexus.

Instructions

1. Find the genitofemoral nerve on the anterior surface of the psoas [Fig. 13.5] and trace it through that muscle to the lumbar ventral rami.
2. Carefully complete the removal of the psoas from the transverse processes of the lumbar vertebrae, disentangling the ventral rami of the lumbar nerves from the substance of the psoas.
3. Expose the lumbar plexus and its branches.

contribution from the subcostal nerve. Although these nerves do not form dorsal and ventral divisions as in the brachial plexus, the major nerves arising from the lumbar plexus can be recognized as belonging to either the dorsal or ventral divisions [Fig. 13.7].

The **iliohypogastric nerve** (L. 1, T. 12) emerges at the lateral border of the psoas and passes inferolaterally between the quadratus lumborum and the kidney. It pierces the transversus abdominis, a short distance superior to the iliac crest, and runs in the abdominal wall.

The **ilio-inguinal nerve** (L. 1) is a branch of the iliohypogastric and takes the same course as the iliohypogastric, but at a slightly lower level. It has no lateral cutaneous branch.

The **genitofemoral nerve** (L. 1, 2; ventral divisions) passes forwards and emerges on the anterior surface of the psoas. It runs inferiorly on that muscle and divides into femoral and genital branches. The **femoral branch** follows the lateral side of the external iliac artery into the femoral sheath. It pierces the anterior wall of the sheath and the fascia lata to supply the skin over the femoral triangle. The **genital branch** pierces the psoas sheath and runs to the deep inguinal ring. It supplies the **cremaster muscle** and the skin of the scrotum in the male. In the female, it sends sensory fibres to the round ligament of the uterus and to the skin of the labium majus.

The **lateral cutaneous nerve of the thigh** (L. 2, 3; dorsal divisions) emerges from the lateral border of the psoas above the iliac crest. It passes obliquely across the iliacus towards the anterior superior iliac spine and enters the thigh, posterior to the lateral end of the inguinal ligament.

The **femoral nerve** (L. 2, 3, 4; dorsal divisions) emerges from the lateral border of the psoas below the iliac crest. It descends in the groove between the psoas and iliacus (posterior to the iliac fascia) and enters the thigh, lateral to the femoral sheath. In the abdomen, it supplies the psoas and iliacus.

The **obturator nerve** (L. 2, 3, 4; ventral divisions) leaves the medial border of the psoas on the base of the sacrum and enters the lesser pelvis.

An **accessory obturator nerve** may arise from the obturator nerve or from the third and fourth lumbar nerves. It runs to the thigh along the medial side of the psoas, gives branches to the hip joint, and sometimes to the pectineus, and joins the obturator nerve.

Lumbosacral trunk

The inferior division of the fourth lumbar ventral ramus descends through the psoas on the fifth lumbar transverse process. It unites with the ventral ramus of the fifth lumbar nerve to form the **lumbosacral trunk**. It enters the lesser pelvis on the base of the sacrum, posterior to the common iliac vessels and psoas.

➲ The roots of the obturator nerve, femoral nerve, and the fourth lumbar contribution to the lumbosacral trunk run anterior to the fifth lumbar transverse process. Any or all of them may be damaged in injuries of this process.

Subcostal and lumbar vessels

The **subcostal artery** is the last parietal branch of the thoracic aorta. It enters the abdomen with the subcostal nerve behind the lateral arcuate ligament. The **subcostal vein** lies superior to the artery and enters the azygos vein on the right side and the hemiazygos vein on the left side. Sometimes the azygos and hemiazygos veins are formed by the union of the subcostal and ascending lumbar veins.

Lumbar arteries

The first four pairs of lumbar arteries arise from the posterior surface of the abdominal aorta on the lumbar vertebral bodies. They curve over the vertebral bodies, passing deep to the fibrous arches which give origin to the psoas major muscle. They run posterior to the sympathetic trunk on both sides, and the cisterna chyli and inferior vena cava on the right [Fig. 13.1]. The upper one or two lumbar arteries are also deep to the azygos or hemiazygos vein and the crura of the diaphragm. At the root of the transverse process, each lumbar artery gives off a posterior branch, then passes posterior to the quadratus lumborum to supply the transversus abdominis and the internal oblique muscles. The **posterior branch** of the lumbar arteries accompanies the dorsal ramus of the spinal nerve. It sends a **spinal branch** through the intervertebral foramen to the contents of the vertebral canal and ends by supplying the erector spinae muscle and the overlying skin.

A small **fifth** pair of lumbar **arteries** arise from the median sacral artery or from the iliolumbar arteries.

Lumbar veins

The lumbar veins accompany the lumbar arteries. The first and second lumbar veins join the ascending lumbar vein on the lumbar transverse process. The third and fourth lumbar veins enter the inferior vena cava, the left veins passing posterior to the aorta. The fifth lumbar vein enters the iliolumbar vein.

The **ascending lumbar vein** runs vertically upwards, uniting the lateral sacral, iliolumbar, and upper four lumbar veins to the subcostal vein. It ascends in the psoas major, anterior to the lumbar transverse processes. It communicates with the **internal vertebral venous plexuses** through the intervertebral foramina [Fig. 13.8].

It is an advantage to remove the pelvis and lower limb from the trunk at this stage, but this can only be done without damage if the erector spinae muscle and the lumbar vertebral canal have been dissected. If this has not been done by the dissectors of the head and neck, then the appropriate pages of Vol. 3 of this manual should be read and the dissections carried out on the lumbar and sacral regions only.

Dissection 13.4 explores the intervertebral joints.

Intervertebral joints

Examine the intervertebral joints between the lumbar vertebrae using the dry bones [see Figs. 1.3, 1.4],

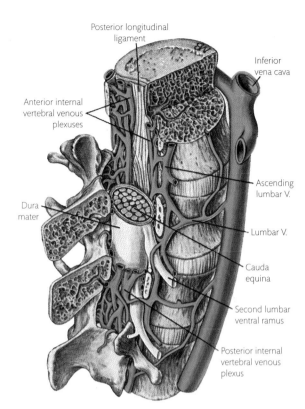

Fig. 13.8 Internal vertebral venous plexuses and their communications with the inferior vena cava at the level of the lumbar vertebrae.

Labels on figure:
Posterior longitudinal ligament
Inferior vena cava
Anterior internal vertebral venous plexuses
Dura mater
Ascending lumbar V.
Lumbar V.
Cauda equina
Second lumbar ventral ramus
Posterior internal vertebral venous plexus

DISSECTION 13.4 Intervertebral joints

Objective

I. To study the intervertebral joints.

Instructions

1. Cut through the intervertebral disc between the third and fourth lumbar vertebrae and all the other soft tissue structures on each side of the vertebral column at this level.

2. Identify the joints between the articular processes of the third and fourth lumbar vertebrae, and divide the ligaments uniting them. This separates the pelvis and lower limbs from the remainder of the trunk.

and compare them with those in the cervical and thoracic regions. Review the structure of the intervertebral disc and the arrangement of the ligaments uniting these vertebrae [Chapter 1].

See Clinical Applications 13.1, 13.2, and 13.3 for the practical implications of the anatomy in this chapter.

CLINICAL APPLICATION 13.1 Aortic aneurysm

An aneurysm is an abnormal bulge in the wall of an artery. Aortic aneurysms can be the result of a congenital or an acquired weakness in the wall of the aorta. Pulsation of the aneurysm can be felt a little to the left of the midline in the abdomen. Sudden rupture of an aortic aneurysm is associated with severe pain and high mortality. Aneurysms are treated by surgical repair.

CLINICAL APPLICATION 13.2 Renal vein entrapment syndrome

A 32-year-old woman presented with frequent bouts of haematuria and pain in the left flank. An ultrasound of the abdomen, followed by CT, revealed compression of the left renal vein between the origin of the superior mesenteric artery and the aorta [see Fig. 13.1A]. A diagnosis of left renal vein entrapment was made.

Study question 1: can a similar problem arise at the right renal vein? Explain your answer. (Hint: what is the course of the left renal vein?) (Answer: no, because the right renal vein enters the inferior vena cava without crossing the aorta. The left renal vein crosses the aorta posterior to the superior mesenteric artery and is susceptible to compression between the two arteries.)

Study question 2: apart from the left kidney, what other organs could be affected in this disease? (Answer: the left suprarenal and left gonad could be affected by back pressure in the veins, as the left suprarenal and left gonadal veins drain into the left renal vein.)

CLINICAL APPLICATION 13.3 Psoas abscess

A 15-year-old boy with a known history of tuberculosis presented with fever, pain on the right side of the abdomen, and a limp due to pain in the right hip. On examination, a soft, round swelling was found in the right femoral region. Further investigation revealed a psoas abscess on the right side.

Study question 1: what are the attachments of the psoas major muscle? What is its covering? (Answer: the psoas major arises in the abdomen from the sides of the last thoracic and the lumbar vertebrae, and is inserted into the lesser trochanter of the femur. The psoas is enclosed in a sheath of fascia—the psoas fascia. The fascia is fused above with the periosteum of the vertebral column and the anterior layer of the thoracolumbar

fascia. Below, the psoas fascia is fused with the arcuate line of the bony pelvis and the iliac fascia. This long, tubular fascial sheath forms a route along which infected material from the vertebral column may travel to the groin. In this patient, tuberculosis of the lumbar or lower thoracic vertebral column gave rise to an abscess which tracked inferiorly within the psoas sheath, deep to the inguinal ligament and presented as a swelling in the anterior part of the thigh.)

Study question 2: what is the action of the psoas on the hip joint? (Answer: the psoas flexes the hip joint. Any inflammation of the muscle or its fascia will cause pain in the joint because of the close proximity between the two.)

CHAPTER 14
MCQs for part 3: The abdomen

The following questions have four options each. You are required to choose the most correct answer.

1. **The arcuate line on the rectus sheath represents the**
   A. superior edge of the posterior layer of the rectus sheath
   B. inferior edge of the posterior layer of the rectus sheath
   C. superior edge of the anterior layer of the rectus sheath
   D. inferior edge of the anterior layer of the rectus sheath

2. **The free posterior border of the falciform ligament contains obliterated**
   A. right umbilical vein
   B. left umbilical vein
   C. right umbilical artery
   D. left umbilical artery

3. **The following statements are true about the splenic artery, EXCEPT**
   A. it is tortuous
   B. it is the largest branch of the coeliac trunk
   C. it runs along the superior border of the pancreas
   D. it forms an anterior relation of the stomach

4. **The vertebral level of origin of the superior mesenteric artery is**
   A. T. 12
   B. L. 1
   C. L. 2
   D. L. 3

5. **Appendices epiploicae are present on the**
   A. caecum
   B. appendix
   C. sigmoid colon
   D. rectum

6. **The hepatic veins drain into the**

    A. inferior vena cava
    B. right branch of the portal vein
    C. left branch of the portal vein
    D. trunk of the portal vein

7. **The sympathetic trunk enters the abdomen**

    A. between the costal and sternal attachments of the diaphragm
    B. through the aortic opening
    C. posterior to the medial arcuate ligament
    D. posterior to the lateral arcuate ligament

8. **Which of the following nerves emerges at the medial border of the psoas major muscle?**

    A. femoral
    B. obturator
    C. ilio-inguinal
    D. genitofemoral

9. **The tail of the pancreas lies in the**

    A. lienorenal ligament
    B. gastrosplenic ligament
    C. gastrophrenic ligament
    D. greater omentum

10. **Which of the following arteries blocks the ascent of the horseshoe kidney?**

    A. superior mesenteric
    B. inferior mesenteric
    C. left colic
    D. superior rectal

11. **Which of the following arteries supplies the vermiform appendix?**

    A. coeliac
    B. superior mesenteric
    C. inferior mesenteric
    D. lumbar

12. **The structure related posteriorly to the epiploic foramen is the**

    A. common bile duct
    B. proper hepatic artery
    C. portal vein
    D. inferior vena cava

13. **The lesser omentum is attached to the**

    A. lesser curvature of the stomach and the anterior abdominal wall
    B. liver and the anterior abdominal wall
    C. greater curvature of the stomach and the anterior abdominal wall
    D. lesser curvature of the stomach and liver

14. The epididymis

A. lies anteromedial to the testis

B. is connected to the testis by efferent ductules

C. is continuous with the vas deferens at the head

D. is not covered by the tunica vaginalis testis

15. The superior suprarenal artery is a branch of the

A. inferior phrenic artery

B. renal artery

C. aorta

D. lumbar artery

Please go to the back of the book for the answers.

PART 4

The pelvis and perineum

CHAPTER 15

Introduction to the pelvis and perineum

Bony pelvis

The bones of the pelvis are the two hip bones, the sacrum, and the coccyx. They are united by four joints: paired synovial sacro-iliac joints posterosuperiorly, the pubic symphysis antero-inferiorly, and the sacrococcygeal joint posteriorly. In the erect position, the upper margin of the pubic symphysis and the anterior superior iliac spines are in the same coronal plane [Figs. 15.1, 15.2].

The pelvis consists of two parts: the greater pelvis and the lesser pelvis. They are separated by the superior aperture of the lesser pelvis, an oblique plane passing from the sacral promontory at the back to the upper surface of the pubic symphysis in front [see Fig. 1.1]. The greater pelvis is bounded by the iliac fossae and is part of the abdomen. The lesser pelvis is simply referred to as the pelvis.

Overview of the pelvis and perineum

Begin by reviewing the bony walls of the lesser pelvis. In the sagittal plane, the cavity of the lesser pelvis is curved [Figs. 15.3A, 15.3B]. It has a long, posterosuperior wall formed by the sacrum and coccyx, and a short antero-inferior wall formed by the pubic bones and pubic symphysis. Due to the forward tilt of the pelvis, the antero-inferior wall lies below the level of the coccyx [Fig. 15.3]. More laterally, the anterior wall is formed inferiorly by the two **rami of the pubis** and the **ischium**

which together surround the **obturator foramen**. The foramen is filled almost completely by the **obturator membrane**, except at the anterior superior margin where the membrane is deficient. The obturator vessels and nerve leave the lesser pelvis through this deficiency—the **obturator canal** [Fig. 15.1A].

Superiorly, the lateral wall is completed by the medial wall of the acetabulum and, above this, by a small part of the ilium. Posteriorly, this part of the ilium curves medially to meet the sacrum at the **sacro-iliac joint** [Figs. 15.1, 15.2, 15.4]. The posterolateral wall of the lesser pelvis is the space between the hip bone laterally and the sacrum and coccyx medially. This space is bridged by the **sacrotuberous** and **sacrospinous ligaments** which divide it into the **greater** and **lesser sciatic foramina** [Figs. 15.5, 15.6].

The superior aperture of the bony pelvis is also known as the **linea terminalis**. It is formed by the anterior margin of the base of the sacrum, the **arcuate line** of the ilium, the **pecten pubis**, the **pubic crest**, and the **pubic symphysis**. It separates the greater pelvis from the lesser pelvis [Figs. 15.1A, 15.1B].

Inferiorly is the **inferior aperture of the pelvis**. This diamond-shaped aperture is bound by the **pubic symphysis** in front, the **coccyx** behind, and the **ischial tuberosities** at the lateral angles. The anterolateral margins of the inferior aperture are formed by the **ischiopubic rami**, and the posterolateral margins are formed by the **sacrotuberous ligaments** [Fig. 15.6]. These boundaries are also the skeletal boundaries of the perineum [Fig. 15.7].

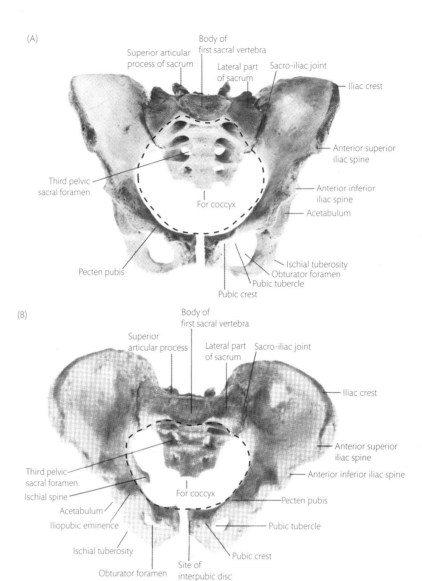

(A)

Superior articular
process of sacrum

Body of
first sacral vertebra

Lateral part
of sacrum

Sacro-iliac joint

Iliac crest

Anterior superior
iliac spine

Anterior inferior
iliac spine

Acetabulum

Third pelvic
sacral foramen

For coccyx

Ischial tuberosity
Obturator foramen
Pubic tubercle

Pecten pubis

Pubic crest

(B)

Superior
articular process

Body of
first sacral vertebra

Lateral part
of sacrum

Sacro-iliac joint

Iliac crest

Anterior superior
iliac spine

Anterior inferior iliac spine

Third pelvic
sacral foramen

Ischial spine

Acetabulum

Iliopubic eminence

For coccyx

Pecten pubis

Pubic tubercle

Ischial tuberosity

Obturator foramen

Site of
interpubic disc

Pubic crest

Fig. 15.1 (A) The female pelvis, seen from in front. (B) The male pelvis, seen from in front. The inlet of the pelvis is marked with a red dotted line.

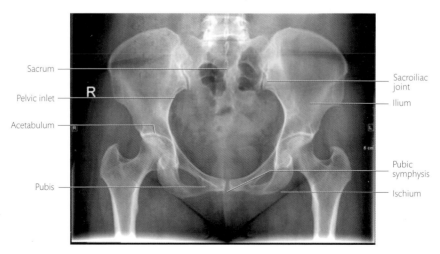

Sacrum

Pelvic inlet

Acetabulum

Pubis

Sacroiliac joint

Ilium

Pubic symphysis

Ischium

R

Fig. 15.2 Anteroposterior radiograph of the female pelvis.

(A)

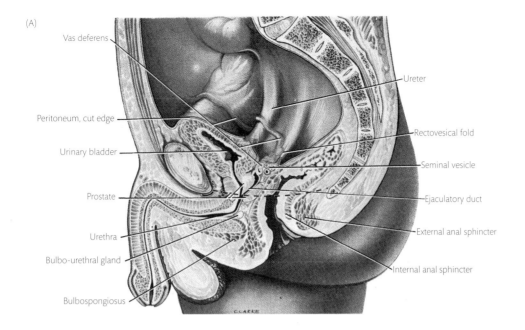

Vas deferens

Peritoneum, cut edge

Urinary bladder

Prostate

Urethra

Bulbo-urethral gland

Bulbospongiosus

Ureter

Rectovesical fold

Seminal vesicle

Ejaculatory duct

External anal sphincter

Internal anal sphincter

(B)

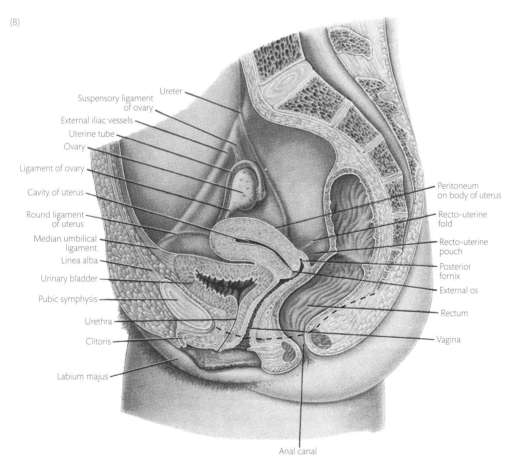

Ureter

Suspensory ligament of ovary

External iliac vessels

Uterine tube

Ovary

Ligament of ovary

Cavity of uterus

Round ligament of uterus

Median umbilical ligament

Linea alba

Urinary bladder

Pubic symphysis

Urethra

Clitoris

Labium majus

Peritoneum on body of uterus

Recto-uterine fold

Recto-uterine pouch

Posterior fornix

External os

Rectum

Vagina

Anal canal

Fig. 15.3 (A) Median section through the male pelvis. (B) Median section through the female pelvis. The red dotted line indicates the junction of the pelvis and the perineum.

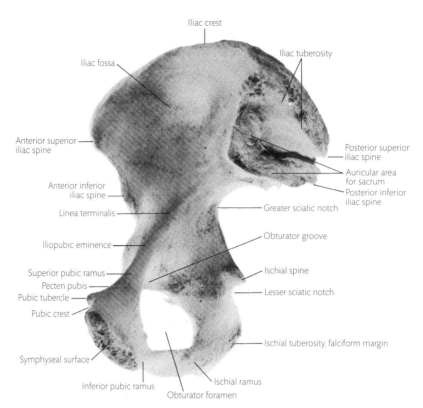

Iliac crest

Iliac fossa

Iliac tuberosity

Anterior superior
iliac spine

Posterior superior
iliac spine

Auricular area
for sacrum
Posterior inferior
iliac spine

Anterior inferior
iliac spine

Linea terminalis

Greater sciatic notch

Iliopubic eminence

Obturator groove

Superior pubic ramus

Ischial spine

Pecten pubis

Pubic tubercle

Lesser sciatic notch

Pubic crest

Ischial tuberosity, falciform margin

Symphyseal surface

Inferior pubic ramus

Ischial ramus

Obturator foramen

Fig. 15.4 The right hip bone, seen from the medial side.

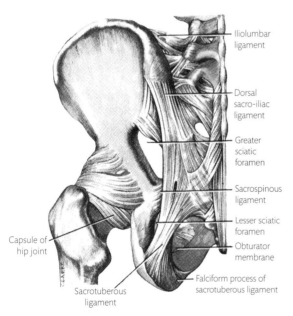

Iliolumbar
ligament

Dorsal
sacro-iliac
ligament

Greater
sciatic
foramen

Sacrospinous
ligament

Lesser sciatic
foramen

Obturator
membrane

Capsule of
hip joint

Falciform process of
sacrotuberous ligament

Sacrotuberous
ligament

Fig. 15.5 Dorsal view of the pelvic ligaments and the hip joint.

The inferior aperture of the pelvis transmits the urethra, the vagina (in the female), and the anal canal. The anterior half of the inferior aperture is closed by the **urogenital diaphragm**, and the posterior half by the **levator ani muscles** [Fig. 15.8]. The walls of the lesser pelvis are lined by muscles—the **piriformis** on the sacrum [see Fig. 18.6], the **coccygeus** on the sacrospinous ligament, and the **obturator internus** on the antero-lateral wall [see Fig. 17.8].

The V-shaped floor of the pelvis—the **pelvic diaphragm**—is formed by the **levator ani**. The two levator ani muscles run postero-inferiorly from the anterolateral walls of the lesser pelvis to the midline. Together they divide the cavity of the bony pelvis into an upper part—the **pelvic cavity** which contains the pelvic viscera—and a lower part which forms part of the **perineum** [Fig. 15.3].

The perineum lies inferior to the pelvic cavity, separated from it by the levator ani [Figs. 15.3, 15.9]. It lies between the upper parts of the thighs and the lower parts of the buttocks and is almost completely hidden by them in the erect posture. The perineum is considerably wider in the female than the male. In both sexes, it is divided into an anterior **urogenital region** and a posterior **anal region** by a transverse line passing through the ischial tuberosities immediately anterior to the anus [Fig. 15.8].

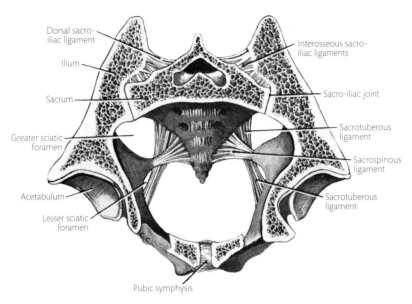

Fig. 15.6 An oblique section through the lesser pelvis to show the ligaments and sacro-iliac joints.

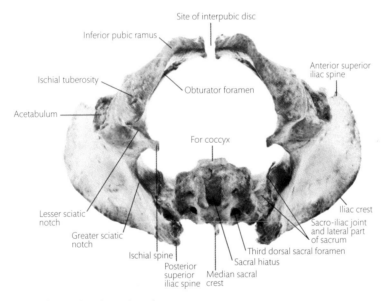

Fig. 15.7 The inferior aperture of the male pelvis without the coccyx.

The **parietal pelvic fascia** lines the walls of the pelvic cavity. It covers the internal surface of the piriformis, coccygeus, and obturator internus and the superior surface of the levator ani muscles. The parietal pelvic fascia is part of the fascial envelope of the abdomen. It is continuous with the visceral pelvic fascia around the pelvic viscera where these structures lie on or pierce—the levator ani [Fig. 15.9].

The **pelvic peritoneum** passes over the superior surfaces of the pelvic viscera and dips between them to form pouches [Fig. 15.3]. Elsewhere the peritoneum is separated from the parietal pelvic fascia by fatty extraperitoneal tissue which contains blood vessels and autonomic nerve plexuses. The **sacral plexus** and its branches lie external to the parietal pelvic fascia [see Fig. 15.13].

Dissection 15.1 explores the vertebropelvic ligaments.

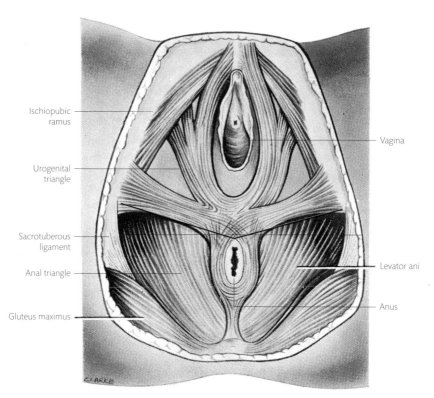

Fig. 15.8 Boundaries and subdivisions of the female perineum. The red line marks the boundary between the urogenital and anal triangles.

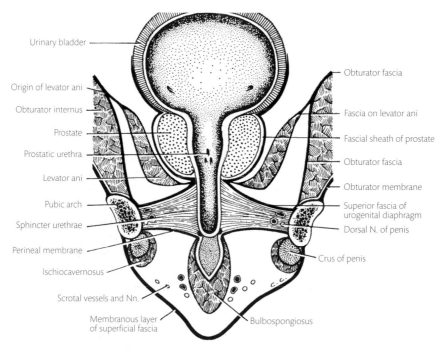

Fig. 15.9 A schematic coronal section through the male pelvis and perineum to show the arrangement of the parietal and visceral pelvic fasciae (red).

DISSECTION 15.1 Vertebropelvic ligaments

Objectives

I. To define the iliolumbar, sacrotuberous, and sacrospinous ligaments.   II. To identify the dorsal sacral
foramina, the pudendal nerve, the internal pudendal
artery, and the nerve to the obturator internus.

Instructions

1. Expose the iliolumbar ligaments and the ligaments
   on the posterior surface of the sacro-iliac joints by
   removing the overlying erector spinae muscles and
   the posterior layer of the thoracolumbar fascia.

2. Expose the dorsal sacral foramina and the dorsal
   rami of the sacral nerves passing through them together with small blood vessels [Fig. 15.10].

3. Define the attachments of the sacrotuberous ligament. Then cut across the ligament at its middle,
   and separate it from the underlying sacrospinous
   ligament. Note any small nerves between them.

4. Define the sacrospinous ligament and the spine of
   the ischium.

5. Find the pudendal nerve, the internal pudendal
   vessels, and the nerve to the obturator internus
   winding over the ligament and the adjacent part
   of the spine.

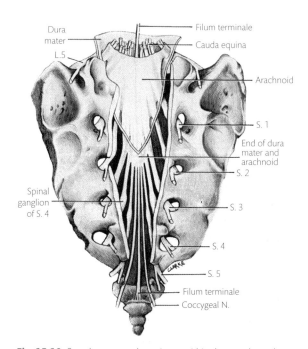

Fig. 15.10 Sacral nerves and meninges within the sacral canal.

Vertebropelvic ligaments

These important ligaments unite the bony pelvis to
the vertebral column. The **iliolumbar ligament**
is a strong, triangular ligament which is attached to
the thick transverse process of the fifth lumbar vertebra and the inner lip of the iliac crest posteriorly.
Its lower fibres descend to the lateral part of the sacrum as the **lateral lumbosacral ligament**. The
horizontal part gives origin to part of the quadratus
lumborum and to the anterior and middle layers of
the **thoracolumbar fascia** which enclose it. Anteriorly, the ligament is covered by the psoas and
posteriorly by the erector spinae. The iliolumbar ligament plays an important part in maintaining the
fifth lumbar vertebra in position [Fig. 15.5]. It resists
the tendency of the weight of the body to force the
fifth lumbar vertebra antero-inferiorly on the sloping superior surface of the sacrum [see Fig. 7.6].

The **sacrotuberous ligament** has a wide origin from the dorsal surfaces of the sacrum and coccyx and from the posterior superior and posterior
inferior iliac spines. It passes downwards, laterally,
and forwards, at first narrowing and then expanding again, to be attached to the medial margin of
the ischial tuberosity. It is partly continuous with
the tendon of the biceps femoris, and its anterior margin curves forwards on the ischial ramus
as the **falciform process**. This ligament forms
part of the boundary of the greater and lesser
sciatic foramina and of the perineum [Figs. 15.6,
15.7]. The sacrotuberous ligament is pierced by the
perforating cutaneous nerve, the coccygeal
and fifth sacral ventral rami, and branches of the
coccygeal plexus.

The **sacrospinous ligament** is the fibrous
dorsal part of the **coccygeus muscle**. It extends
as a thin, triangular sheet from the lateral margins
of the coccyx and the last piece of the sacrum to
the ischial spine. It separates the greater and lesser
sciatic foramina [Figs. 15.5, 15.6]. Part of the sacrospinous ligament is covered posteriorly by the
sacrotuberous ligament, and has the **perineal
branch of the fourth sacral** and the **perforating cutaneous nerves** between them.

The sacrotuberous and sacrospinous ligaments
bind the sacrum to the ischium and hold down
the posterior part of the sacrum. Along with the
iliolumbar ligament, they prevent the weight of
the body from depressing the anterior part of the

pelvis. At the same time, these ligaments allow some movement at the sacro-iliac joints, making them resilient to sudden increased loading as when a person jumps from a height and lands on the feet [see Fig. 7.6].

Sciatic foramina

The **greater sciatic foramen** is bound by the greater sciatic notch of the hip bone and the sacrotuberous and sacrospinous ligaments. It lies superior to the pelvic diaphragm and is continuous anteriorly with the pelvic cavity. This foramen is almost completely filled by the piriformis as it leaves the pelvis to enter the gluteal region. The greater sciatic foramen also transmits vessels and nerves to the buttock, the posterior aspect of the thigh, and the perineum. The **superior gluteal vessels** and **nerve** emerge through the greater sciatic foramen, superior to the piriformis. The large **sciatic nerve**, **nerve to quadratus femoris**, **inferior gluteal vessels** and **nerve**, and **posterior cutaneous nerve of the thigh** emerge inferior to the piriformis.

The **lesser sciatic foramen** is bound by the lesser sciatic notch and the sacrotuberous and sacrospinous ligaments. The **tendon of the obturator internus** enters the gluteal region through it. Just as the greater sciatic foramen is continuous anteriorly with the pelvic cavity, the lesser sciatic foramen is continuous anteriorly with the perineum. (The greater sciatic foramen lies superior to the pelvic diaphragm and the lesser sciatic foramen lies inferior to it.) The pudendal nerve, the internal pudendal artery, and the nerve to the obturator internus, which pass from the pelvis to the ischioanal fossa in the perineum, emerge through the greater foramen, run a short course in the gluteal region, and enter the lesser sciatic foramen, hooking over the sacrospinous ligament and the ischial spine [Figs. 15.5, 15.6].

Position of the pelvic viscera

Use Figs. 15.3A and 15.3B to study the general arrangement of the pelvic viscera in the male and female. (This is just an introduction to the pelvic viscera which will be covered in detail later.)

In both sexes, part of the **sigmoid colon** may be lifted out of the pelvis, but its inferior part is attached to the posterosuperior wall of the pelvis by the medial limb of the sigmoid mesocolon. The sigmoid colon is continuous with the rectum on the third piece of the sacrum. The **rectum** follows the concavity of the sacrum, the coccyx, and the posterior part of the levator ani. Inferiorly, it turns sharply downwards and backwards as the **anal canal**.

The **urinary** bladder lies in the antero-inferior part of the pelvic cavity, posterosuperior to the pubic bones and symphysis. Between the bladder and the rectum is a transverse septum of connective tissue. The ureters pass antero-inferiorly through this septum to the bladder. In the male, the septum is small and contains the **vas deferens**, **seminal vesicle**, and **ureter**. Each vas deferens runs postero-inferiorly from the deep inguinal ring across the anterolateral part of the pelvis, immediately inferior to the peritoneum. It passes over the ureter and runs medially on the posterior surface of the bladder, superior to the seminal vesicle. Near the midline, the vas deferens turns acutely downwards [see Fig. 17.12] and ends by uniting with the duct of the seminal vesicle to form the **ejaculatory duct**. The ejaculatory duct runs through the prostate and ends in the prostatic urethra.

In the female, the connective tissue septum between the bladder and rectum is large and extends upwards into the lesser pelvis. The superior part of the septum contains the **uterus** in the midline, the **uterine tube** in the free margin, and an **ovary** close to each lateral extremity [Figs. 15.3A, 15.11]. The **broad ligament of the uterus** is a double fold of peritoneum surrounding the uterine tubes and the ovaries. The **vagina** lies inferiorly and slopes antero-inferiorly, posterior to the bladder and urethra, and anterior to the rectum. It opens on the perineum between the urethra and rectum.

The rounded upper end or **fundus of the uterus** is continuous with the **body of the uterus**. The body is continuous with the narrower posteroinferior third—the **cervix** or **neck of the uterus**. The neck is partly inserted into the anterior wall of the vagina.

Each **uterine tube** extends laterally from the junction of the fundus and body to the lateral wall of the pelvis [Fig. 15.12]. At the lateral end, the

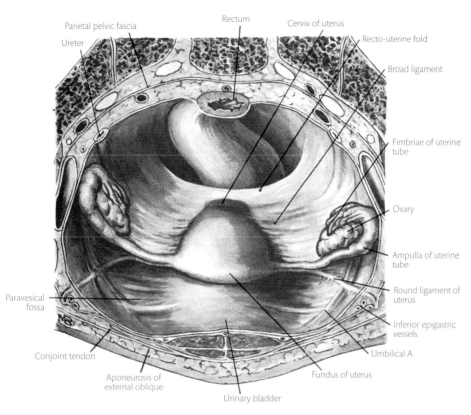

Parietal pelvic fascia

Rectum

Cervix of uterus

Ureter

Recto-uterine fold

Broad ligament

Fimbriae of uterine tube

Ovary

Ampulla of uterine tube

Round ligament of uterus

Paravesical fossa

Inferior epigastric vessels

Conjoint tendon

Umbilical A.

Aponeurosis of external oblique

Fundus of uterus

Urinary bladder

Fig. 15.11 The peritoneum of the lesser pelvis in the female.

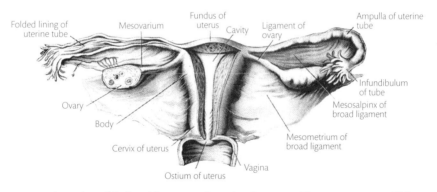

Folded lining of uterine tube

Mesovarium

Fundus of uterus

Cavity

Ligament of ovary

Ampulla of uterine tube

Infundibulum of tube

Ovary

Mesosalpinx of broad ligament

Body

Mesometrium of broad ligament

Cervix of uterus

Vagina

Ostium of uterus

Fig. 15.12 The posterosuperior surface of the broad ligament and associated structures. The vagina, uterus, and left uterine tube have been opened, and the left ovary is sectioned parallel to the broad ligament.

uterine tube expands to form the **ampulla** and recurves upon itself to end as the funnel-shaped **infundibulum**. The infundibulum is directed medially towards the ovary and opens into the peritoneal cavity.

Attached to the uterus at the tubo-uterine junction are two ligaments: (1) the **round ligament of the uterus**, which curves anterolaterally to the deep inguinal ring; and (2) the **ligament of the ovary**, which passes to the medial end of the ovary. In addition, a ridge of the pelvic fibrous tissue curves posterosuperiorly from the cervix of the uterus towards the lateral part of the sacrum. This is the **uterosacral ligament**.

The ureter in the female follows the same course as in the male but passes postero-inferior to the ovary and lateral to the uppermost part of the vagina, deep in the genital septum.

Pelvic peritoneum

The parietal peritoneum from the abdomen passes into the lesser pelvis over the margins of the superior aperture. It covers the superior surfaces of the pelvic organs—the rectum, uterus, and bladder—and dips between them, producing peritoneal pouches and fossae. Anteriorly and posteriorly, the arrangement of this peritoneum is virtually identical in the two sexes. It differs in the intermediate region because of the presence of the large genital septum in the female.

Use Figs. 15.3A and 15.3B to trace the peritoneum in the pelvis. The posterosuperior surface of the lesser pelvis is covered with the peritoneum down to the second piece of the sacrum, except where the medial limb of the sigmoid mesocolon is attached [see Fig. 11.13]. Inferior to this, the peritoneum passes in front of the rectum as it lies on the sacrum. The peritoneum covers the front and sides of the upper third of the **rectum**. On the middle third of the rectum, the peritoneum turns forwards from the anterior surface to run upwards over the genital septum. In doing so, the peritoneum forms the **recto-uterine pouch** in the female, and the **rectovesical pouch** in the male. In the female, the peritoneum in the median plane passes from the recto-uterine pouch on to the superior part of the posterior wall of the vagina, the superior surface of the cervix, and body of the uterus. It then turns over the fundus of the uterus to cover the inferior surface of the body of the uterus [Fig. 15.3B]. Anteriorly, at the junction of the body and cervix of the uterus, the peritoneum bends forwards onto the superior surface of the bladder, thus forming the **uterovesical pouch** of the peritoneum. The peritoneum on the superior surface of the bladder continues forwards and passes on to the posterior surface of the anterior abdominal wall.

Lateral to the uterus, the peritoneum passes from the cervix as the **recto-uterine fold** on the uterosacral ligament, and from the body of the uterus as a double layer—the **broad ligament**. The broad ligament encloses the uterine tube, the connective tissue of the septum (**parametrium**), the round ligament of the uterus, and the ligament of the ovary. It is thickened laterally where the uterosacral ligament passes posteriorly and the round ligament of the uterus passes anteriorly.

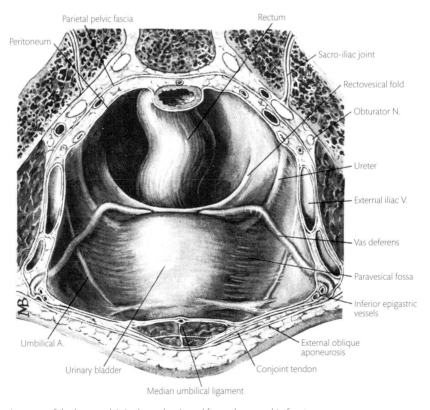

Fig. 15.13 The peritoneum of the lesser pelvis in the male, viewed from above and in front.

The superior layer of the broad ligament runs back as a short **mesovarium** and covers the ovary. The part of the broad ligament lateral to the ovary is the **suspensory ligament of the ovary**. The part between the ovary and the uterine tube is the **mesosalpinx** (mesentery of the tube), and the remainder is the **mesometrium** (mesentery of the uterus) [Fig. 15.12].

Thus the uterus and parametrium lie in a transverse peritoneal fold with a free anterior margin. This allows the uterus to expand upwards into the abdominal cavity during pregnancy without disturbing its supporting structures in the base of the broad ligament. The connective tissue which holds the cervix to the wall of the pelvis is especially thickened as the **transverse ligaments of the cervix** around the uterine arteries and as the **uterosacral ligaments**.

Lateral to the bladder, the peritoneum passes forwards on the floor of a shallow **paravesical fossa** on each side [Fig. 15.11]. This fossa is limited laterally by the ridge produced by the round ligament and has the obliterated umbilical artery in its floor.

In the male, the peritoneum from the rectovesical fossa passes on to the superior part of the posterior surface of the bladder between the two vas deferens. Anterior to this, the peritoneum covers the entire superior surface of the bladder. Laterally, the peritoneum arches over the ureter as it runs from the brim of the pelvis to the base of the bladder. The ureter forms the posterior limit of the paravesical fossa in the male. At this point, the ureter is crossed by the vas deferens [Fig. 15.13].

The greater part of the intra-abdominal vas deferens lies immediately inferior to the peritoneum. Anteriorly, it is in the same position as the round ligament of the uterus [Fig. 15.11], but it extends further posteriorly to reach the base of the bladder [Fig. 15.13].

CHAPTER 16
The perineum

Introduction

The perineum lies inferior to the pelvic cavity, between the upper parts of the thighs and the lower parts of the buttocks.

It has a shared boundary with the inferior aperture of the pelvis—the inferior margin of the pubic symphysis, the inferior rami of the pubic bones, the rami and tuberosities of the ischia, the sacrotuberous ligaments, and the coccyx [Figs. 16.1, 16.2]. In both sexes, the perineum is divided into an anterior **urogenital region** and a posterior **anal region** by an imaginary line drawn between the two ischial tuberosities and passing anterior to the anus [see Fig. 15.8].

In the male, the urogenital region contains the urethra, the root of the penis with its muscles, vessels and nerves, and the bulbo-urethral glands. A median cutaneous ridge—the **raphe of the perineum**—extends from the anus over the inferior surface of the scrotum and the ventral surface of the penis. The raphe marks the line of fusion of the structures that form the separate labia in the female [see Fig. 16.5]. In the female, the urogenital region contains the terminal parts of the urethra and vagina, the clitoris, the bulb of the vestibule with its muscles, vessels, and nerves, the greater vestibular glands, and the labia minora and majora [see Fig. 16.8].

The **anal region** transmits the terminal 3–4 cm of the large intestine—the anal canal.

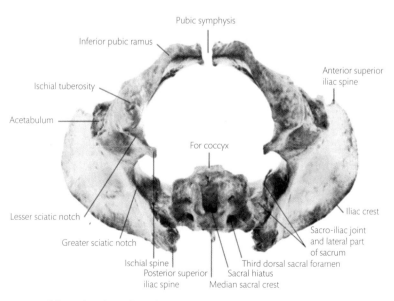

Fig. 16.1 The inferior aperture of the male pelvis without the coccyx.

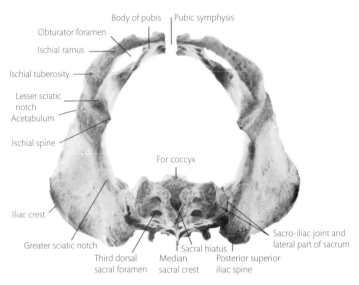

Body of pubis | Pubic symphysis

Obturator foramen

Ischial ramus

Ischial tuberosity

Lesser sciatic notch
Acetabulum

Ischial spine

For coccyx

Iliac crest

Sacro-iliac joint and lateral part of sacrum

Greater sciatic notch
Third dorsal sacral foramen
Sacral hiatus
Median sacral crest
Posterior superior iliac spine

Fig. 16.2 The inferior aperture of the female pelvis without the coccyx.

Female external genital organs

It is useful to have a thorough understanding of the external genitalia before dissecting the region. (The male external genitalia is described in Chapter 9.) The female external genitalia, or **vulva**, consists of: the mons pubis, labia majora, labia minora, clitoris, and vestibule [Fig. 16.3].

1. The **mons pubis** lies anterior to the pubic bones. It is a protrusion of hairy skin overlying subcutaneous fat. The hairs cease abruptly at a horizontal line where the mons meets the anterior abdominal wall. (In the male, the corresponding pubic hairs extend upwards towards the umbilicus.)

2. The labia majora are a pair of rounded folds which extend postero-inferiorly from the mons. They decrease in size posteriorly. The lateral parts of the

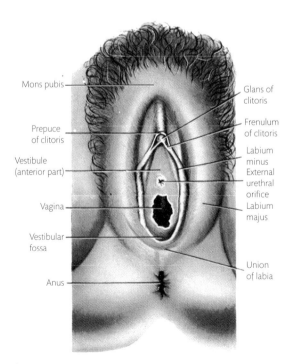

Mons pubis

Prepuce of clitoris

Vestibule (anterior part)

Vagina

Vestibular fossa

Anus

Glans of clitoris

Frenulum of clitoris

Labium minus
External urethral orifice

Labium majus

Union of labia

Fig. 16.3 The female external genital organs.

skin of the labia are hairy, but the medial surfaces are smooth and lubricated by sebaceous glands.

3. The **labia minora** are a pair of smooth cutaneous folds. Anteriorly, each fold splits into two as it approaches the clitoris. The smaller posterior parts fuse with each other and are attached to the inferior surface of the clitoris as the **frenulum of the clitoris**. The anterior parts pass on either side of the clitoris and unite to form a hood over the tip of the clitoris—the **prepuce of the clitoris**. Posteriorly, the labia minora are united by a transverse fold—the **frenulum of the labia**.

4. The **clitoris** is an erectile structure which closely resembles the penis but is not traversed by the urethra. It has a root, body, and glans.

5. The **vestibule of the vagina** lies between the two labia minora. It contains the orifices of the urethra, the vagina, and the **ducts** of the two **greater vestibular glands**. A shallow vestibular fossa lies between the vaginal orifice and the frenulum of the labia minora.

6. The vaginal orifice lies in the posterior part of the vestibule. Prior to sexual intercourse, it is partly closed by a thin membrane (the **hymen**) attached to the margins of the orifice. When ruptured, the position of the hymen is marked by small, rounded tags—the **carunculae hymenales**.

7. The **urethral orifice** lies immediately anterior to the vaginal orifice, 2 cm posterior to the clitoris. Its margins are raised, puckered, and palpable.

The general arrangement of the perineum

The urogenital region

The **urogenital region** has three layers of fascia with two spaces, or pouches, between them. The two spaces are the **superficial perineal space**, or **superficial perineal pouch**, and the **deep perineal space** or **deep perineal pouch**. The three fascial layers are: (1) a superficial **membranous layer**; (2) the **inferior fascia of the urogenital diaphragm** or **perineal membrane**; and (3) the **superior fascia of the urogenital diaphragm**. The superficial perineal space is the space between the membranous superficial layer and the perineal membrane. The deep perineal space is the space between the perineal membrane and the superior fascia of the urogenital diaphragm. These layers are most obvious in the male.

The first layer—the superficial membranous layer—is continuous anteriorly with the membranous layer of the superficial fascia of the anterior abdominal wall [see Fig. 8.4; Fig. 16.4B]. In the perineum, it is attached laterally to the pubic tubercles, the body of the pubis, the ischiopubic rami, and the ischial tuberosities. Between the attachments to the pubic bones, it forms the fascial sheath and fundiform ligament of the penis, and the **dartos** layer in the scrotum. Anterior to the anal orifice, this membranous layer turns superiorly to fuse with the posterior border of the second layer—the **perineal membrane**. The superficial perineal space lies between these two layers of fascia and is closed posteriorly by the fusion of these layers.

In the midline, immediately anterior to the anus is the **central perineal tendon**, a fibrous mass to which a number of perineal muscles are attached.

In the male, the **superficial perineal pouch** (space) contains the **root of the penis** and the associated muscles, vessels, and nerves. The root of the penis comprises of: (1) the two **crura of the penis**; and (2) the median **bulb of the penis**. Each crus is attached to the everted margins of the ischiopubic rami and is covered by the **ischiocavernosus** muscle. The bulb of the penis is attached to the inferior surface of the perineal membrane. It is covered by the **bulbospongiosus** muscle. The urethra pierces the perineal membrane and enters the bulb of the penis. The **superficial transverse perineal** muscles lie transversely across the posterior margin of the superficial perineal space [Figs. 16.5, 16.6].

The deep perineal pouch (superior to the perineal membrane) contains a thin layer of muscle stretched across the pubic arch [Figs. 16.4A, 16.7]. The main part of this muscle surrounds the urethra and forms the voluntary **sphincter urethrae**. The posterior fibres of the muscle run transversely as the **deep transverse perineal** muscles. This layer of muscle fills the **deep perineal space**, which is limited superiorly by the third layer of fascia—the **superior fascia of the urogenital diaphragm**. The superior fascia of the urogenital diaphragm is attached laterally to the pubic arch and fuses anteriorly and posteriorly with the perineal membrane, thus closing the deep perineal space. Anteriorly, the perineal membrane and superior fascia of the urogenital diaphragm do not reach the pubic symphysis. A small space exists between the

(A)

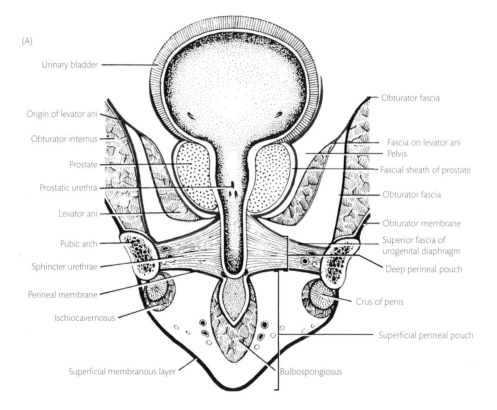

Urinary bladder

Origin of levator ani

Obturator internus

Prostate

Prostatic urethra

Levator ani

Pubic arch

Sphincter urethrae

Perineal membrane

Ischiocavernosus

Superficial membranous layer

Obturator fascia

Fascia on levator ani
Pelvis

Fascial sheath of prostate

Obturator fascia

Obturator membrane

Superior fascia of
urogenital diaphragm

Deep perineal pouch

Crus of penis

Superficial perineal pouch

Bulbospongiosus

(B)

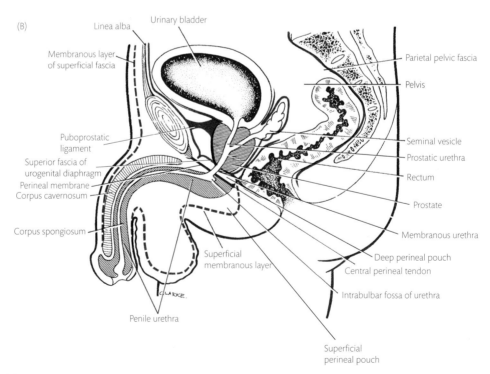

Linea alba

Urinary bladder

Membranous layer
of superficial fascia

Puboprostatic
ligament

Superior fascia of
urogenital diaphragm

Perineal membrane

Corpus cavernosum

Corpus spongiosum

Superficial
membranous layer

Penile urethra

Parietal pelvic fascia

Pelvis

Seminal vesicle

Prostatic urethra

Rectum

Prostate

Membranous urethra

Deep perineal pouch

Central perineal tendon

Intrabulbar fossa of urethra

Superficial
perineal pouch

Fig. 16.4 (A) A schematic coronal section through the male pelvis and perineum to show the arrangement of the pelvic and perineal fasciae. (B) A schematic median section through the male pelvis to show the parietal and visceral pelvic fascia.

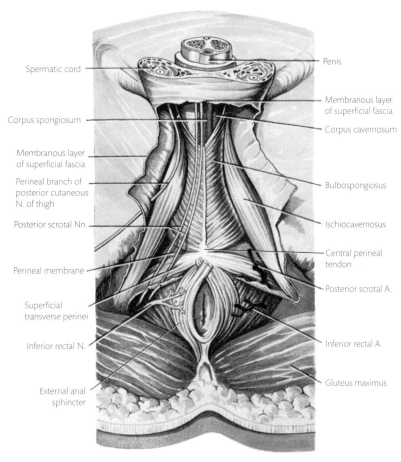

Spermatic cord

Corpus spongiosum

Membranous layer
of superficial fascia

Perineal branch of
posterior cutaneous
N. of thigh

Posterior scrotal Nn.

Perineal membrane

Superficial
transverse perinei

Inferior rectal N.

External anal
sphincter

Penis

Membranous layer
of superficial fascia

Corpus cavernosum

Bulbospongiosus

Ischiocavernosus

Central perineal
tendon

Posterior scrotal A.

Inferior rectal A.

Gluteus maximus

Fig. 16.5 Contents of the superficial perineal pouch and ischioanal fossa in the male. The penis and scrotum have been removed.

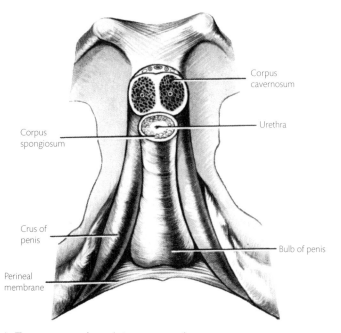

Corpus
cavernosum

Urethra

Corpus
spongiosum

Crus of
penis

Bulb of penis

Perineal
membrane

Fig. 16.6 The root of the penis. The corpora are shown in transverse section.

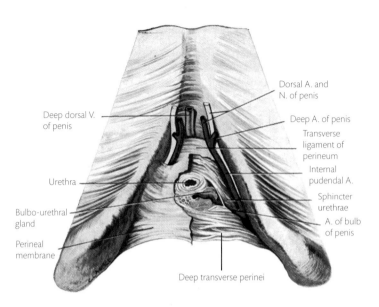

Fig. 16.7 Diagram showing the perineal membrane (right) and contents of the deep perineal pouch (left) in the male perineum.

inferior margin of the pubic symphysis and the anterior margin of the perineal membrane. The **deep dorsal vein of the penis** or **clitoris** enters the pelvis through this space [Fig. 16.7]. The perineal membrane, the superior layer of the urogenital diaphragm, and the muscle enclosed by them together constitute the **urogenital diaphragm**. This diaphragm closes the urogenital part of the inferior aperture of the pelvis [Figs. 16.4A, 16.4B].

The female superficial perineal pouch has the same elements as in the male, but the midline structures are split by the vestibule of the vagina. The superficial **membranous fascia** is poorly defined and is confined to the labia majora. The bulbospongiosus muscles, the urogenital diaphragm, and the bulb of the vestibule (which corresponds to the bulb of the penis) are split into right and left halves by the vestibule of the vagina [Figs. 16.8, 16.9]. They are less well formed and more difficult to define than in the male. The two crura of the clitoris are attached to the ischiopubic rami and covered by the ischiocavernosus muscle, as in the male.

The anal region

The anal region is triangular in shape and extends from the interischial line (posterior margin of the urogenital diaphragm) to the coccyx. The inferior aperture of the pelvis in this region is closed by the right and left **levator ani muscles** [Figs. 16.5, 16.8]. The muscles slope downwards, backwards, and medially from the lateral pelvic wall and are inserted into the central perineal tendon, the anal canal, and the **anococcygeal ligament** which stretches from the anal canal to the coccyx. The anal canal lies in the midline. On each side of the anal canal between the levator ani muscle and the lower part of the lateral wall of the pelvis is a space—the **ischioanal fossa** [Fig. 16.10]. The ischioanal fossa is filled with fatty superficial fascia which permits distension of the **anal canal**. The anal canal is surrounded by the voluntary **external anal sphincter**.

General features of the penis and male urethra

The penis consists of a root and a body. The root of the penis is in the perineum. The body is free and pendulous. The **body of the penis** contains three cylindrical masses of spongy, fibro-elastic, erectile tissue. They are the paired dorsally placed **corpora cavernosa** and the median ventral **corpus spongiosum**. The corpora cavernosa are bound together side by side by a thick sheath of tough fibrous tissue—the **tunica albuginea** [see Fig. 9.8]. The distal end of the corpus cavernosa are embedded in the **glans penis** which is the enlarged end of the corpus spongiosum. Proximally, at the root of the penis, the corpora cavernosa separate and form the crus of the penis. Each crura is attached to the everted inferomedial surface of the ischiopubic ramus [Fig. 16.6].

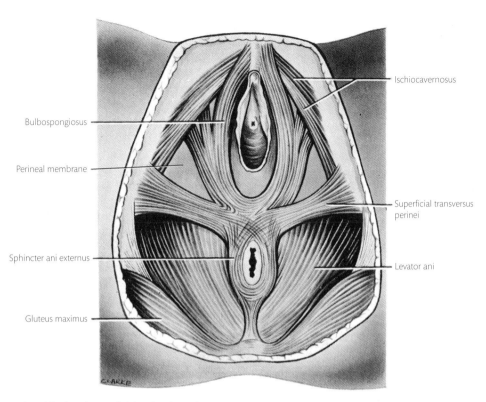

Fig. 16.8 Muscles of the female superficial perineal pouch.

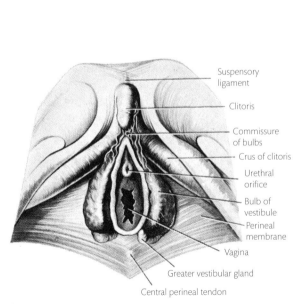

Fig. 16.9 Superficial perineal space in the female. The muscles have been removed to show the deeper structures.

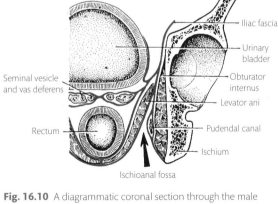

Fig. 16.10 A diagrammatic coronal section through the male pelvis to show the pelvic and perineal fasciae around the levator ani, obturator internus, and pelvic viscera.

In the body of the penis, the **corpus spongiosum** lies between and inferior to the corpora cavernosa. It consists of delicate erectile tissue and a thin **tunica albuginea**. Proximally, the corpus spongiosum expands to form the **bulb of the penis** which is attached to the perineal membrane [Fig. 16.6]. Distally, it expands to form the glans penis. The corpus spongiosum transmits the penile part of the urethra.

The male **urethra** is approximately 20 cm long. It extends from the most inferior part of the

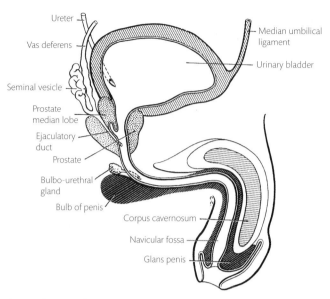

Fig. 16.11 A diagrammatic mid-sagittal section showing the bladder, urethra, and penis.

urinary bladder (the neck of the bladder) to the tip of the glans penis [Figs. 16.4B, 16.11]. It is arbitrarily divided into three parts: **prostatic part**, **membranous part**, and **penile part**. The **prostatic urethra** is 3 cm long and runs from the base of the prostate to a point anterior to the apex. (This part of the urethra lies in the pelvis and will be seen later.) The **membranous urethra** is 2–2.5 cm long and is within the urogenital diaphragm. It is surrounded by the sphincter urethrae. The **penile urethra** extends from where the urethra pierces the perineal

membrane to the external urethral orifice in the glans. As the urethra pierces the perineal membrane, it enters the bulb of the penis—the bulbar part of the penile urethra. In the bulb, the wall of the urethra dilates posteriorly to form the **intrabulbar fossa** [Fig. 16.4B]. The urethra then passes forwards through the corpus spongiosum and opens on the apex of the glans. In the glans, the urethra is expanded to form the **navicular fossa**.

Dissection 16.1 gives instructions on examining the urethra and the os of the cervix.

DISSECTION 16.1 Examination of the perineum

Objectives

I. To explore the urethra in the male and female.   II. To examine the cervix of the uterus.

Instructions

1. In the male, pass a greased catheter gently along the spongy part of the **urethra** in a plane parallel to the perineum. Direct the point towards the inferior surface of the penis to avoid entering recesses in the superior wall of the urethra. Palpate the tip of the catheter through the corpus spongiosum to follow its progress. The progress will be arrested in the intrabulbar fossa, midway between the root of the scrotum and the anus.

2. With the catheter in position, note that it is easily palpated in the spongy urethra.

3. In the female, identify the urethral orifice, and pass a catheter through the **urethra** into the bladder. Note that the catheter is readily palpable through the anterior vaginal wall.

4. If possible, introduce a speculum into the vagina and examine the **cervix** of the uterus as it projects through the anterior wall of the uppermost part of the vagina. The opening of the cervix—the **os uteri**—faces postero-inferiorly. It is a small, circular aperture in the cervix. In women who have had vaginal deliveries, the os is elongated transversely, with lips that are cleft or scarred.

The anal region

Superficial fascia

The superficial fascia in the **anal region** contains much lobulated fat which extends upwards into the ischioanal fossa.

Anal canal

The anal canal extends postero-inferiorly from the lower extremity of the rectum to the anus. It is 4 cm long and the superior part lies in the pelvic cavity. The circular muscle layer of the intestine is thickened in this part to form the involuntary **internal anal sphincter**. The lower parts of the levator ani muscles lie on either side of it. The inferior part of the anal canal lies in the perineum and is surrounded by the voluntary **external anal sphincter** [Fig. 16.12].

Anococcygeal ligament

This is a poorly defined fibro-fatty raphe permeated with muscle fibres from the levator ani and exter-

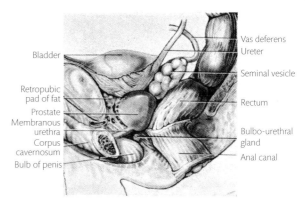

Bladder
Retropubic pad of fat
Prostate
Membranous urethra
Corpus cavernosum
Bulb of penis

Vas deferens
Ureter
Seminal vesicle
Rectum
Bulbo-urethral gland
Anal canal

Fig. 16.12 Diagram of male pelvic organs from the left side.

nal anal sphincter. It extends from the anus to the tip of the coccyx and helps to support the lower part of the rectum which lies on it.

Dissection 16.2 explores the ischioanal fossa.

External anal sphincter

The external anal sphincter has three parts which are indistinctly separate from each other. (1) The **subcutaneous part** surrounds the anal orifice. It

---

DISSECTION 16.2 Ischioanal fossa

Objectives

I. To uncover the anococcygeal ligament and central perineal tendon.   II. To identify and trace the inferior rectal vessels and nerves, and the perineal branch of the fourth sacral nerve.   III. To explore the ischioanal fossa.   IV. To identify and trace the pudendal nerve, internal pudendal vessels, inferior rectal nerves, and arteries in the ischioanal fossa.   V. To identify the initial segment of the posterior scrotal vessels and nerves.

Instructions

1. Make a transverse cut through the skin between the ischial tuberosities, immediately anterior to the anus. Make a median skin incision from the coccyx to the transverse incision, encircling the anus. Reflect the flaps of skin.

2. Note the radiating strands of muscle passing outwards from the anus. These are the terminal fibres of the longitudinal muscle of the intestine.

3. Remove the fascia from the external anal sphincter, the anococcygeal ligament, the margins of the anus, and the central perineal tendon.

4. Find the inferior rectal vessels and nerve on the medial side of the ischial tuberosity. Trace them through the ischioanal fossa to the anal canal [Fig. 16.5].

5. Trace the perineal branch of the fourth sacral nerve over the surface of the levator ani from the side of the coccyx. It supplies the external anal sphincter and the overlying skin.

6. With the body in the prone position, identify the sacrotuberous ligament deep to the inferior border of the gluteus maximus.

7. Expose the posterior scrotal or posterior labial vessels and nerves near the lateral part of the posterior margin of the perineal membrane [Fig. 16.5] and follow them into the superficial perineal space.

8. Complete the exposure of the **inferior rectal vessels** and **nerve**, following them to the lateral wall of the ischioanal fossa. Remove the fat from the ischioanal fossa. Find and follow the pudendal nerve and vessels in the **pudendal canal** on the lateral wall [Fig. 16.10].

has no bony attachments, but its fibres decussate anterior and posterior to the anus [Figs. 16.5, 16.8]. (2) The **superficial part** is oval in shape. Its fibres arise from the coccyx and anococcygeal ligament and pass anteriorly around the anus to the central perineal tendon. (3) The **deep part** arises from the central perineal tendon. It encircles the upper half of the anal canal and is fused with the puborectalis part of the levator ani.

Nerve supply: the perineal branch of the fourth sacral nerve and the inferior rectal nerves. **Actions**: the subcutaneous and superficial parts close the anus. The deep part acts with the puborectalis to draw the anal canal forwards to increase the angle between the anal canal and the rectum [see Fig. 17.5]. All parts of the external anal sphincter are formed of striated muscle fibres and are under voluntary control.

Ischioanal fossa

The ischioanal fossa is a fat-filled, wedge-shaped space, lateral to the anus and levator ani. The base of the fossa is the perineal skin. The upper edge lies where the levator ani muscle arises from the fascia covering the obturator internus. The lateral wall is the fascia covering the medial surface of the obturator internus. The obturator fascia is split to form the **pudendal canal** in which the pudendal nerve, internal pudendal artery and nerve to the obturator internus lie [Fig. 16.10]. The superomedial wall is the fascia covering the inferior surface of the levator ani. Posteriorly, the fossa is continuous with the **lesser sciatic foramen**. Anteriorly, it is continuous with a narrow space, which extends forwards between the levator ani and obturator internus, superior to the urogenital diaphragm. The fossa is wide and deep posteriorly but becomes narrow and more shallow anteriorly.

Vessels and nerves of the ischioanal fossa

The ischioanal fossa contains the pudendal nerve, the internal pudendal vessels, the nerve to the obturator internus, and the perineal branch of the fourth sacral nerve. The pudendal nerve, internal pudendal vessels, and the nerve to the obturator internus enter it through the lesser sciatic foramen. They run anteriorly on the lateral wall of the fossa in the pudendal canal. The **inferior rectal nerve** and **artery** are branches of the pudendal nerve and internal pudendal artery. (The inferior rectal nerve may arise directly from the third and fourth sacral nerves in the pelvis.) The inferior rectal vessels and

nerve pierce the medial wall of the pudendal canal, pass through the fat of the ischioanal fossa, and supply the levator ani, the external anal sphincter, the anal canal, and the overlying skin. The nerve communicates with the other cutaneous nerves of the perineum. The **artery** sends branches over the margin of the gluteus maximus into the buttock and anastomoses with the other rectal arteries in the anorectal wall. The pudendal nerve ends by dividing into the **perineal nerve** and the **dorsal nerve of the penis** or **clitoris** in the pudendal canal. These nerves continue through the pudendal canal with the internal pudendal vessels. The perineal branch of the fourth sacral nerve enters the ischioanal fossa at the side of the coccyx. It supplies the external anal sphincter and the skin posterior to the anus.

Superficial fascia

The membranous superficial fascia of the perineum forms the floor of the superficial perineal pouch [see Fig. 8.4; Fig. 16.4]. In the male, a median fibrous septum extends superiorly from the membranous layer to the raphe between the bulbospongiosus muscles [Fig. 16.5]. In the female, the membranous layer is split in the midline by the vestibule. In both sexes, the membranous layer continues forwards into the anterior abdominal wall. The fatty layer (which lies superficial to the membranous layer) is absent from the labium minus.

Superficial perineal pouch

Dissection 16.3 describes the dissection of the superficial vessels and nerves and muscles of the superficial perineal pouch.

Nerves and vessels of the superficial perineal space

The **lateral** and **medial posterior scrotal** or **posterior labial nerves** (S. 3, 4) arise from the perineal branch of pudendal nerve. They cross the anterior part of the ischioanal fossa, enter the superficial perineal pouch, and supply the skin of the urogenital region, including the scrotum or labium majus.

The **perineal branch of the posterior cutaneous nerve of the thigh** (S. 3) pierces the deep fascia anterolateral to the ischial tuberosity. It runs anteromedially across the pubic arch and supplies

DISSECTION 16.3 Superficial perineal pouch-1

Objectives

I. To explore the continuity of the superficial perineal space with the space in the anterior abdominal wall.   II. To uncover the membranous layer of the superficial fascia.   III. To dissect the muscles of the superficial perineal pouch.

Instructions

1. Explore the superficial perineal space from above by passing a finger down, deep to the membranous layer of the superficial fascia of the anterior abdominal wall.

2. In the female, remove the fat from the labium majus and expose the membranous layer. Incise it and explore the posterior part of the superficial perineal pouch. Note the posterior limit where the membranous layer passes superiorly to fuse with the perineal membrane.

3. In the male, expose the membranous layer of the superficial fascia in the perineum. Make an incision into it and explore one side of the superficial perineal space. Note the incomplete septum between the two sides and the continuity of the space into the anterior abdominal wall. (Note that, if the spongy part of the urethra ruptures into this space, urine will track forwards deep to the membranous layer into the anterior abdominal wall.)

4. Divide the membranous layer in the median plane, posterior to the scrotum or the frenulum of the labia. Carry the incision posterolaterally to each ischial tuberosity. Reflect the fascia, taking care not to damage the posterior scrotal or labial nerves and vessels which lie immediately deep to it. Confirm the attachments of the fascia.

5. Follow the posterior scrotal or posterior labial vessels and nerves through the superficial perineal space to the scrotum or labium majus.

6. Identify the **perineal branch** of the **posterior cutaneous nerve of the thigh**, 2–3 cm anterior to the ischial tuberosity. Follow its branches to the scrotum or labium majus.

7. Expose the structures in the superficial perineal space [Fig. 16.5]. These are: (1) the **ischiocavernosus muscle** which covers the inferior surface of each crus of the penis or clitoris; (2) the **bulbospongiosus muscle**: in the male, this muscle passes anterosuperiorly round each side of the bulb of the penis to meet dorsally. In the female, these muscles are smaller and surround the sides of the vestibule; (3) the **superficial transverse perineal muscles** which extend from the central perineal tendon to the ischial tuberosities in both sexes. Part of the perineal membrane can be seen in the interval between these three muscles [Figs. 16.5, 16.6].

the lateral and anterior parts of the scrotum or labium majus.

Two **posterior scrotal** or **posterior labial arteries** arise from the internal pudendal artery in the anterior part of the pudendal canal. One of them may give rise to a small **perineal artery** which runs on the superficial transverse perineal muscle to the central tendon of the perineum [Fig. 16.5].

Dissection 16.4 explores the deeper structures in the superficial perineal pouch.

Superficial perineal muscles

Each **superficial transverse perineal muscle** is a small muscle that arises from the medial side of the ischial tuberosity and joins its fellow in the central perineal tendon. In the female, it is very small, pale in colour, and difficult to define.

The **bulbospongiosus muscles** are different in the two sexes. In the male [Fig. 16.5], they arise from the central perineal tendon and the median raphe that stretches anteriorly from the central perineal tendon. The fibres curve anterosuperiorly round the bulb and posterior part of the corpus spongiosum. The posterior fibres pass round the bulb to the perineal membrane. The middle fibres form the largest part. They encircle the corpus spongiosum and unite, dorsal to it. The anterior fibres pass round the corpus spongiosum and the corresponding corpus cavernosum to join on the dorsal surface of the penis. The anterior fibres constitute the **bulbocavernosus**. In the female, the fibres arise from the central perineal tendon. They sweep round the sides of the vestibule, inferior to the greater vestibular glands and the bulbs of the vestibule, and are inserted into the sides and dorsum of the clitoris [Figs. 16.8, 16.9].

The **ischiocavernosus muscles** arise from the ramus of the ischium, close to the ischial tuberosity.

DISSECTION 16.4 Superficial perineal pouch-2

Objective

I. To remove the muscles of the superficial perineal pouch and expose the deeper structures.

Instructions

1. Place a finger in the ischioanal fossa and push gently forwards. It will pass easily above the urogenital diaphragm, lateral to the levator ani. The **urogenital diaphragm** can now be felt easily between the finger and thumb. Note that it is a tough, rigid structure in both the male and female, though it is difficult to define by dissection.

2. Divide the posterior scrotal or labial vessels and nerves and turn them aside.

3. Separate the superficial perineal muscles and expose part of the perineal membrane between them.

4. Cut the transverse perineal muscles from the central perineal tendon. Turn them aside, and expose the deep branches of the perineal nerve.

5. In the male, separate the two bulbospongiosus muscles along the raphe. Turn them away from the bulb of the penis and follow the fibres to their termination.

6. In the female, lift the bulbospongiosus muscles [Fig. 16.8] from the underlying bulb of the vestibule on each side of the vaginal orifice.

7. In both sexes, strip the ischiocavernosus muscles from the crura of the penis or clitoris and expose the crura.

They run forwards on the crus of the penis or clitoris and are inserted into the crus anteriorly.

Nerve supply: all three muscles are supplied by the perineal branch of the pudendal nerve. **Actions**: the transverse perineal muscles help to steady the central perineal tendon and, through it, the posterior part of the perineal membrane. The central perineal tendon supports the structures superior to it, i.e. the prostate or vagina. The ischiocavernosus may assist with erection by compressing the deep vein leaving the crus. The bulbospongiosus in the male compresses the bulb and corpus spongiosum, thus emptying the urethra of any residual urine or semen. Its anterior fibres can assist with erection by compressing the deep dorsal vein of the penis and impeding venous drainage from the cavernous tissue. In the female, the bulbospongiosus is a sphincter of the vagina and is assisted by the underlying erectile tissue of the bulb.

Central tendon of the perineum

The central perineal tendon is an indefinite mass of fibrous tissue between the anal canal and the bulb of the penis in the male or the vagina in the female. It gives attachment to the superficial and deep transverse perinei muscles, the bulbospongiosus, the superficial and deep parts of the external anal sphincter, the longitudinal muscle of the rectum, and some of the anterior fibres of the levator ani [Fig. 16.9]. The tendon is an important structure in the female as it supports the uterus.

↪ Tearing or stretching of the central perineal tendon in childbirth removes support from the posterior wall of the vagina and allows prolapse of the uterus through the vaginal orifice.

Crus of the penis and clitoris

These paired bodies of erectile tissue are parts of the root of the penis or clitoris [Figs. 16.6, 16.9]. The crura are divergent posterior parts of the corpora cavernosa. They are attached to the everted medial surfaces of the pubic arch and the adjacent parts of the perineal membrane. Each crus is covered by, and gives attachment to, the corresponding ischiocavernosus muscle. The deep artery and vein of the penis or clitoris enter and leave through the superior surface. At their distal ends, the corpora cavernosa are inserted into the glans of the penis or clitoris [see Figs. 9.9, 9.10]. (The glans penis is the expanded end of the corpus spongiosum. The glans clitoris is a separate structure united to the bulbs of the vestibule by connective tissue and a narrow strip of erectile tissue.)

Bulb of the penis

The bulb of the penis is the expanded proximal part of the corpus spongiosum. It is attached to the inferior surface of the perineal membrane and is covered by the bulbospongiosus muscles [Figs. 16.5, 16.6]. The urethra pierces the perineal membrane to enter the bulb. The **ducts of the bulbo-urethral glands** and the arteries of the bulb pierce the perineal membrane, close to the urethra, and enter the bulb. The artery of the bulb is a branch of the internal pudendal artery [Fig. 16.7].

Bulb of the vestibule

The bulbs of the vestibule are paired oval masses of erectile tissue on either side of the vestibule. They are attached to the perineal membrane and overlap the greater vestibular glands posteriorly [Fig. 16.9]. The bulbs narrow anteriorly and are united by a plexus of veins, known as the **commissure of the bulbs**, which lies between the urethra and the clitoris. The commissure is attached to the glans of the clitoris by a thin strip of erectile tissue. This strip of erectile tissue, the glans, the commissure, and the bulbs together correspond to the corpus spongiosum and glans penis of the male. Each bulb is covered by the bulbospongiosus muscle [Fig. 16.8].

Greater vestibular glands

The greater vestibular glands lie on either side of the vestibule between the perineal membrane and the bulb of the vestibule [Fig. 16.9]. Each gland has a long duct that opens in the vestibule at the side of the vaginal orifice, between the hymen and the labium minus.

Dissection 16.5 explores the perineal membrane.

Perineal membrane (inferior fascia of the urogenital diaphragm)

The perineal membrane is a triangular sheet of fibrous tissue. The posterior margin extends transversely between the two ischial tuberosities through the central perineal tendon. The truncated apex almost reaches the pubic symphysis. Laterally, the perineal membrane is attached to the pubic arch [Figs. 16.6, 16.7, 16.9]. Its posterior margin is fused with the membranous layer of the superficial perineal fascia and with the superior fascia of the urogenital diaphragm. Thus both superficial and deep **perineal spaces** are closed posteriorly [Fig. 16.4B]. Anteriorly, the truncated margin of the perineal membrane fuses with the superior fascia of the urogenital diaphragm and closes the deep perineal space. At the anterior margin, the perineal membrane is thickened to form the **transverse perineal ligament** which is separated from the pubic symphysis by a small gap. The **deep dorsal vein of the penis** or **clitoris** enters the pelvis through this gap [Fig. 16.7].

In the anatomical position, the perineal membrane lies horizontally between the superficial and deep perineal pouches. The **urethra** and **vagina** pierce the membrane in the median plane. In the male, the urethra is 2.5 cm from the pubic symphysis and is accompanied by the ducts of the bulbourethral glands and the arteries of the bulb. In the female, the urethra is closer to the symphysis and anterior to the vagina. The **arteries of the bulbs** accompany the vagina through the perineal membrane. The internal pudendal arteries and the dorsal nerves of the penis or clitoris pierce the membrane anterolaterally [Figs. 16.7, 16.13].

DISSECTION 16.5 Perineal membrane

Objective

I. To complete the exposure of the perineal membrane.

Instructions

1. Remove the superficial perineal muscles, and detach one crus of the penis carefully from the ischiopubic ramus. Turn it forwards to expose the deep artery and vein on its superior surface.

2. In the male, find and trace the dorsal artery and nerve of the penis. They lie close to the deep artery [Fig. 16.7] and pass into a position lateral to the **deep dorsal vein** on the dorsum of the penis. Trace the deep dorsal vein proximally till it disappears into the pelvis between the pubic symphysis and the anterior margin of the perineal membrane.

3. In the male, detach the bulb of the penis from the central perineal tendon. Turn it forwards to expose the **urethra** and the **artery of the bulb** piercing the perineal membrane and entering the bulb. The ducts of the bulbo-urethral glands lie at the sides of the urethra but are difficult to identify.

4. Expose as much of the perineal membrane as possible without damage to the urethra and the artery to the bulb.

5. In the female, raise the posterior end of the bulb of the vestibule to expose the greater vestibular gland. Follow it forwards to its duct, and find the artery of the bulb. Divide this artery, and turn the bulb forwards to expose as much of the perineal membrane as possible.

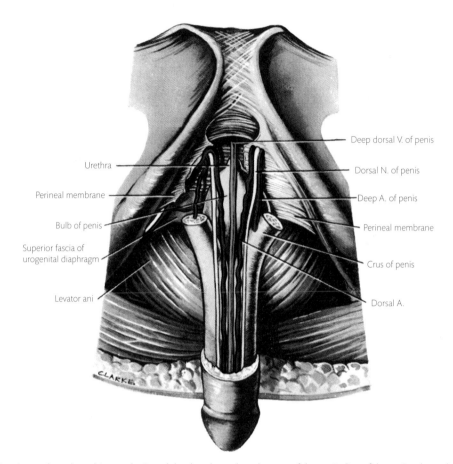

Urethra

Perineal membrane

Bulb of penis

Superior fascia of
urogenital diaphragm

Levator ani

Deep dorsal V. of penis

Dorsal N. of penis

Deep A. of penis

Perineal membrane

Crus of penis

Dorsal A.

Fig. 16.13 Drawing to show the pubic symphysis and the dorsal vessels and nerves of the penis. Part of the perineal membrane and sphincter urethrae muscle have been removed on the right side.

Dissection 16.6 explores the deep perineal pouch.

Deep perineal pouch

The deep perineal pouch or urogenital diaphragm lies between the perineal membrane and the superior fascia of the urogenital diaphragm [Figs. 16.4A, 16.4B]. It contains the sphincter urethrae, the deep transverse perineal muscles in both sexes, and the bulbo-urethral glands in the male [Fig. 16.7]. The space is traversed by the urethra and vagina and transmits

---

DISSECTION 16.6 Deep perineal pouch

Objective

I. To cut the perineal membrane and expose the contents of the deep perineal pouch.

Instructions

1. Separate the perineal membrane from the pubic arch on the side from which the crus of the penis or clitoris was removed. Carefully reflect the membrane medially. This exposes a thin sheet of muscle—the **sphincter urethrae**—anteriorly and the **deep transverse perinei muscles** posteriorly.

They are difficult to dissect and differentiate from each other.

2. Follow the **internal pudendal artery** and the dorsal nerve of the penis or clitoris forwards in this deep perineal space and through the perineal membrane. Identify the branches of the artery—the deep and dorsal arteries of the penis or clitoris. Find and trace the artery of the bulb.

3. In the male, look for the **bulbo-urethral gland** posterolateral to the urethra on the superior surface of the deep transverse perineal muscle.

the internal pudendal vessels and the dorsal nerves of the penis or clitoris. The part of the male urethra in the deep perineal pouch is the membranous urethra. It is the least distensible part of the male urethra. It is 2–2.5 cm long and is continuous above with the prostatic urethra through the superior fascia of the urogenital diaphragm, and below with the penile part of the urethra through the perineal membrane [Fig. 16.4].

The **sphincter urethrae** consists of transverse muscle fibres which arise from the medial surface of the ischiopubic ramus. In the male, the fibres pass medially to encircle the urethra and unite with the fibres from the opposite side, anterior and posterior to the urethra. The most posterior fibres form the **deep transverse perinei muscle** [Fig. 16.7]. In the female, the arrangement is the same, but the posterior fibres are attached to the vaginal wall. **Nerve supply**: small branches of the perineal nerve. **Action**: voluntary constriction of the urethra.

Female urethra

The female urethra is 4–5 cm long and 6 mm wide. It is dilatable and extends from the neck of the bladder through the pelvic cavity and urogenital diaphragm to open immediately anterior to the vaginal orifice. Throughout its length, it is attached to the anterior wall of the vagina [see Fig. 17.4].

Internal pudendal artery

The internal pudendal artery arises in the pelvis from the internal iliac artery. It enters the gluteal region through the greater sciatic foramen and leaves it almost immediately through the lesser sciatic foramen to enter the ischioanal fossa. In the ischioanal fossa, it runs in the **pudendal canal** [Fig. 16.10]. It enters the deep perineal space at the posterior border of the perineal membrane and runs forwards with the dorsal nerve of the penis or clitoris. One to 2 cm posterior to the pubic symphysis, it pierces the perineal membrane either before or after dividing into the dorsal and deep arteries of the penis or clitoris [Figs. 16.7, 16.13].

Branches

The inferior rectal, perineal, and posterior scrotal or labial branches of the internal pudendal artery are described earlier.

The **artery of the bulb** arises in the posterior part of the deep perineal space. It passes medially and supplies the sphincter urethrae and the bulbourethral gland in the male. It then pierces the perineal membrane to enter and supply the bulb of

the penis in the male and the bulb of the vestibule in the female [Fig. 16.7].

The **deep artery of the penis** or **clitoris** enters the crus and supplies the crus and corpus cavernosum. The **dorsal artery** passes anterosuperiorly on to the dorsum of the penis or clitoris [Fig. 16.13].

Pudendal nerve [S. (1), 2, 3, 4]

The pudendal nerve arises from the sacral plexus in the pelvis. It leaves the pelvis through the greater sciatic foramen and enters the ischioanal fossa through the lesser sciatic foramen. In the ischioanal fossa, it gives off the **inferior rectal nerve**, runs anteriorly in the pudendal canal, and divides into the perineal nerve and the dorsal nerve of the penis or clitoris.

The **perineal nerve** passes with the internal pudendal artery to the posterior margin of the urogenital diaphragm. It gives off two **posterior scrotal** or **labial nerves** and divides into small terminal branches. These branches enter the superficial and deep perineal pouches to supply the muscles, the bulb of the penis, or the bulb of the vestibule.

The **dorsal nerve of the penis** or **clitoris** runs in the pudendal canal and in the deep perineal space close to the pubic arch. It gives a branch to the crus of the penis or clitoris and then runs with the dorsal artery of the penis or clitoris [Figs. 16.13, 16.14]. From the dorsal surface of the

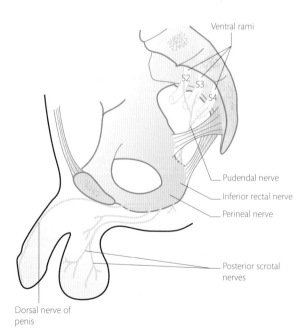

Fig. 16.14 Course and branches of the pudendal nerve.

penis, the nerve sends branches round the side of that organ to its ventral surface. It thus supplies all the skin of the penis and clitoris and the glans.

The pudendal nerve also carries **autonomic nerve fibres** to the erectile tissue of the penis and clitoris.

Bulbo-urethral glands

These small glands lie posterolateral to the membranous urethra in the male [Fig. 16.7]. The long ducts pierce the perineal membrane with the urethra and open into the spongy part of the urethra in the bulb of the penis [Fig. 16.11].

Lymph vessels of the perineum

The numerous and important lymph vessels of the perineum cannot be demonstrated by dissection.

Lymph from all the perineal structures, including the inferior parts of the anal canal, vagina, and urethra, drain to the **medial superficial inguinal lymph nodes**. Lymph from the upper parts of the anal canal, vagina, and urethra drains superiorly into the pelvis [see Fig. 18.2]. Some deep lymphatics run along the internal pudendal vessels and the deep dorsal vein of the penis to nodes in the pelvis. (The testicular lymph vessels drain to the lumbar lymph nodes.)

➲ It is important to remember that enlargement of the medial superficial inguinal lymph nodes may be the first sign of infection in the perineum.

Dissection 16.7 examines the perineal surface of the levator ani.

See Clinical Applications 16.1–16.4 for the practical implications of the anatomy in this chapter.

DISSECTION 16.7 Perineal surface of the levator ani

Objective

I. To study the levator ani from the inferior aspect.

Instructions

1. Remove the exposed muscles of the deep perineal space and the superior fascia of the urogenital diaphragm.

2. Remove the fat and fascia deep to the urogenital diaphragm to expose the perineal surface of the **levator ani** as much as possible [Fig. 16.13]. Note that the anterior part of this muscle has a free medial border separated from its fellow by a gap. The most medial fibres of the levator ani are inserted into the central tendon of the perineum.

3. Confirm the gap between the margins of the levator ani which transmits the urethra in the male and the urethra and vagina in the female. Note that some of the fibres which pass to the central perineal tendon turn round the posterior vaginal wall and form a partial sphincter for it. In the male, the prostate lies on the medial margins of the levator ani, with its apex projecting downwards in the gap between them. These parts of the levator ani are known as the **levator prostatae**.

4. Trace the more posterior fibres of the levator ani to the sides of the anal canal, deep to the external anal sphincter. Some of the fibres of the levator join the longitudinal muscle layer of the intestine and extend to the perianal skin.

5. Confirm the origin of the levator ani from the fascia covering the obturator internus muscle. Note that each levator ani muscle forms a continuous sheet with the corresponding sacrospinous ligament. The right and left parts of the levator ani meet at the insertion into the central perineal tendon, anal canal, and anococcygeal ligament. Thus together, they form a fibromuscular floor for the pelvis—the **pelvic diaphragm**.

6. Note that the pelvic floor is deficient anteriorly where the two levator ani muscles separate, but this gap is filled by the urogenital diaphragm inferiorly.

CLINICAL APPLICATION 16.1 Rupture of the penile urethra

Rupture of the bulbar part of the penile urethra results in a circumscribed swelling of the perineum, scrotum, and lower anterior abdominal wall from extravasation of urine.

Study question 1: using your knowledge of the anatomy of the fasciae in this region, explain how urine tracks into the scrotum. (Answer: the superficial membranous fascia extends over the scrotum [Fig. 16.4B] and allows urine from the ruptured site to enter the scrotum.)

Study question 2: what feature of the perineal fascia prevents urine from tracking into the ischioanal fossa? (Answer: the superficial membranous layer fuses with the posterior margin of the perineal membrane and prevents spread of extravasated urine posteriorly.)

Study question 3: explain why urine spreads into the anterior abdominal wall, but not into the thighs.

(Answer: continuation of the superficial membranous layer of the perineum with the membranous layer of the superficial fascia of the anterior abdominal wall allows for extravasated urine to spread into the anterior abdominal wall. The attachments of the membranous layer of superficial fascia to the fascia lata of the thigh, prevent spread of urine into the thigh.)

CLINICAL APPLICATION 16.2 Urethral stricture

Strictures, or narrowing, of the urethra can occur following instrumentation, infection, or trauma. Micturating cystourethrogram (MCUG) is a procedure where the urinary bladder is filled with iodinated contrast and radiographs are taken as the patient micturates. Fig. 16.15 is an MCUG of a patient with strictures in the membranous and bulbar urethra (straight arrows). Back pressure has resulted in a circumscribed dilatation in the prostatic urethra (curved arrow).

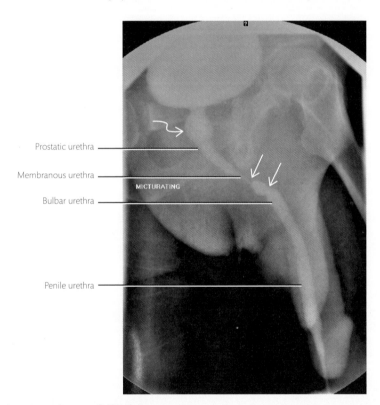

Prostatic urethra
Membranous urethra
MICTURATING
Bulbar urethra

Penile urethra

Fig. 16.15 Micturating cystourethrogram (MCUG) showing strictures in the bulbar and membranous urethrae (straight arrows), and dilatation in the prostatic urethra (curved arrow).

CLINICAL APPLICATION 16.3 Fistula *in ano*

Infections in the fat of the ischioanal fossa can result in the formation of a 'perianal abscess'. Such an abscess may either burst medially into the anal canal or inferiorly to the outside through the perineal skin. An abscess may also drain in both directions, i.e. into the anal canal and the perineal skin. When this happens, a track may be formed, leading from the skin to the anal canal. This is known as **fistula *in ano***.

CLINICAL APPLICATION 16.4 Episiotomy

Episiotomy is a surgical incision of the perineum and posterolateral wall of the vagina to enlarge the vaginal orifice during childbirth. An episiotomy is done to reduce the risk of uncontrolled tearing of the perineal tissue. A mediolateral episiotomy extends downwards and laterally from the inferior margin of the vaginal orifice. Care is taken to avoid injury to the central perineal tendon and muscles of the anal sphincter which lie in the midline.

CHAPTER 17
The pelvic viscera

Ovaries

The ovaries are pinkish-white, ovoid structures, approximately 3 cm long, 1.5 cm wide, and 1 cm thick. Between the two ovaries, they usually produce one mature **ovum** per menstrual cycle. This ovum is released into the peritoneal cavity. In women after the menopause, the entire ovary shrinks following the loss of hormonal stimulation.

Each ovary lies near the lateral wall of the pelvic cavity in a slight depression between the ureter posteromedially, the external iliac vein laterally, and the obturator nerve posterolaterally. The uterine tubes in the free margin of the broad ligament lie anterior to the ovary [Figs. 17.1, 17.2]. The lateral end of the **uterine tube** curves round the lateral end of the ovary and is attached to the ovary by one or more of the **fimbriae** [see Fig. 15.11]. The ovary is attached to the superior surface of the

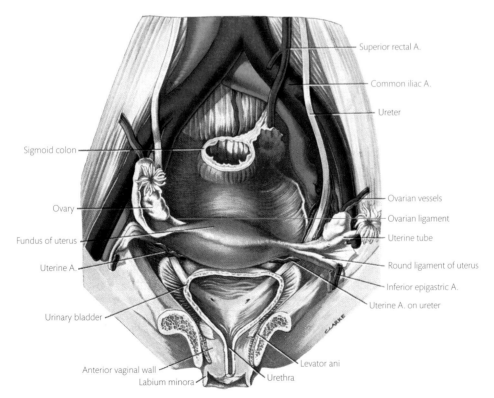

Fig. 17.1 The female pelvis, seen from the front, after removal of the greater part of the bodies of the pubic bones and the anterior parts of the bladder and urethra.

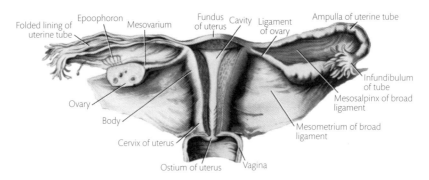

Fig. 17.2 The posterosuperior surface of the broad ligament and associated structures. The vagina, uterus, and left uterine tube have been opened, and the left ovary is sectioned parallel to the broad ligament.

The pelvic viscera

256

broad ligament by a short fold of peritoneum—the **mesovarium**. The ovarian vessels run through the mesovarium and enter the **hilus** of the ovary. The medial end of the ovary is attached to the uterus by the **ligament of the ovary**. When the **vermiform appendix** is pelvic in position, it may be very close to the right ovary.

During pregnancy, the broad ligament and ovary are carried superiorly with the expanding uterus. When these structures return to the pelvis after the birth of the child, the ovary may return to a site other than that described above [see Fig. 15.11; Fig. 17.1].

Vessels and nerves

Each **ovarian artery** arises from the aorta below the renal artery [see Fig. 11.59]. It descends on the posterior abdominal wall, crosses the external iliac artery, and enters the suspensory ligament of the ovary. It sends branches through the mesovarium to the ovary and continues medially in the broad ligament to supply the uterine tubes. It ends by anastomosing with the uterine artery.

The **ovarian veins** leave the hilus as a **pampiniform plexus of veins** on the ovarian artery. A single ovarian vein is formed near the superior aperture of the pelvis. The right ovarian vein ascends to drain into the inferior vena cava, and the left into the left renal vein.

The **lymph vessels** from the ovary unite with those from the uterine tube and the fundus of the uterus. They ascend with the vein and end in the lumbar lymph nodes which lie between the bifurcation of the aorta and the renal arteries.

The surface of the ovary is covered by cuboidal epithelium which is continuous with the peritoneum of the mesovarium.

Uterine tubes

Each uterine tube is approximately 10 cm long. It is arbitrarily divided into an **intramural part** (within the wall of the uterus), an **isthmus**, an **ampulla**, and an **infundibulum**. The isthmus, ampulla, and infundibulum lie in the free margin of the broad ligament. The isthmus begins at the junction of the body and fundus of the uterus and is 2–3 cm long. It continues laterally with the expanded and slightly convoluted **ampulla** which passes towards the lateral pelvic wall. Here it curves over the lateral extremity of the ovary and expands into the funnel-shaped **infundibulum**. The infundibulum opens into the peritoneal cavity. The tubal opening is surrounded by a fringe of finger-like processes known as the **fimbriae**. One or two of the fimbriae are attached to the ovary—the **ovarian fimbriae**. Near the time of ovulation, the tube becomes turgid and the infundibulum moves medially over the ovary. The discharged ovum is carried into the tube by the action of the ciliated lining of the tube. The fimbriae are continuous with the numerous longitudinal folds of mucous membrane that virtually fill the infundibulum and ampulla [Figs. 17.2, 17.3].

Dissection 17.1 describes the dissection of the uterine tube and ovarian artery.

Blood vessels and lymphatics of the uterine tube

The blood vessels of the uterine tube are branches of the ovarian and uterine vessels. The lymph vessels join those of the ovary and pass to the lumbar nodes.

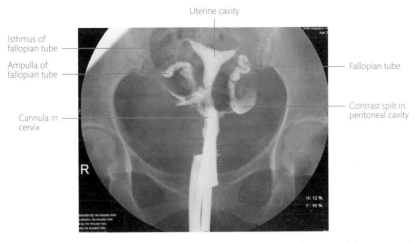

Uterine cavity

Isthmus of
fallopian tube

Ampulla of
fallopian tube

Cannula in
cervix

Fallopian tube

Contrast spilt in
peritoneal cavity

R

Fig. 17.3 Image of a hysterosalpingogram. This is a radiological procedure done to assess the cavity of the uterus and patency of the uterine tubes. The dye—an iodinated contrast—is injected into the cervix through a cannula. The spill of contrast into the peritoneal cavity demonstrates the patency of the tubes.

DISSECTION 17.1 Uterine tube and ovarian artery

Objectives

I. To study the external and internal features of the uterine tube.   II. To identify and trace the ovarian artery.

Instructions

1. Open one uterine tube longitudinally. Note the folds of its mucous membrane, the thinness of its wall, and the variations in its internal diameter.

2. Trace the ovarian vessels to the ovary and uterine tube. Follow them to their origins and terminations. Note the course of the ovarian artery in the broad ligament and its anastomosis with the uterine artery near the uterus.

Ligament of the ovary

The ligament of the ovary is a band of connective tissue and smooth muscle which extends from the medial end of the ovary to the superior surface of the junction of the uterine tube and uterus. It forms a ridge on the superior surface of the broad ligament [Fig. 17.2].

Round ligament of the uterus

The round ligament of the uterus consists of the same tissue as the ligament of the ovary. It arises from the tubo-uterine junction on the inferior sur-face. The round ligament passes to the side wall of the pelvis, forming a ridge on the inferior surface of the broad ligament. It then sweeps forwards, immediately deep to the peritoneum, to the deep inguinal ring. Here it hooks round the lateral side of the inferior epigastric vessels, traverses the inguinal canal, and spreads out to its attachment in the labium majora [Fig. 17.1]. The ligament of the ovary and the round ligament of the uterus together represent the remains of the **gubernaculum**.

Pelvic parts of the ureters

The ureter is 25 cm long and half of it lies in the pelvis. The pelvic part of each ureter begins at the brim of the pelvis where the ureter crosses the origin of the external iliac artery [see Figs. 15.11, 15.13; Fig. 17.4]. It ends in the bladder by entering its posterosuperior angle. From its origin on the external iliac artery, the pelvic part of the ureter runs postero-inferiorly on the front of the internal iliac artery. It is deep to the peritoneum of the lateral wall of the pelvis and postero-inferior to the ovary in the female [Fig. 17.5]. At the level of the ischial spine, it curves anteromedially above the levator ani and runs forward to the bladder. In the female, it passes immediately lateral to the **lateral fornix of the vagina**, inferior to the broad ligament and the uterine artery [see Fig. 17.18]. In the male, it remains in contact with the peritoneum initially and then runs deep to the vas deferens before it reaches the bladder [Figs. 17.4, 17.6].

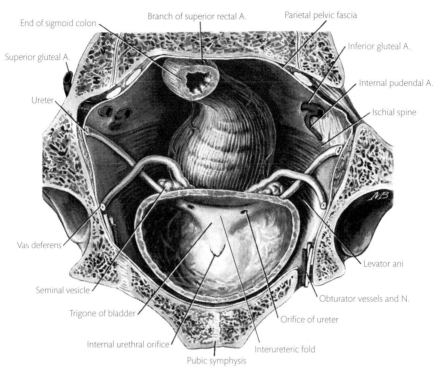

Branch of superior rectal A.

Parietal pelvic fascia

End of sigmoid colon

Inferior gluteal A.

Superior gluteal A.

Internal pudendal A.

Ureter

Ischial spine

Vas deferens

Levator ani

Seminal vesicle

Obturator vessels and N.

Trigone of bladder

Orifice of ureter

Internal urethral orifice

Interureteric fold

Pubic symphysis

Fig. 17.4 The male pelvis, seen from above and in front.

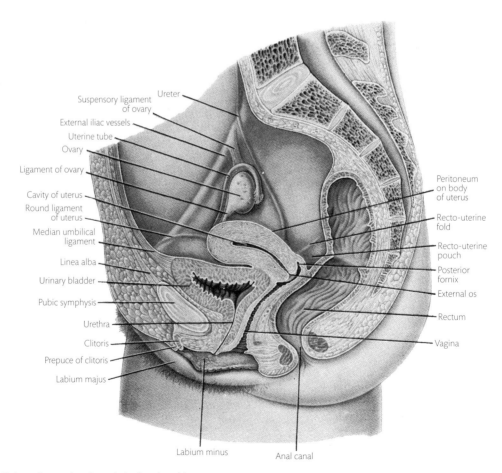

Suspensory ligament of ovary

Ureter

External iliac vessels

Uterine tube

Ovary

Ligament of ovary

Peritoneum on body of uterus

Cavity of uterus

Recto-uterine fold

Round ligament of uterus

Recto-uterine pouch

Median umbilical ligament

Posterior fornix

Linea alba

External os

Urinary bladder

Rectum

Pubic symphysis

Urethra

Vagina

Clitoris

Prepuce of clitoris

Labium majus

Labium minus

Anal canal

Fig. 17.5 A median section through the female pelvis.

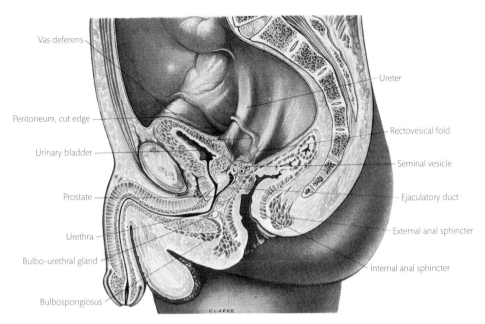

Vas deferens

Peritoneum, cut edge

Urinary bladder

Prostate

Urethra

Bulbo-urethral gland

Bulbospongiosus

Ureter

Rectovesical fold

Seminal vesicle

Ejaculatory duct

External anal sphincter

Internal anal sphincter

Fig. 17.6 A section through the male pelvis.

In both sexes, the ureters pass obliquely through the bladder wall in an inferomedial direction. The ureteric opening in the bladder is at the upper angles of the **trigone of the bladder** [Fig. 17.4].

Dissection 17.2 describes the dissection of the bladder, the ligaments of the bladder, and structures in the broad ligament.

Internal surface of the urinary bladder

The internal surface of the contracted bladder is ridged by folds of mucous membrane. On the posterior wall is a smooth triangular area—the **trigone of the bladder**. At the inferior angle of the trigone is the median **internal urethral orifice**. At the

DISSECTION 17.2 Pelvic viscera

Objectives

I. To study the peritoneal coverings and the external and internal surfaces of the bladder. II. To identify the median umbilical, puboprostatic, and pubovesical ligaments of the bladder. III. To expose the ligament of the ovary and round ligament of the uterus, the uterine artery, and the ureter in the broad ligament.

Instructions

1. Remove the peritoneum from the superior surface of the bladder, stopping short of the depths of the uterovesical pouch in the female.

2. Identify and follow the median umbilical ligament upwards [Fig. 17.7] from the apex of the bladder.

3. Remove the fat from the retropubic space and from the paravesical fossae. Push a finger inferiorly between the bladder and the pubis till resistance of the puboprostatic or pubovesical ligaments is felt. Carry the finger round the side of the bladder and note the presence of loose connective tissue here.

4. Place a finger in the ischioanal fossa, and note that a finger in the pelvic cavity is separated from it by the levator ani muscle and its fascia. As far as possible, explore the relation of the pelvic cavity to the ischioanal fossa and perineum by passing the fingers forwards and backwards.

5. Displace the apex of the bladder posteriorly and expose the puboprostatic or pubovesical ligaments.

6. In the male, trace the vas deferens and ureter to the base of the bladder on both sides.

7. In the female, expose the ligament of the ovary, the round ligament of the uterus, and the ureter on the side on which the uterine tube was opened. Identify the uterine artery crossing above the ureter at the side of the vaginal fornix.

8. Make an incision through the bladder wall along the lateral margins of the superior surface [Fig. 17.7]. Carry these to the lateral extremities of the base, then fold back the superior wall of the bladder and examine the internal surface [Figs. 17.1, 17.4].

Pelvic parts of the ureters

259

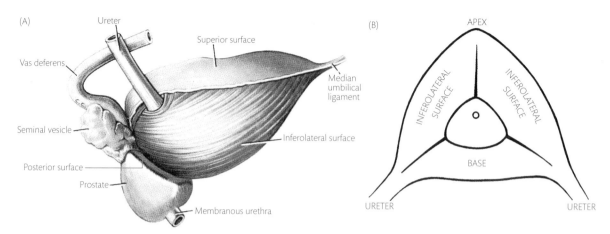

Fig. 17.7 (A) Lateral view of the urinary bladder, prostate, and seminal vesicle. (B) Urinary bladder, as seen from below. The enclosed area in the centre marks the position of the prostate.

superolateral angles of the trigone are the small, obliquely placed **ureteric orifices**. The two ureteric orifices are joined by a well-defined **interureteric fold**. This fold forms the superior margin of the trigone [Fig. 17.4].

Orifices of the ureters

Pass a fine seeker into each ureteric orifice. It passes obliquely through the bladder wall into the ureter [Fig. 17.4]. As a result of the obliquity, compression of the intramural parts of the ureters occur during bladder contraction, preventing urinary reflux into the ureter. This is important in children, as reflux is associated with urinary infection and renal scarring.

Internal urethral orifice

The internal urethral orifice is a Y-shaped slit at the inferior angle of the trigone. In the male, the mucous membrane between the limbs of the Y bulges forwards to form the **uvula of the bladder**. The bulge is produced by the median lobe of the prostate gland which lies immediately below the trigone [Fig. 17.4].

Retropubic space

The retropubic space is the space between the anterior surface of the bladder and the pelvic surface of the pubic bones and symphysis pubis. It is filled with loose fatty connective tissue—the **retropubic

pad of fat—which extends posterolaterally on the sides of the bladder as far as the ureters. Posterior to the bodies of the pubic bones, the space is limited inferiorly by the strong puboprostatic ligaments which pass to the neck of the bladder and to the base of the prostate in the male, and the pubovesical/pubo-urethral ligaments which pass to the neck of the bladder and the urethra in the female. Superiorly, the space is continuous with loose extraperitoneal tissue which extends up the anterior abdominal wall to the level of the umbilicus, between the lateral umbilical ligaments. This arrangement permits the bladder to expand superiorly between the anterior abdominal wall and its peritoneum.

Further dissection of the pelvic viscera requires hemisection of the pelvis. Study the anatomy of the pubic symphysis before proceeding with the dissection.

Pubic symphysis

The pubic symphysis unites the two hip bones anteriorly. It is a secondary cartilaginous joint. The articular surfaces of the pubic bones are covered with hyaline cartilage and united by a disc of fibrous tissue which has a central slit-like cavity. The disc is surrounded by ligaments. Anteriorly, the ligament is very strong and is fused superficially with the abdominal aponeuroses. Inferiorly, it forms the strong **arcuate ligament**—a curved band which rounds off the apex of the pubic arch and extends along the inferior pubic rami. The deep dorsal vein of the penis or clitoris enters the pelvis between the arcuate and transverse perineal ligament.

The pubic symphysis permits a small amount of movement between the hip bones and absorbs shocks transmitted from the femora. In common with many other tissues, the disc contains more tissue fluid in the later stages of pregnancy and may permit a slight increase in range of movement in childbirth [Figs. 17.4, 17.5, 17.8].

Dissection 17.3 gives instructions for hemisectioning the pelvis.

Urinary bladder

When empty, the urinary bladder lies in the antero-inferior part of the lesser pelvis [see Figs. 15.11, 15.13]. The empty bladder has the shape of a three-sided pyramid, with its apex directed anteriorly and the base posteriorly [Fig. 17.7]. It becomes spherical when distended [Fig. 17.9]. The bladder lies relatively free in the surrounding loose extraperitoneal tissue, except at its inferior part—the **neck**. The neck is held firmly in place by the **puboprostatic ligament** in the male and the **pubovesical liga-**

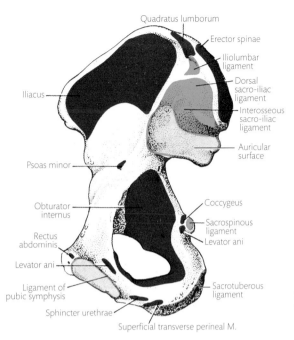

Fig. 17.8 The medial aspect of the right hip bone. Red: muscle attachments. Blue: ligamentous attachments.

ments in the female. Thus the bladder is free to expand superiorly in the extraperitoneal tissue of the anterior abdominal wall, stripping the peritoneum from the transversalis fascia. ➲ This feature permits

---

DISSECTION 17.3 Hemisection of the pelvis

Objective

I. To separate the two halves of the pelvis by a midline cut.

Instructions

1. Expose the superior, anterior, and arcuate parts of the superficial ligament of the pubic symphysis.

2. In the male, make a median section through the penis, opening the entire length of the spongy urethra. Examine the internal surface of the urethra. Note any recesses or lacunae in its dorsal wall, especially in the glans penis. Identify the intrabulbar fossa [see Fig. 16.4B] and the continuity of the membranous and bulbous parts of the urethra.

3. Pass a probe through the urethra into the bladder. In the female, the probe should be inserted into the external orifice. In the male, the probe should be inserted from the opening of the membranous part, through the membranous and prostatic urethra, into the bladder.

4. Cut through the pubic symphysis in the median plane, and extend the incision into the urethra by cutting down on the probe. Remove the probe and continue the median incision to the anterior surfaces of the sacrum and coccyx. In the perineum, this incision should pass through the middle of the central perineal tendon, the anal canal, and the anococcygeal ligament. In the pelvis, the incision should pass through the bladder, the internal urethral orifice, the uterus and vagina in the female, the prostate in the male, and the rectum in both sexes.

5. Make a median saw cut through the fourth and fifth lumbar vertebrae, the sacrum, and the coccyx to meet the knife cut through the soft tissues. Avoid carrying the saw into the soft tissues of the pelvis.

6. Separate the two halves of the pelvis; wash out the rectum and vagina with a jet of water, and examine the cut surfaces of all the tissues [Figs. 17.5, 17.6].

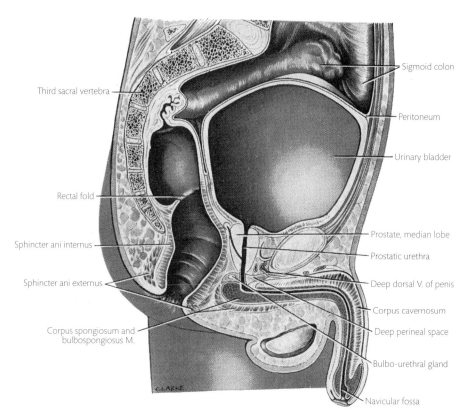

Third sacral vertebra

Rectal fold

Sphincter ani internus

Sphincter ani externus

Corpus spongiosum and
bulbospongiosus M.

Sigmoid colon

Peritoneum

Urinary bladder

Prostate, median lobe

Prostatic urethra

Deep dorsal V. of penis

Corpus cavernosum

Deep perineal space

Bulbo-urethral gland

Navicular fossa

Fig. 17.9 A section through the male pelvis. The urinary bladder and rectum are distended. Note that the distending bladder peels the peritoneum from the anterior abdominal wall.

the introduction of a catheter into the distended bladder—suprapubic cystostomy—through the anterior abdominal wall without involving the peritoneal cavity. In the child, the bladder is an abdominal organ, even when empty. It begins to enter the enlarging pelvis at 6 years of age but is not entirely pelvic in position till after puberty [Fig. 17.10] [Figs. 17.3, 17.4, 17.5].

The empty bladder has four surfaces—superior, posterior or fundus or base, and two inferolateral surfaces [Figs. 17.7A, 17.7B]. Its superior surface is covered with **peritoneum**. At the posterior border of the superior surface, the peritoneum is continued on to the junction of the body and cervix of the uterus in the female [Fig. 17.5]. In the male, the peritoneum is reflected over the superior surface of the vas deferens [Fig. 17.6].

The apex of the bladder is continuous with the **median umbilical ligament**, posterior to the upper margin of the pubic symphysis. This ligament is the fibrous remnant of the intra-abdominal part of the **allantois**—a tubular structure which extends from the bladder into the umbilical cord in the embryo [Fig. 17.7]. ⊃ The allantois may remain

patent in part, or rarely throughout its length. If it is completely patent, urine may be discharged through the umbilicus when the umbilical cord is cut at birth.

The two **inferolateral surfaces** form the sides of the bladder [Figs. 17.7A, 17.7B, 17.11]. They lie on the retropubic fat, parallel to the levator ani muscles, and form a boundary of the retropubic space. They meet each other at a blunt edge, which slopes postero-inferiorly from the apex to the most inferior part or neck of the bladder [Figs. 17.5, 17.6].

The triangular **base** or **fundus** of the bladder faces posteriorly [Figs. 17.7, 17.11]. It is separated from the superior surface by the posterior border. The ureters join the bladder at the lateral ends of the posterior border [Figs. 17.4, 17.11, 17.12]. In the female, the base of the bladder is in contact with the cervix of the uterus and the upper part of the vagina [Fig. 17.5]. In the male, the two seminal vesicles and the ampullae of the vas deferens between them cover all but a small part of the base [Figs. 17.6, 17.11, 17.13].

Dissection 17.4 gives instructions to examine the vas deferens, seminal vesicle, prostate, and prostatic urethra.

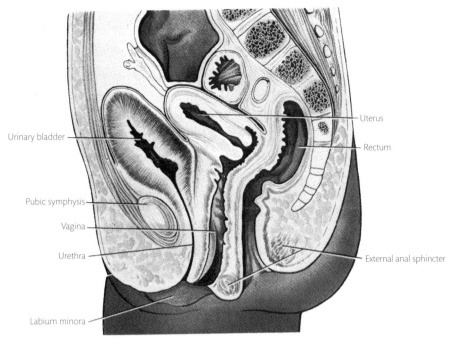

Fig. 17.10 A median section through the lower abdomen and pelvis of a newborn female child. Note that the urinary bladder and uterus lie in the abdomen.

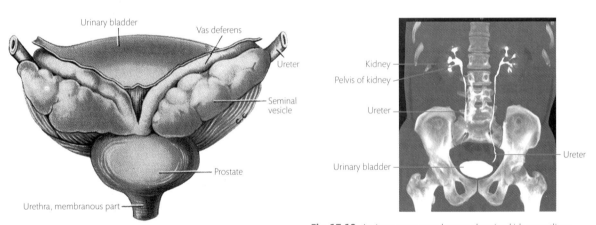

Fig. 17.11 The posterior surfaces of the urinary bladder, prostate, and seminal vesicles.

Fig. 17.12 An intravenous pyelogram showing kidney outlines, calyces, pelvis of the kidney, ureters, and urinary bladder.

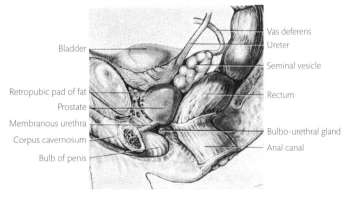

Fig. 17.13 Male pelvic organs from the left side.

DISSECTION 17.4 Vas deferens, seminal vesicle, prostate, and prostatic urethra

Objectives

I. To examine the terminal part of the vas deferens and seminal vesicle.   II. To examine the prostate, prostatic urethra, and openings in the prostatic urethra.

Instructions

1. Pull the half bladder medially and expose the structures on its lateral aspect: the obliterated umbilical artery, the superior vesical branches passing to the bladder, the obturator vessels and nerve, and the superior part of the levator ani.

2. Identify the prostate. It is a firm structure traversed by the urethra and separated from the rectum only by the rectovesical septum.

3. In the male, follow the **vas deferens** to the base of the bladder. Separate it from the adjoining **seminal vesicle**, and follow both to the base of the prostate [Fig. 17.11]. Note the visceral pelvic fascia surrounding these structures and passing to the prostate. Follow this fascia inferiorly to the superior fascia of the urogenital diaphragm on the side where the diaphragm is intact.

4. Find the **deep dorsal vein of the penis** entering the pelvis anteriorly. It joins the plexus of veins in the angle between the bladder and the prostate [Fig. 17.14].

Follow the prostatic fascia on to the back of the pubic bone and symphysis as the puboprostatic ligament.

5. Pull the bladder and prostate medially to expose the medial margin of the levator ani, immediately inferolateral to the prostate. This part of the levator ani is the **levator prostatae muscle**. The urethra and apex of the prostate descend to the urogenital diaphragm through the gap between the medial margins of the levator ani muscles.

6. The upper and lower parts of the **prostatic urethra** lie at an angle to each other. A median ridge—the **urethral crest**—extends the length of the posterior wall of the prostatic urethra [Fig. 17.15]. The **prostatic sinus** is a groove on either side of the urethral crest. Immediately inferior to the angle, a small hillock—the **seminal colliculus**—projects forwards from the **urethral crest**. On the apex of the colliculus is the opening of the **prostatic utricle**, a small blind median pouch which extends posterosuperiorly into the prostate.

7. On each side of the opening of the utricle are smaller openings of the **ejaculatory ducts**. Attempt to pass a fine seeker into the latter opening. At the junction of the vas deferens and seminal vesicle, find the beginning of the ejaculatory duct and trace it through the posterior part of the prostate [see Fig. 16.11].

Vas deferens

The vas deferens is the thick-walled, muscular part of the duct of the testis. It begins as the continuation of the tail of the epididymis at the inferior pole of the testis and ascends through the spermatic cord and inguinal canal to the deep inguinal ring. At the deep inguinal ring, it leaves the other constituents of the spermatic cord and runs over the external iliac vessels to the lateral wall of the lesser pelvis, immediately deep to the peritoneum. In the pelvis, it crosses the ureter near the posterolateral angle of the bladder [Figs. 17.6, 17.7A], runs medially on the base of the bladder, superior to the seminal vesicle, and bends inferiorly to lie between the seminal vesicles. It expands to form the sac-like **ampulla of the vas deferens** on the base of the bladder [Fig. 17.11]. Along with the seminal vesicle, it is enclosed in the upper part of the **rectovesical sep-**

tum. The vas then narrows rapidly and joins the duct of the seminal vesicle to form the **ejaculatory duct**, immediately posterior to the neck of the bladder. The thick **muscular wall** of the vas deferens makes it readily palpable in the spermatic cord. [see Fig. 15.13; Figs. 17.4, 17.11; see also Fig. 18.1].

Seminal vesicle

The seminal vesicles are paired glands bound to the base of the bladder by the fascia of the rectovesical septum. Each seminal vesicle is a dilated, sac-like tube, approximately 15 cm long and folded upon itself. The narrow duct lies posterior to the neck of the bladder and the rest of the gland extends superolaterally to a point near the entry of the ureter into the bladder. The duct lies below the terminal part of the vas deferens and lateral to the ampulla of the vas [Figs. 17.6, 17.7A, 17.11, 17.13].

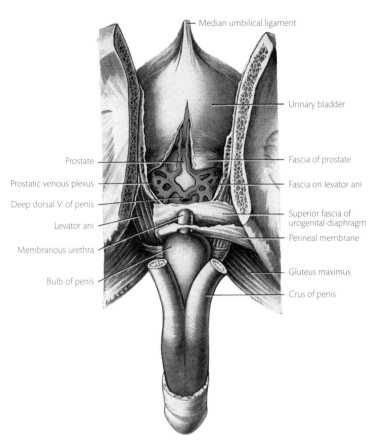

Median umbilical ligament

Urinary bladder

Prostate

Fascia of prostate

Prostatic venous plexus

Fascia on levator ani

Deep dorsal V. of penis

Superior fascia of urogenital diaphragm

Levator ani

Perineal membrane

Membranous urethra

Gluteus maximus

Bulb of penis

Crus of penis

Fig. 17.14 The retropubic space, seen from the front.

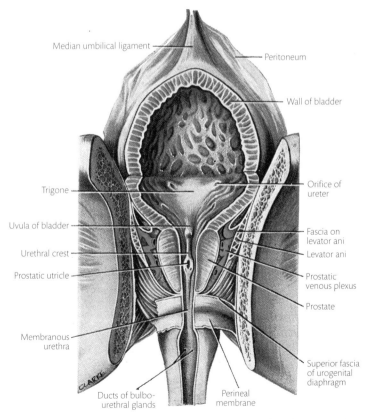

Median umbilical ligament

Peritoneum

Wall of bladder

Trigone

Orifice of ureter

Uvula of bladder

Fascia on levator ani

Urethral crest

Levator ani

Prostatic utricle

Prostatic venous plexus

Prostate

Membranous urethra

Superior fascia of urogenital diaphragm

Ducts of bulbo-urethral glands

Perineal membrane

Fig. 17.15 Urinary bladder and urethra, seen from the front, in the male. The contents of the deep perineal space have been removed, except for the membranous urethra.

Ejaculatory duct

Each ejaculatory duct is formed by the union of the vas deferens with the duct of the seminal vesicle, immediately posterior to the neck of the bladder. The duct passes antero-inferiorly through the upper posterior half of the prostate, along the side of the prostatic utricle, to open into the prostatic urethra on the seminal colliculus [Fig. 17.6].

Prostate

The prostate gland resembles a compressed inverted cone, approximately 3 cm from apex to base and 3.5 cm across the base [Figs. 17.7A, 17.11]. The complex glandular elements are buried in a firm, dense fibromuscular **stroma** which makes it firm to touch.

The **apex** of the prostate is directed inferiorly between the medial margins of the levator ani muscles and rests on the superior fascia of the urogenital diaphragm. The urethra traverses the prostate from the base to a point immediately anterosuperior to the apex [Fig. 17.6].

The convex **inferolateral surfaces** of the prostate lie between the medial margins of the levator ani muscles (the levator prostatae). These two surfaces meet in the rounded **anterior surface** which lies behind the lower part of the pubic symphysis.

The **posterior surface** of the prostate is nearly flat. It is easily palpated by a finger in the rectum because only the rectovesical fascial septum intervenes [Figs. 17.13, 17.16] and the prostate is firm to touch. A peripheral groove between the base of the prostate and the bladder lodges part of the **prostatic plexus of veins** and has the **ejaculatory ducts** entering it posteriorly. The prostate has a thin **capsule** of fibromuscular tissue but is also enclosed in a loose **sheath** of visceral pelvic fascia. Between the pelvic fascia and the capsule at the front and sides of the gland is the **prostatic venous plexus**. This plexus drains the prostate, the bladder, and the deep dorsal vein of the penis [Fig. 17.14].

The **median lobe** of the prostate is the part of the gland that lies posterior to the urethra and above the ejaculatory ducts. Superiorly, it is in direct contact with the inferior part of the trigone of the bladder and pushes the trigone upwards to produce the **uvula of the bladder**. Laterally, there is no separation of the median lobe from the remainder of the prostate which is arbitrarily divided into **right** and **left lobes** by the urethra [Fig. 17.16]. ⊃ Hypertrophy of the prostate is a common cause of obstruction of the urethra in elderly men.

Blood and lymph vessels of the bladder, prostate, seminal vesicles, and vas deferens

The bladder, prostate, seminal vesicles, and vas deferens are supplied by three irregular branches of each internal iliac artery. The **superior vesical**

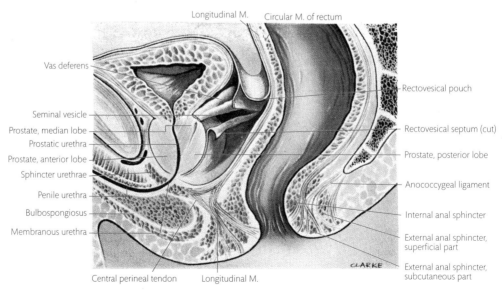

Fig. 17.16 A median section of the male pelvis.

branches of the umbilical arteries supply the anterosuperior part of the bladder and sometimes the superior part of the seminal vesicles and vas deferens [see Fig. 18.1].

The **inferior vesical arteries** supply the base of the bladder and are joined by branches from the middle rectal arteries. They also supply the prostate (and its contained structures), the seminal vesicles, the ampullae of the vas deferens, and the greater part of the length of the vas through a slender branch—the **artery of the vas deferens**.

Veins corresponding to the arteries drain to the internal iliac veins. In addition, the anterosuperior part of the bladder may drain to the external iliac vein. Veins of the bladder, prostate, and deep dorsal vein of the penis drain through the prostatic plexus to the **inferior vesical veins** which drain to the internal iliac veins. The prostatic plexus also communicates through the **lateral sacral veins** and pelvic sacral foramina with the **internal vertebral venous plexus** in the vertebral canal [see Fig. 13.8].

The **lymph vessels** from the superior part of the bladder drain to the external iliac nodes. Those from the inferior part of the bladder drain to the internal iliac nodes. Some vessels from the neck of the bladder pass directly to sacral or common iliac nodes.

The **nerve supply** of the pelvic viscera is from the inferior hypogastric plexus which contains sympathetic, parasympathetic, and sensory nerve fibres.

Puboprostatic and pubovesical ligaments

The puboprostatic and pubovesical ligaments are fibro-elastic condensations of the pelvic fascia which support the bladder. They may contain some smooth muscle fibres. They pass from the back of the body of the pubis, close to the median plane, to the anterior surface of the sheath of the prostate and the neck of the bladder in the male or to the neck of the bladder and the urethra in the female. They are united across the median plane by a thin fascial layer and extend laterally to fuse with the fascia over the medial margins of the levator ani muscles. These ligaments are important in maintaining the posi-

tion of the bladder, prostate, and urethra. In the female, the upper part of the S-shaped urethra is convex anteriorly. Inferiorly, the urethra curves forwards below the pubic symphysis. Both parts are held against the pubis by the **pubo-urethral ligament**.

Male urethra

The parts of the male urethra have been described, and the entire length has been opened. The mucous membrane of the urethra is pitted by minute recesses—the **urethral lacunae**—which face distally [see Fig. 16.4B; Figs. 17.15, 17.16].

Prostatic part

The prostatic part is approximately 3 cm long and runs through the prostate from its base to a point just anterosuperior to its apex. It is the widest and most dilatable part of the urethra and is concave anteriorly. On the posterior wall of the prostatic urethra is a narrow median ridge—the **urethral crest**—with a groove on each side—the **prostatic sinus** [Fig. 17.15]. The crest extends inferiorly from the internal urethral orifice to a rounded eminence—the **seminal colliculus**—on the middle of the crest. The crest then rapidly diminishes and is absent in the membranous urethra.

The **seminal colliculus** has three small openings on it—the median prostatic utricle and paired slit-like **ejaculatory ducts** on each side. Numerous **ducts of the prostate gland** open in the prostatic sinuses [Fig. 17.15].

The **prostatic utricle** is approximately 1 cm long. It is a blind sac which extends posterosuperiorly into the prostate. It represents the remains of the fused parts of the **paramesonephric ducts** of the embryo which form the vagina in the female.

Membranous part

This is the narrowest, shortest (2–2.5 cm), and least distensible part of the urethra. It pierces the superior and inferior fasciae of the urogenital diaphragm and is surrounded by the sphincter urethrae between them.

Immediately below the inferior fascia of the urogenital diaphragm (the perineal membrane), the urethra inclines forwards and enters the corpus spongiosum obliquely, leaving its anterior wall uncovered for a short distance. It is this part which may be ruptured during catheterization, if entry into the membranous part is attempted before the tip has reached the correct position [Figs. 17.15, 17.16].

Penile part

The penile part is approximately 16 cm long. It begins on the upper aspect of the bulb of the penis. In the bulb, the urethra first bulges backwards to form the **intrabulbar fossa** [see Fig. 16.4B]. It then passes through the corpus spongiosum. In the glans penis, it expands dorsoventrally to form the slit-like **fossa navicularis**.

Vessels and nerves

The nerves, blood supply, and lymphatic drainage of the urethra are the same as the surrounding structures: the prostate (prostatic part), the urogenital diaphragm (the membranous part), and the penis (the penile part). Most of the lymph drains to the internal iliac nodes. Lymph from the distal part of the penile urethra drains to the deep inguinal lymph nodes.

Female urethra

The female urethra is 4 cm long. It is wider and more distensible than the male urethra. The mucous membrane is pitted by small **urethral lacunae** which face inferiorly. On each side of the urethra are a number of small mucous glands—the **paraurethral glands**. The paraurethral ducts open near the margin of the external urethral orifice.

The female urethra is S-shaped when seen from the side. The superior part is convex anteriorly; the inferior part curves forwards below the pubic symphysis. Each part is held in position by a **pubourethral ligament** which also supports the anterior vaginal wall to which the urethra is closely applied [Figs. 17.1, 17.5].

Vessels of the female urethra

The blood supply to the female urethra is derived from the vaginal and internal pudendal vessels. Lymph vessels pass to the sacral and internal iliac nodes. A few lymph vessels pass to the superficial inguinal nodes with the other lymph vessels of the vulva.

Dissection 17.5 explores the uterus, vagina, and female urethra.

DISSECTION 17.5 Uterus, vagina, and female urethra

Objective

I. To examine the body and cervix of the uterus, the vagina, and the female urethra.

Instructions

1. Lift the divided **uterus** and confirm that the body is covered with peritoneum on its superior and inferior aspects. Compare this with the fixity of the **cervix** which is attached to the lateral pelvic wall by the broad ligament and to the sacrum by the **uterosacral ligament**.

2. The part of the cervix which projects into the upper anterior wall of the vagina is surrounded on all sides by a narrow, slit-like part of the vaginal cavity—the **fornices of the vagina**.

3. If there is no fat in the upper thin part of the broad ligament, transilluminate it and attempt to see the remnant of the mesonephric duct and tubules (the epoophoron [Fig. 17.2]) of the embryo. This is sometimes visible between the ovary and the uterine tube. It corresponds to the efferent ductules of the testis and the epididymis which degenerate in the female.

4. Note the position of the vagina. Examine the interior of the vagina. Compare the laxity of the tissue which separates it from the rectum with the dense tissue which binds it to the bladder, urethra, and central perineal tendon.

5. Confirm the attachment of the bladder and urethra to the pubis by the pubovesical and pubourethral ligaments. Note how the urethra could be bruised against the pubis by the fetal head during childbirth.

Uterus

The uterus is a thick-walled, firm, muscular organ, 7–8 cm long. It has an upper part—the **body**—and a lower part—the **cervix** or **neck**. The cervix is cylindrical and nearly half of it is inserted into the uppermost part of the anterior wall of the vagina. A narrow constriction—the **isthmus**—joins the body of the uterus to the cervix. The uterine tubes are attached at the lateral margin of the upper part of the body. The rounded part of the body that projects beyond the attachment of the tubes is the **fundus of the uterus** [Figs. 17.1, 17.2].

Body of the uterus

The body is 5 cm wide and 2.5 cm thick and extends from the cervix to the fundus. The fundus lies in the free edge of the broad ligament. The inferior or **vesical surface** of the body is nearly flat and overlies the superior surface of the bladder. The peritoneum from the upper surface of the bladder is reflected on to the junction of the body and cervix of the uterus and forms the **uterovesical pouch of peritoneum** between the uterus and bladder. This pouch is usually empty.

The convex superior or **intestinal surface** of the uterus is covered with peritoneum. The peritoneum extends posteriorly over the supravaginal part of the cervix and the posterior fornix of the vagina to the rectum and forms the recto-uterine pouch [Fig. 17.5]. Loops of the ileum and sigmoid colon lie in this pouch.

The broad ligament of the uterus is a double fold of peritoneum attached to the uterus on each side. The uterine vessels pass between the layers of the broad ligament. The **ligament of the ovaries** and the **round ligament of the uterus** also lie in the broad ligament and are attached to the uterus, superior and inferior to the tubo-uterine junction [Fig. 17.2].

The **cavity of the uterus** is a triangular slit between the walls. The uterine tubes enter the upper angles of the cavity, near the fundus. The apex of the triangular cavity is continuous with the cervical canal [Fig. 17.2].

Cervix

The cervix is 2.5 cm long and the lower half is inserted into the anterior wall of the vagina. The part of the vaginal cavity which encircles the **vaginal part** of the cervix is known as the **vaginal fornix**. For descriptive purposes, the fornix is arbitrarily divided into anterior, posterior, and right lateral and left lateral fornices. The anterior fornix is shallow [Figs. 17.17, 17.18].

The posterosuperior surface of the **supravaginal part** of the cervix and the adjacent posterior vaginal fornix are covered with peritoneum. The antero-inferior surface of the cervix is directly in contact with the upper part of the base of the bladder [Fig. 17.17].

The **canal of the cervix** is spindle-shaped. It is continuous anterosuperiorly with the cavity of the body of the uterus. Usually there is no demarcation between the cervix and the body of the uterus, except in the pregnant uterus where the cervix remains small and is not dilated until childbirth. Inferiorly, the cervical canal opens into the vagina through the external os of the uterus. In women who have not had vaginal deliveries, the uterine os is circular. After vaginal delivery, it becomes a narrow, transverse slit with short anterior and long posterior lips [Figs. 17.2, 17.3, 17.17, 17.18].

The cervix, unlike the body of the uterus, is held in position by a number of ligaments. These ligaments are principally condensations of fascia in the base of the broad ligament. The main mass of condensed fascia surrounds the uterine artery and forms the **transverse ligament of the cervix**. It passes from the cervix and the lateral fornix of the vagina to the lateral wall of the pelvis. A similar condensation in each recto-uterine fold forms the **uterosacral ligaments**. Thus the cervix remains in position, while the body of the uterus expands upwards in pregnancy.

The uterus overlies the posterior part of the superior surface of the bladder. When the bladder is empty, the cervix is tilted forwards at right angles to the vagina [Fig. 17.17]. This angulation is known as **anteversion** of the uterus. The body of the uterus is slightly bent downwards at the isthmus on the firmer, more fibrous cervix [Fig. 17.5]. This angulation is known as **anteflexion** of the uterus. The body of the uterus, enclosed between the layers of the **broad ligament**, is freely mobile. As the bladder fills, the uterus is raised and may be forced back till it lies in line with the vagina when the bladder is fully distended. ⊃ In certain pathological conditions, the uterus may be permanently pushed back, a condition known as retroverted uterus. If the body of the uterus is bent backwards on itself at the isthmus, the condition is known as retroflexed uterus. Fig. 17.19 is an MRI of a fetus *in utero*.

Vessels of the uterus

The **uterine artery** is a branch of the internal iliac artery. It runs medially in the root of the broad ligament to the lateral fornix of the vagina, superior to the ureters [Fig. 17.18]. It then turns to run superiorly along the lateral sides of the uterus. At the tubo-uterine junction, it turns laterally in the broad ligament to supply the uterine tubes and

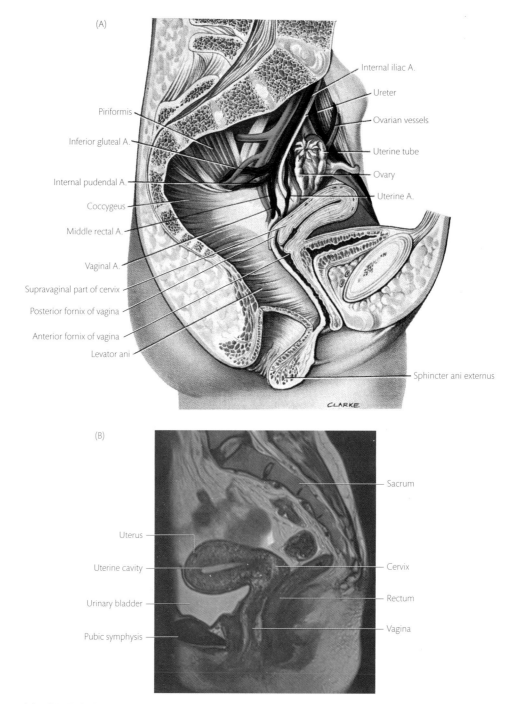

(A)

Piriformis

Inferior gluteal A.

Internal pudendal A.

Coccygeus

Middle rectal A.

Vaginal A.

Supravaginal part of cervix

Posterior fornix of vagina

Anterior fornix of vagina

Levator ani

Internal iliac A.

Ureter

Ovarian vessels

Uterine tube

Ovary

Uterine A.

Sphincter ani externus

CLARKE.

(B)

Uterus

Uterine cavity

Urinary bladder

Pubic symphysis

Sacrum

Cervix

Rectum

Vagina

Fig. 17.17 (A) Left half of a female pelvis. The greater part of the rectum has been removed. The uterus is anteverted and anteflexed. (B) A T2W mid-sagittal image of the female pelvis.

ends by anastomosing with the ovarian artery. Large branches of the artery pass into the muscle of the uterus and send smaller vessels into the uterine mucosa.

The **lymph** from the uterus drains by a number of routes [see Fig. 18.2]. (1) From the cervix, body, and fundus, lymph drains laterally through the broad ligament (occasionally interrupted by small para-uterine nodes in the broad ligament) to the external iliac nodes. (2) From the fundus, lymph drains with the ovarian lymph vessels to the lumbar nodes, and along the round ligaments of the

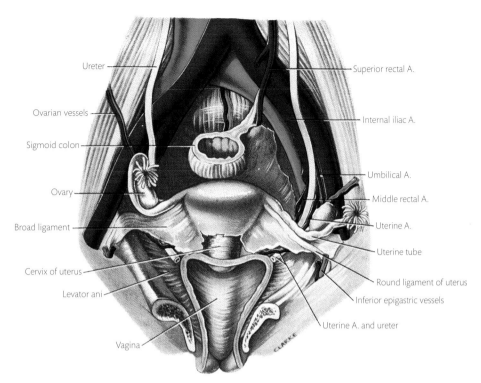

Ureter

Ovarian vessels

Sigmoid colon

Ovary

Broad ligament

Cervix of uterus

Levator ani

Vagina

Superior rectal A.

Internal iliac A.

Umbilical A.

Middle rectal A.

Uterine A.

Uterine tube

Round ligament of uterus

Inferior epigastric vessels

Uterine A. and ureter

Fig. 17.18 Female pelvis from the front. The uterus has been displaced backwards, and the bladder, urethra, and anterior wall of the vagina removed.

uterus to the superficial inguinal nodes. (3) From the cervix, lymph drains to the internal iliac and sacral nodes.

The **nerves** of the uterus come from the inferior hypogastric plexus. Many of the post-ganglionic parasympathetic nerve fibres arise in large pelvic ganglia close to the cervix.

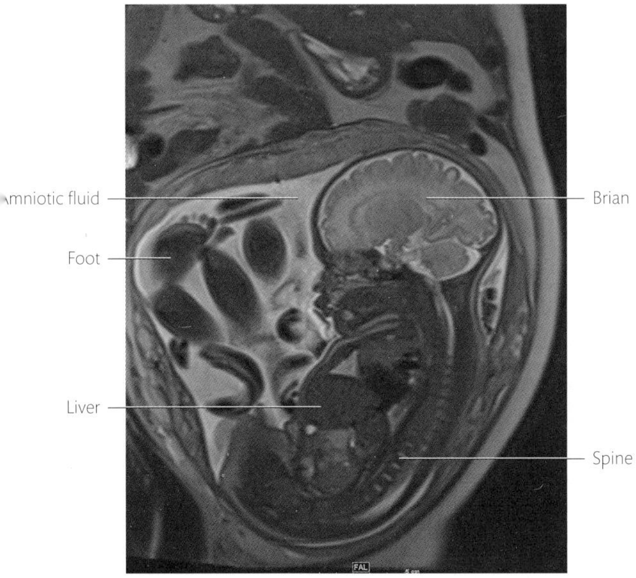

Vagina

The vagina descends antero-inferiorly from the fornix to the vestibule between the labia minora. It passes between the medial borders of the two levator ani muscles and pierces the urogenital diaphragm and sphincter urethrae. The anterior wall is 7.5 cm long and the posterior wall, which extends above the cervix to the posterior fornix, is 9 cm long. The cervix projects into a slightly enlarged part of the cavity of the vagina and separates the two walls which are otherwise in contact with each other [Fig. 17.17].

The **anterior wall** of the vagina is in contact with the base of the bladder and the terminal parts of the ureters. It is tightly bound to the neck of the bladder and to the urethra and, through them, to the pubis through the pubovesical and pubo-urethral ligaments.

The **posterior fornix** is covered with peritoneum. Injuries to this part of the vagina may involve

Amniotic fluid

Foot

Liver

Brian

Spine

Fig. 17.19 Fetal MRI—a T2W image of a fetus *in utero*.

the peritoneal cavity. More inferiorly, the **posterior wall** of the vagina is separated from the lowest part of the rectum only by loose areolar tissue. At the **lateral fornices**, the **lateral walls** of the vagina give attachment to the base of the broad ligament. The uterine vessels and ureters are contained in the base of the broad ligament, in close relation to the lateral fornix. Inferiorly, the lateral walls of the vagina are in contact with the levator ani muscles, the urogenital diaphragm, the great vestibular glands, and the bulb of the vestibule [Fig. 17.18]. At the margin of the orifice of the vagina, the mucous membrane may extend inwards as a circumferential fold—**the hymen**. The hymen is usually an incomplete ring which is torn at first sexual intercourse. It may rupture earlier during non-sexual physical activity. The remnants of the torn hymen are the **carunculae hymenales**. ➲ Rarely, the hymen may be a complete membrane which prevents the discharge of the menstrual flow at puberty.

Vessels of the vagina

The **vaginal artery**, which corresponds to the inferior vesical artery in the male, supplies the vagina. It is supplemented by twigs from the uterine artery, the middle rectal artery, and arteries of the bulbs of the vestibule. The **veins** of the vagina form submucous and adventitial plexuses and drain into the internal iliac veins.

DISSECTION 17.6 Rectum

Objectives

I. To examine the internal surface of the rectum.   II. To identify and trace the superior rectal artery.

Instructions

1. Confirm the relation of the peritoneum to the upper two-thirds of the **rectum**.

2. Examine the mucous membrane of the rectum, noting the position of one right and two left transverse folds.

3. Find the **superior rectal artery**, the continuation of the inferior mesenteric artery from the abdomen. Trace it on to the posterior surface of the upper part of the rectum, and follow its branches downwards on the posterolateral surfaces to the lowest part of the rectum [see Fig. 17.21].

4. Strip the remaining peritoneum and fascia from the external surface of the rectum to expose the outer longitudinal layer of muscle.

The **lymph vessels** of the upper part of the vagina drain with the uterine vessels to the internal and external iliac nodes. The middle part of the vagina drains with the vaginal vessels to the internal iliac nodes. The inferior part of the vagina drains either to the sacral and common iliac nodes, or with the vessels of the vulva to the superficial inguinal nodes [see Fig. 18.2].

See Dissection 17.6 for instructions on dissecting the rectum.

Rectum

The rectum begins as the continuation of the sigmoid colon on the pelvic surface of the third piece of the sacrum. It is approximately 12 cm long. In spite of its name, the rectum is not straight. In the sagittal plane, it follows the curve of the sacrum and coccyx and continues antero-inferiorly on the **anococcygeal ligament** and parts of the levator ani muscles. It ends by turning postero-inferiorly as the **anal canal**, 2–3 cm anterior to the tip of the coccyx. The anorectal junction is immediately posterior to the **central perineal tendon** and to the apex of the prostate in the male. The lower part of the rectum is frequently more distended than the remainder and is known as the **ampulla** [Fig. 17.5]. In the coronal plane, the rectum deviates from the midline in three lateral curves. The upper and lower curves are convex to the right; the middle one is convex to the left [Fig. 17.20].

Peritoneum covers the front and sides of the upper third of the rectum. At the junction of the middle and lower thirds, the peritoneum is reflected anteriorly. In the male, this peritoneum forms the floor of the **rectovesical pouch** and passes on to the back of the bladder. In the female, it forms the floor of the **recto-uterine pouch** and passes on to the posterior fornix of the vagina [Figs. 17.5, 17.6].

The upper two-thirds of the rectum is in contact anteriorly with coils of the sigmoid colon and ileum. The lower third is separated from the vagina by loose areolar tissue in the female. In the male, the lower third of the rectum is related to the base of the bladder, the seminal vesicles, the vas deferens, and the prostate but is separated from them by the rectovesical septum. Small weak bundles of the longitudinal muscle of the rectum pass forwards to the apex of the prostate in the male [Fig. 17.16], and to the back of the vagina in the female. These fibres constitute the **recto-urethralis muscle**.

Posteriorly, in the midline, a layer of pelvic fascia separates the rectum from the sacrum,

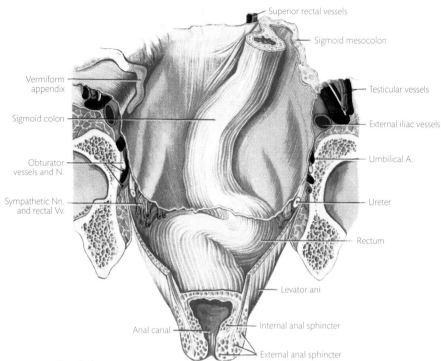

Superior rectal vessels

Sigmoid mesocolon

Vermiform appendix

Testicular vessels

Sigmoid colon

External iliac vessels

Obturator vessels and N.

Umbilical A.

Sympathetic Nn. and rectal Vv.

Ureter

Rectum

Levator ani

Anal canal

Internal anal sphincter

External anal sphincter

Fig. 17.20 The rectum seen from in front.

coccyx, and anococcygeal ligament in the median plane. On each side, posterolateral to the rectum is a branch of the superior rectal artery, the piriformis, the coccygeus, and the levator ani [Fig. 17.21]. The pelvic fascia around the rectum contains the median sacral vessels, the sympathetic trunks on each side, and the ganglion impar on the coccyx. Lateral to these are the lateral sacral vessels and the lower sacral and coccygeal nerves.

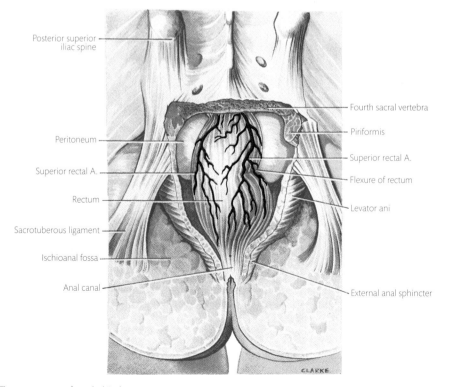

Posterior superior iliac spine

Fourth sacral vertebra

Piriformis

Peritoneum

Superior rectal A.

Superior rectal A.

Flexure of rectum

Rectum

Levator ani

Sacrotuberous ligament

Ischioanal fossa

Anal canal

External anal sphincter

CLARKE

Fig. 17.21 The rectum seen from behind.

Laterally, the upper part of the rectum is in contact with the peritoneum, and the lower part is in contact with the fat and fascia over the coccygeus and the levator ani muscles. Some of this fascia is condensed around the middle rectal artery as it passes to the rectum and provides support for the rectum.

Rectal and vaginal examinations

In the male, the posterior surface of the prostate, seminal vesicles, and the terminal parts of the vas deferens can be palpated by a finger in the rectum. In the female, the firm cervix may be palpated through the rectal and vaginal walls. The cervix and body of the uterus may also be examined by bimanual palpation, with two fingers in the vagina and a hand on the anterior abdominal wall.

Examine the internal surface of the anal canal by following Dissection 17.7.

Anal canal

The anal canal is the terminal part of the large intestine. It is approximately 4 cm long and descends postero-inferiorly from the anorectal junction. It is surrounded by the internal and external anal sphincters and the levator ani muscles. The ischioanal fossae lie lateral and inferior to the levator ani muscles. The anal canal ends at the anus.

The **internal anal sphincter** is a thickening of the circular smooth muscle of the intestine. It surrounds the upper two-thirds of the anal canal. The **external anal sphincter** surrounds the lower two-thirds of the anal canal. (The external anal sphincter overlaps the internal sphincter in the middle third of the anal canal.) The fibres of the **puborectalis** part of the levator ani sweep round the sides and posterior aspect of the anorectal junction. When they contract, they pull the upper part of the anal canal anteriorly and increase the angulation between the rectum and the anal canal. In doing this, the puborectalis also acts as a sphincter. Some of the more vertical fibres of the levator ani muscles join the longitudinal muscle of the intestine and run through the external sphincter to the perineal skin. As such the longitudinal muscle and the levator ani are attached to the skin inferiorly. Longitudinal muscle bundles of the rectum also pass forwards into the central perineal tendon and to the apex of the prostate or posterior vaginal wall. These form the **recto-urethralis** muscle [Fig. 17.16]. Figs. 17.22A and 17.22B are axial and sagittal images through the male pelvis, showing the pelvic viscera and puborectalis.

Internal features of the rectum and anal canal

The **rectum** is surrounded by a fascial layer internal to the pelvic fascia. The mucosa of the rectum is raised into three **transverse folds**, one opposite the concavity of each rectal flexure. The right fold is the largest and lies at the level of the rectovesical or recto-uterine pouch. The two left folds are approximately 4 cm above and below the right one.

Near the mucocutaneous junction, the mucosa of the anal canal forms a series of longitudinal ridges (**anal columns**) which are united to each other inferiorly by horizontal folds (**anal valves**). The anal valves and columns together form a series of small pockets—the **anal sinuses**—at the inferior end of the groove between two columns.

The **anal valves** lie at the level formerly occupied by the anal part of the **cloacal membrane**.

DISSECTION 17.7 Anal canal

Objective

I. To examine the internal surface of the anal canal.

Instructions

1. Examine the lining of the **anal canal**. Identify, if possible, the junction of the mucous membrane and skin, usually below the middle of the canal. The **mucous membrane** is thrown into a number of longitudinal folds—the anal columns. These folds are united inferiorly by small, horizontal, semilunar folds—the anal valves. Between the valves and the lower end of the folds are small pockets lined by mucous membrane—the **anal sinuses**.

2. The lowest part of the anal canal is lined first by true skin. Superior to this, the anal canal is lined by skin devoid of hair follicles and glands. Above the valves, the anal canal is lined by mucosa.

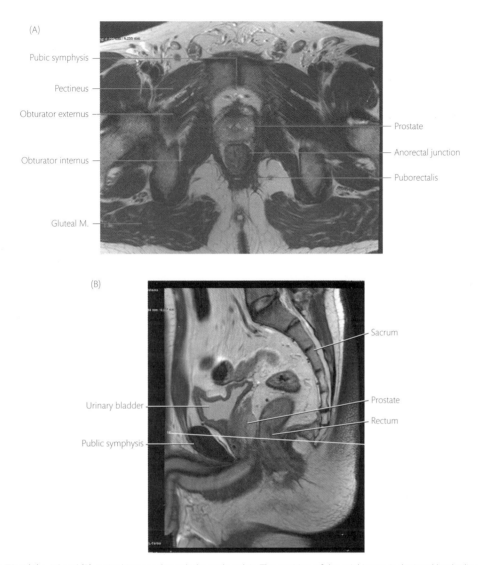

(A)

Pubic symphysis

Pectineus

Obturator externus

Obturator internus

Gluteal M.

Prostate

Anorectal junction

Puborectalis

(B)

Sacrum

Urinary bladder

Prostate

Rectum

Public symphysis

Fig. 17.22 T2W (A) axial and (B) sagittal images through the male pelvis. The position of the axial image is depicted by the line on the sagittal image.

In the embryo, the cloacal membrane temporarily closes the anal end of the alimentary canal. ⮑ If the membrane persists at birth, it results in a condition known as imperforate anus.

The anal valves are liable to be torn by the passage of a hard faecal mass, thus allowing infection from the gut to spread into the wall of the anal canal (fissure *in ano*).

Arteries and veins of the rectum

Five **rectal arteries** anastomose with each other to supply the rectum. They are the superior rectal artery (a continuation of the inferior mesenteric artery), two middle rectal arteries from the internal iliac arteries, and two inferior rectal arteries from the internal pudendal arteries in the ischioanal fossa. The **veins** form submucous and adventitial plexuses. They drain along the corresponding arteries to the internal iliac veins and the portal vein.

An extensive asymmetrical **plexus of veins** links the superior rectal veins, which are indirect tributaries of the portal vein, with the middle and inferior rectal veins, which are indirect tributaries of the inferior vena cava. ⮑ When distended, this plexus can give rise to haemorrhoids. (See Chapter 11 for discussion on porto-systemic anastomosis and Chapter 18 for more on haemorrhoids.)

Lymph vessels

[See Fig. 18.2.]

(1) From the lower part of the anal canal and the surrounding perianal skin, lymph drains to the medial **superficial inguinal lymph nodes**.

(2) From the upper part of the anal canal, lymph drains either across the ischioanal fossa with the inferior rectal blood vessels or laterally with the middle rectal vessels to the **internal iliac nodes**.

(3) Other lymph vessels pass from the rectum to the **sacral** and **common iliac lymph nodes**.

(4) Some lymph ascends with the inferior mesenteric vessels to **inferior mesenteric** and **lumbar nodes**.

See Clinical Applications 17.1–17.5 for the practical implications of the anatomy in this chapter.

CLINICAL APPLICATION 17.1 Tubal pregnancy

The ovum is fertilized in the ampulla of the uterine tube, and development begins as it slowly passes to the uterus. If passage is delayed along the tube, the ovum may adhere to the wall of the tube and implant in it. This is the most common type of **ectopic gestation**. Unlike the uterus, the tube is too thin-walled to withstand the invading ovum. It can rupture and lead to severe intraperitoneal bleeding—one cause of acute abdominal emergency in women of childbearing age. Very rarely, a fertilized ovum may escape into the peritoneal cavity and implant on the peritoneal surface of any of the pelvic viscera or pelvic walls.

CLINICAL APPLICATION 17.2 Double J stent

A double J ureteric stent is a soft tube placed within the ureter to ensure its patency and prevent or relieve a block in the ureter. The tube has a curl at both ends designed to prevent the stent from moving down into the bladder or up into the kidney. Fig. 17.23 is a plain X-ray of a patient with a stent in the left ureter.

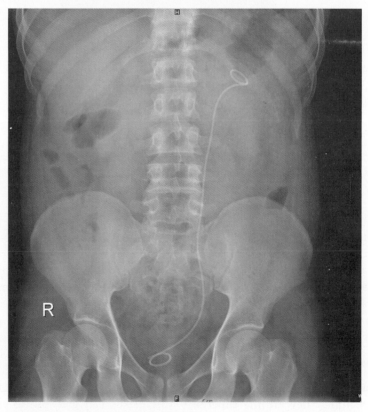

Fig. 17.23 A plain kidneys, ureters, and bladder (KUB) radiograph showing a double J stent in the left ureter, with the superior end in the left renal pelvicalyceal system and the lower end in the bladder.

CLINICAL APPLICATION 17.3   Benign prostatic hyperplasia

Benign prostatic hyperplasia (BPH) is one of the most common benign tumours in adult males. Hyperplasia affects the glandular epithelium as well as the fibromuscular stroma of the prostate. Sex steroids, particularly oestrogen, and a testosterone metabolite—dihydrotestosterone—have been implicated in the development of prostatic hyperplasia. BPH typically causes an enlargement of the lateral lobes. When hyperplasia affects the median lobe of the prostate, it results in elevation of the mucosa of the trigone. Prostatic hyperplasia primarily causes narrowing of the prostatic urethra and bladder outflow obstruction, resulting in bladder hypertrophy. Hydroureters (dilatation of ureters) occur because the bladder loses its compliance, i.e. the ability to keep the pressures low (normal <10 cm). This leads to two types of symptoms: (1) symptoms of storage such as frequency, urgency, and urge leak; and (2) symptoms of emptying such as hesitancy, poor flow, intermittency, and incomplete emptying.

Patients present with sudden painful retention of urine requiring urgent urinary catheterization. Digital rectal examination in BPH typically reveals an enlarged, firm prostate gland. In prostatic cancer, however, the gland may be nodular and hard. Two main groups of drugs are used in the medical management of BPH: (1) 5-alpha-reductase inhibitors which prevent the conversion of testosterone to its metabolite dihydrotestosterone. It decreases the size of the enlarged prostate by reducing the hyperplasia; (2) alpha receptor blockers relax the tone of the smooth muscle of the prostatic stroma and bladder neck and improve bladder emptying.

Surgical removal of the prostate is carried out endoscopically. Transurethral resection of the prostate (TURP) aims to relieve the obstruction by removing the hyperplastic prostatic tissue. In this procedure a resectoscope is passed through the urethra and strips of prostatic tissue are removed from between the bladder neck and the verumontanum. Using laser, the hyperplastic prostatic tissue can be either vaporized or enucleated.

CLINICAL APPLICATION 17.4   Access to the pelvic peritoneal cavity in women

The recto-uterine perineal pouch (of Douglas) is the most dependent part of the peritoneal cavity in women. Free fluid in the peritoneal cavity tends to collect in the recto-uterine pouch. The posterior fornix of the vagina is separated from this part of the peritoneal cavity only by the vaginal wall. The proximity of the recto-uterine pouch to the posterior fornix of the vagina is made use of in some clinical settings. **Culdocentesis** is a diagnostic procedure in which a needle is inserted into the recto-uterine pouch through the vaginal wall at the posterior fornix. Blood, pus, or other abnormal fluid collections can be aspirated for testing. Incision into the peritoneal cavity through the posterior fornix is called **posterior colpotomy**. It can be done to drain such fluid collections or as an adjunct to laparoscopic pelvic surgery.

CLINICAL APPLICATION 17.5   Pelvic organ prolapse

Pelvic organ prolapse involves protrusion of parts of one or more of the surrounding organs through the vaginal wall. It could be a part of the bladder (cystocele), the rectum (rectocele), the small bowel (enterocele), or the descent of the uterus through the vaginal orifice (uterine prolapse). Pelvic organ prolapse occurs due to breakdown in normal support mechanisms of the pelvic organs, either by actual tear, neuromuscular dysfunction, or both.

Study question 1: name the supports of the pelvic viscera. (Answer: the main supports for the pelvic organs are the muscles and connective tissue of the pelvic floor, the fibromusular tissue of the vaginal wall, and thickenings of the endopelvic connective tissue. The levator ani and perineal body play an important role in supporting the uterus. These are often damaged due to trauma during childbirth and can be largely prevented by pelvic floor strengthening exercises. Endopelvic connective tissue is condensed to form the transverse cervical (cardinal), pubocervical, and uterosacral ligaments. The normal processes of pregnancy and labour result in stretching and weakening of these ligaments.)

Study question 2: what is the normal position of the uterus and how does this play a role in its support? (Answer: in the nulliparous state, the long axis of the uterus usually is at an angle of about 90° (anteversion) with that of the vagina. Furthermore, the body of the uterus lies at an angle of about 125° (anteflexion) with the cervix. The fact that the uterus is not in line with the vaginal canal decreases the likelihood of prolapse. The round ligament of the uterus helps maintain this position, although this too may be stretched during labour.)

CHAPTER 18
The pelvic wall

Vessels of the lesser pelvis

The parietal layer of the pelvic fascia lines the walls of the pelvis. The nerves of the pelvis lie posterior to the parietal fascia. The arteries and veins of the pelvis lie internal (anterior) to the fascia, between the fascia and the parietal peritoneum.

Dissect the internal iliac vessels using the instructions given in Dissection 18.1.

Superior rectal artery

The superior rectal artery is the continuation of the inferior mesenteric artery. It begins on the middle of the left common iliac artery and descends in the medial limb of the sigmoid mesocolon. On the third piece of the sacrum, it divides

---

DISSECTION 18.1 Internal iliac artery and vein

Objectives

I. To study the internal iliac artery and its branches.
II. To study the internal iliac vein and its tributaries.

Instructions

1. Move the pelvic viscera medially away from the pelvic walls and follow the internal iliac vessels and their branches or tributaries [see Fig. 17.17A; Fig. 18.1]. If necessary, remove the veins to get a clearer view of the arteries.

2. Note any parts of the hypogastric plexus that are exposed with the vessels.

---

into two branches. These branches descend first on the back and then on the sides of the rectum. Each then divides into three or four branches which pierce the circumference of the rectum and descend in the submucosa down to the anal canal [see Fig. 17.21]. In the anal canal, they anastomose with branches of the inferior and middle rectal arteries.

The **superior rectal vein** accompanies the artery. It joins the sigmoid veins to become the inferior mesenteric vein. It drains the rectal venous plexuses and other pelvic plexuses which anastomose with them [Pelvic venous plexuses, p. 281].

Internal iliac artery

The internal iliac artery is the smaller of the two branches of the common iliac artery. (It is large in the fetus when it transmits blood to the placenta through the umbilical artery. At birth, the umbilical arteries are tied and degenerate into fibrous cords up to the level of the superior vesical artery.)

The internal iliac artery supplies most of the walls and contents of the pelvis. It begins as a terminal branch of the common iliac artery, medial to the psoas major and anterior to the sacro-iliac joint. It lies deep to the peritoneum and passes posteriorly into the lesser pelvis, medial to the external iliac vein and the obturator nerve. It lies between the ureter anteriorly and the internal iliac vein posteriorly. At the upper margin of the greater sciatic notch, it ends by dividing into anterior and posterior divisions. The arrangement of its visceral branches is very variable [see Fig. 17.17A; Fig. 18.1].

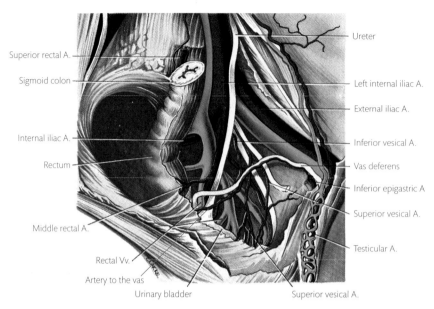

Fig. 18.1 Structures on the lateral wall of the male pelvis.

Branches of the posterior division

The posterior division of the internal iliac artery gives off three branches:

1. The **superior gluteal artery** supplies structures in the gluteal region. It runs between the lumbosacral trunk and the ventral ramus of the first sacral nerve through the uppermost part of the greater sciatic foramen, superior to the piriformis.

2. The **iliolumbar artery** ascends deep to the psoas and divides into two branches: (i) an iliac branch which runs laterally on the abdominal surface of the iliacus; and (ii) a lumbar branch which ascends posterior to the psoas to supply it and the quadratus lumborum. This branch may form the fifth lumbar artery. The corresponding vein joins the common iliac vein.

3. **Lateral sacral arteries**, two on each side, descend in front of the pelvic sacral foramina, through which they send branches to the sacral nerves, the contents of the sacral canal, and the muscles and skin overlying the dorsal sacral foramina.

Branches of the anterior division

The anterior division of the internal iliac artery gives off the following branches:

1. The **superior vesical artery** which runs antero-inferiorly between the bladder and the lateral wall of the pelvis. It gives two or three superior vesical branches to the bladder, ureter, vas deferens, and seminal vesicle [Fig. 18.1]. In the fetus, the superior

vesical arteries are branches of the **umbilical arteries** which supply the placenta. After birth, the distal part of the artery becomes obliterated and forms a fibrous cord—the medial umbilical ligament. This ligament runs from the anterior part of the pelvis through the extraperitoneal tissue of the anterior abdominal wall to the umbilicus. (The umbilical vein does not accompany the artery. In the fetus, it runs from the umbilicus to the liver and forms the ligamentum teres of the liver after birth.)

2. The **inferior vesical artery** in the male runs forwards to the base of the bladder, supplies the postero-inferior part of the bladder, seminal vesicle, and prostate, and sends a long, slender **artery of the vas deferens** on the vas to the testis [Fig. 18.1]. The equivalent artery in the female is the **vaginal artery** [see Fig. 17.17A]. It supplies the vagina, the postero-inferior part of the bladder, and the pelvic part of the urethra.

3. The **middle rectal artery** is a small branch of the internal iliac artery which passes medially to the rectum. It supplies branches to the rectum and to the vagina or seminal vesicle and prostate, and anastomoses with the other rectal arteries [see Fig. 17.17A].

4. The **obturator artery** runs antero-inferiorly with the obturator nerve and vein through the obturator canal to the adductor compartment of the thigh. In the pelvis, it gives small branches to surrounding structures. It also gives a pubic branch which anastomoses with the pubic branch of the inferior epigastric artery on the pelvic surface of

the body of the pubis. This anastomosis may replace part or all of the obturator artery to form the **accessory obturator artery**.

5. The **uterine artery** [see Figs. 17.1, 17.17A, 17.18] may be separate or may arise from the vaginal, umbilical, or middle rectal arteries. It passes medially at the base of the broad ligament to the lateral vaginal fornix. At the lateral fornix, it lies above the ureter. It turns anterosuperiorly to run a tortuous course along the lateral margin of the uterus. It supplies the superior part of the vagina, the uterus, and the medial part of the uterine tube. It ends by anastomosing with the **ovarian artery** in the broad ligament.

In the base of the broad ligament, the uterine artery is surrounded by a condensation of connective tissue which helps to hold the cervix in position by attaching it to the lateral pelvic wall. This mass of connective tissue is the **transverse ligament of the cervix**.

6. The **internal pudendal artery** descends anterior to the piriformis and the sacral plexus. It leaves the pelvis through the lowest part of the greater sciatic foramen, passes over the posterior surface of the ischial spine, and enters the perineum through the lesser sciatic foramen [see Fig. 17.17A].

7. The **inferior gluteal artery** passes postero-inferiorly between the ventral rami of the first and second sacral nerves to enter the gluteal region below the piriformis [see Fig. 17.17A].

Median sacral artery

This small artery arises from the posterior surface of the aorta, immediately above its bifurcation. It descends on the vertebral column, in the midline, to end in a series of arteriovenous anastomoses in the cellular **coccygeal body**, on the front of the coccyx. It gives rise to the fifth lumbar arteries, sends twigs to the back of the rectum, and anastomoses with the lateral sacral arteries [see Fig. 17.1].

Veins of the pelvis

The venous drainage of the pelvis is through the internal iliac veins. The internal iliac vein is posterosuperior to the internal iliac artery and receives tributaries which correspond to many of its branches. Blood from the pelvis also drains into other veins through the following channels. From the rectum, some blood drains into the inferior mesenteric vein through the **superior rectal vein**. Blood from

the ovaries drains into the left renal vein or inferior vena cava. Veins corresponding to the median sacral artery—the **median sacral veins**—drain into the **internal vertebral venous plexus** through the pelvic sacral foramina. The **iliolumbar veins** drain into the common iliac veins. In the fetus, the **umbilical** vein drains into the hepatic portal vein [see Fig. 17.17A; Fig. 18.1].

Pelvic venous plexuses

A number of pelvic venous plexuses lie in relation to the pelvic viscera. They communicate with adjacent plexuses and drain into the internal iliac veins.

The **rectal venous plexuses** lie on the surface and submucosa of the rectum. They drain through the **superior**, **middle**, and **inferior rectal veins** into the inferior mesenteric veins and internal iliac veins. This plexus also communicates with the internal vertebral venous plexus through the pelvic sacral foramina, and with the vesical venous plexus in the male. The rectal veins form a route of communication between the portal and systemic venous systems.

➔ Blockage of the portal vein can lead to distension of the submucosal plexus of rectal veins. When distended, this plexus forms haemorrhoids, or piles, especially on the left lateral and the right anterior and right posterior segments of the rectum. The mucosa of the anal canal is so loosely connected to the muscle layer that it may prolapse through the anus with the dilated submucous veins. Since the rectal plexuses communicate with the other pelvic plexuses, they may be distended whenever pelvic blood flow is increased, as in pregnancy.

In the male, the **vesical venous plexus** is principally found on the base of the bladder around the seminal vesicles, the vas deferens, and the ends of the ureters. It drains through the **inferior vesical veins** to the **internal iliac veins**. The plexus also drains along the rectovesical fold to the anterior surface of the sacrum. From there, it may drain either through the pelvic sacral foramina to the **internal vertebral venous plexus**, or through the lateral sacral veins to the **internal iliac vein**.

➔ The size of the internal vertebral venous plexus is big enough to form an alternative route for drainage of all the blood to the inferior vena cava, when the internal iliac vein is blocked.

The **prostatic venous plexus** lies on the front and sides of the prostate within its fascial sheath. It receives the deep dorsal vein of the penis and drains into the vesical venous plexus [see Figs. 17.14, 17.15].

In the female, the **vesical plexus** surrounds the pelvic part of the urethra and the neck of the bladder. It receives the dorsal vein of the clitoris and drains into the vaginal plexuses. The vaginal plexuses lie on the sides of the vagina and in its mucosa. They communicate with the uterine and rectal plexuses and drain mainly through the **vaginal veins**.

The **uterine plexuses** lie principally at the sides of the uterus between the layers of the broad ligament. They drain through the **uterine veins** which accompany the uterine arteries. They also communicate through the broad ligament with the pampiniform plexus and drain into the **ovarian veins**.

Lymph nodes and vessels of the pelvis

These are numerous and difficult to demonstrate. They lie in groups along the major blood vessels and are named according to the vessels [Fig. 18.2].

The **external iliac nodes** lie along the external iliac artery and drain lymph from the lower limb, abdominal wall, bladder, prostate, and uterus. They drain into the common iliac nodes.

The **internal iliac nodes** lie along the internal iliac artery and its branches. They drain lymph from all the pelvic contents, the deep structures in the perineum through lymph vessels along the internal pudendal vessels, the gluteal region, and the back of the thigh through lymph vessels along the su-

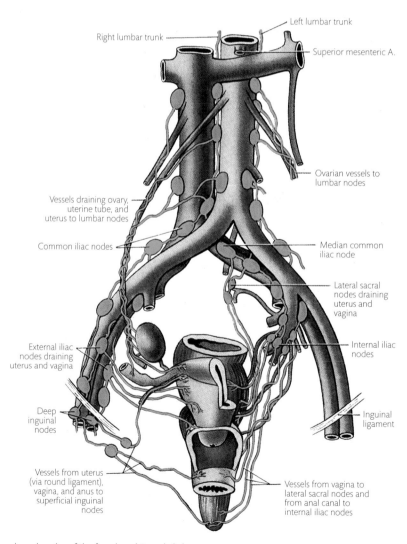

Fig. 18.2 Lymph vessels and nodes of the female pelvis and abdomen.

perior and inferior gluteal vessels. Like the external iliac nodes, they drain to the common iliac nodes.

The **sacral nodes** lie along the median and lateral sacral arteries. They drain the dorsal wall of the pelvis, rectum, neck of the bladder, prostate, or cervix of the uterus. They drain to the common iliac nodes.

In addition to these groups, small nodes lie in the broad ligament and in the fascial sheaths of the bladder and rectum [see Fig. 13.2; Fig. 18.2].

Nerves of the lesser pelvis

Contents of the sacral canal

Dissection 18.2 explores the sacral canal.

The sacral canal contains the following:

1. The **dura mater** and **arachnoid mater** which surround the spinal medulla extend down to the level of the second sacral vertebra. Here they fuse on the filum terminale [Fig. 18.3] which receives a

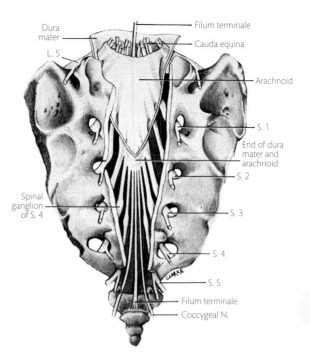

Fig. 18.3 Sacral nerves and meninges within the sacral canal.

DISSECTION 18.2 Sacral canal

Objective

I. To explore the sacral canal and study its contents.

Instructions

1. Explore the **sacral hiatus**. This varies in extent, from a notch between the sacral cornua [see Fig. 7.5] to a large hiatus extending upwards to the second sacral spine.

2. Expose the dura mater and the nerves in the sacral canal by removing the fat and numerous veins (**internal vertebral venous plexus**) which surround them.

3. Identify the leash of nerve roots (**cauda equina** [Fig. 18.3]) which surrounds the filum terminale inside the arachnoid. Follow each **sacral nerve** to its division into dorsal and ventral rami by extending the opening of the canal into each dorsal sacral foramen.

4. Find the end of the dural sac, and trace the fine strand (**filum terminale**) from its caudal extremity to the coccyx where it is close to the fifth sacral and coccygeal nerves.

5. Find the thin, transparent **arachnoid** applied to the internal surface of the dura.

thin covering from them and passes to the back of the coccyx.

2. The roots of five pairs of **sacral nerves** and one pair of **coccygeal nerves** make up the cauda equina in the sacral canal. They pierce the arachnoid and dura and receive a sheath from each of them. The **ventral** and **dorsal roots** of the upper four sacral nerves unite at their spinal ganglia in the lateral part of the sacral canal and divide almost at once into dorsal and ventral rami. The small **dorsal rami** pass through the dorsal sacral foramina. They supply the erector spinae muscle and the skin on the dorsum of the sacrum and the adjacent gluteal region. The large **ventral rami** enter the pelvis through the pelvic sacral foramina to form the greater part of the sacral plexus [Fig. 18.3].

The roots of each **fifth sacral nerve** unite in the lower part of the sacral canal, and their rami leave the canal through its inferior end. The roots of the **coccygeal nerves** unite within the dural sac, pierce it, and leave with the fifth sacral nerve. The dorsal rami of the fifth sacral and coccygeal nerves unite to supply the overlying skin. Their ventral rami run forwards through the sacrotuberous and sacrospinous ligaments and enter the pelvis to form the coccygeal plexus.

3. The **internal vertebral venous plexus** surrounds the dural sac and nerves. It communicates

with the pelvic veins through the pelvic sacral foramina and is directly continuous with the internal vertebral venous plexus in the lumbar region [see Fig. 13.8].

Using the instructions given in Dissection 18.3 trace the nerves of the pelvis.

Lumbosacral trunk

This thick cord of nerves is formed by the ventral ramus of the lower part of the fourth lumbar and the entire fifth lumbar nerves [see Fig. 13.5]. It descends obliquely over the lateral part of the sacrum into the pelvis, posterior to the pelvic fascia. It joins the sacral ventral rami on the front of the piriformis.

Sacral and coccygeal ventral rami

The upper four sacral ventral rami emerge through the pelvic sacral foramina. The fifth and coccygeal ventral rami pierce the sacrospinous ligament and the coccygeus, above and below the transverse process of the coccyx. The first and second sacral ventral rami are large; the remainder diminish rapidly in size from above downwards.

The lumbosacral trunk and the **ventral ramus** of the **first sacral nerve** are separated by the superior gluteal vessels. Both cross the pelvic surface of the **sacro-iliac joint** before uniting on the pi-

riformis, so both may be involved in pathological changes in this joint. The first sacral ventral ramus is separated from the **second sacral ventral ramus** by the inferior gluteal vessels. The lumbosacral trunk and the ventral rami of the first, second, third, and part of the fourth sacral nerves together converge to form **the sacral plexus**. The sacral plexus is a triangular mass of nerve fibres and connective tissue which lies between the piriformis and the pelvic fascia. It terminates by branching into a smaller medial **pudendal nerve** and a larger lateral **sciatic nerve**. Other branches arise from the dorsal and pelvic surfaces of the plexus. The internal pudendal vessels descend over the front of the plexus, and the rectum overlaps the lower part of it. The inferior part of the fourth sacral ventral ramus descends to the coccygeal plexus on the surface of the coccygeus.

Before uniting to form the sacral plexus, each ventral ramus forming the sacral plexus receives a **grey ramus communicans** from the sympathetic trunk and gives rise to certain branches: (1) the first and second sacral ventral rami give twigs to the piriformis; (2) irregular branches from the third and fourth ventral rami supply the coccygeus and levator ani; and (3) **pelvic splanchnic nerves** arise from the second and third, or third and fourth, sacral ventral rami to the inferior hy-

DISSECTION 18.3 Nerves of the pelvis

Objectives

I. To identify and trace the sympathetic trunks.
II. To examine the formation of the sacral and coccygeal plexuses. III. To identify the branches of the sacral plexus.

Instructions

1. Find the sympathetic trunks as they enter the pelvis, posterior to the common iliac vessels. Trace them to their termination in the **ganglion impar** on the coccyx. Note that the **sacral splanchnic** branches are small and that the **grey rami communicantes** are the largest branches. One grey ramus communicans passes to each sacral ventral ramus as it emerges through the pelvic sacral foramen.

2. If the **superior hypogastric plexus** can be found anterior to the common iliac vessels, follow it to the **inferior hypogastric plexus** in the pelvis. Find the **pelvic**

splanchnic nerves from the ventral rami of the second to fourth sacral nerves to the inferior hypogastric plexus.

3. Expose the lumbosacral trunk and each of the five sacral ventral rami in turn. Follow them inferolaterally to the sacral plexus on the piriformis muscle.

4. Find the nerve to the quadratus femoris and obturator internus from the front of the sacral plexus. Follow them till they leave the pelvis through the greater sciatic foramen.

5. Lift the sacral plexus forwards and expose its terminal branches—the sciatic and pudendal nerves. Find the branches that arise from the dorsal surface of the plexus—the superior and inferior gluteal nerves, the perforating cutaneous nerve, and the perineal branch of the fourth sacral nerve.

6. Trace the **fourth sacral ventral ramus**. Part of it joins the fifth and the coccygeal nerve to form the coccygeal plexus on the pelvic surface of the coccygeus.

pogastric plexus. The pelvic splanchnics consist of **preganglionic parasympathetic nerve fibres** to peripheral parasympathetic ganglia innervating the pelvic viscera, the descending colon, the sigmoid colon, and the external genitalia [Fig. 18.4].

Terminal branches of the sacral plexus

The **sciatic nerve** (L. 4, 5; S. 1, 2, 3) is formed on the piriformis and leaves the pelvis through the lower part of the greater sciatic foramen. In the back of the thigh, it divides into the tibial and common fibular nerves. Occasionally, when this division occurs in the pelvis, the common fibular nerve pierces the piriformis to leave the pelvis.

The **pudendal nerve** (S. (1), 2, 3, 4) arises by separate branches from these ventral rami. It leaves the pelvis between the piriformis and coccygeus and turns round the sacrospinous ligament to enter the perineum [Fig. 18.4].

Nerves arising from the pelvic surface of the sacral plexus

The **nerve to the quadratus femoris** (L. 4, 5; S. 1) and the **nerve to the obturator internus** (L. 5; S. 1, 2) arise from the anterior surface of the sacral plexus. They leave the pelvis through the greater sciatic foramen. The nerve to the obturator internus enters the perineum through the lesser sciatic foramen and supplies the obturator internus [Fig. 18.4].

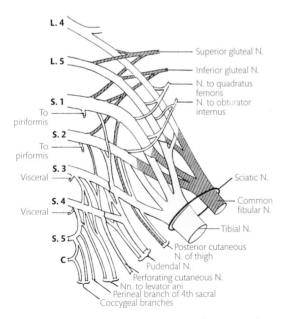

Fig. 18.4 Sacral and coccygeal plexuses. Ventral rami are yellow; ventral divisions are pale yellow; dorsal divisions are orange.

Nerves arising from the dorsal surface of the sacral plexus

The **superior gluteal nerve** (L. 4, 5; S. 1) arises above the piriformis and runs with the superior gluteal vessels to the gluteal region.

The **inferior gluteal nerve** (L. 5; S. 1, 2) and the **posterior cutaneous nerve of the thigh** (S. 1, 2, 3) leave the pelvis immediately superficial to the sciatic nerve.

The **perforating cutaneous nerve** (S. 2, 3) descends on the piriformis and coccygeus. It pierces the coccygeus muscle to reach and pierce the sacrotuberous ligament and gluteus maximus. It supplies the skin over the gluteal region.

The **perineal branch of the fourth sacral nerve** pierces the coccygeus and enters the ischio-anal fossa at the side of the coccyx by passing deep to the sacrotuberous ligament. It runs on the perineal surface of the levator ani to supply the external anal sphincter and the surrounding skin [Fig. 18.4].

Coccygeal plexus (S. 4, 5; Co.)

This minute plexus is made of the ventral rami of part of the fourth and fifth sacral and the coccygeal nerves. It lies on the pelvic surface of the coccygeus. It supplies the coccygeus, part of the levator ani, and the skin between the coccyx and anus [Fig. 18.4].

Obturator nerve (L. 2, 3, 4)

The obturator nerve is formed in the substance of the psoas from the ventral divisions of the second, third, and fourth lumbar ventral rami. It emerges from the medial aspect of the psoas, deep to the common iliac vessels, and crosses the superior aperture of the pelvis, lateral to the internal iliac vessels and the ureter. It runs antero-inferiorly on the obturator internus, anterior to the obturator vessels, and leaves the pelvis through the obturator canal. In the pelvis, it lies posterolateral to the ovary and is crossed by the attachment of the broad ligament [see Fig. 13.5; Fig. 18.1].

Autonomic nerves of the pelvis

The sympathetic trunks

The sympathetic trunks descend in the pelvis between the bodies and the pelvic sacral foramina of the sacrum. On the coccyx, they unite with each other in a median ganglion—the **ganglion impar**. The sympathetic trunks lie posterior to the pelvic fascia. There are four sacral ganglia on each trunk and one common ganglion impar [Fig. 18.5].

Branches

(1) Grey rami communicantes to all the sacral and coccygeal ventral rami.
(2) Small branches to the median sacral artery.

(3) **Sacral splanchnic nerves** from the upper ganglia to the inferior hypogastric plexus, and from the lower ganglia to the rectum.
(4) Twigs to the coccygeal body from the ganglion impar [Fig. 18.5].

Inferior hypogastric plexuses

The two inferior hypogastric (pelvic) plexuses are located around the corresponding internal iliac ar-

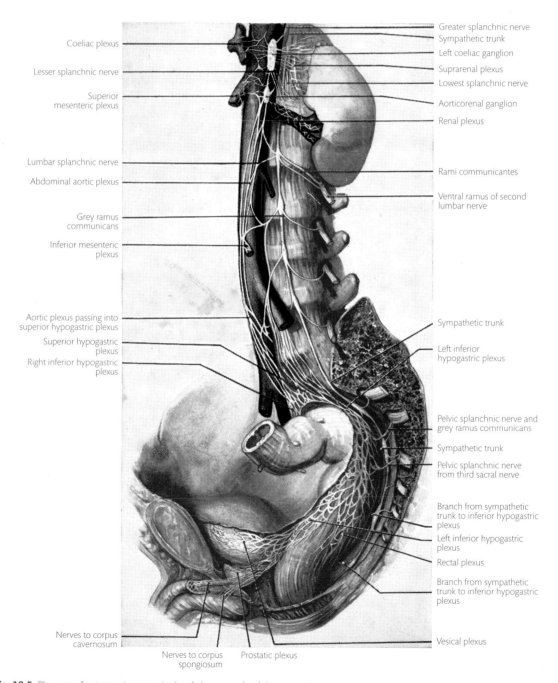

Fig. 18.5 Plexuses of autonomic nerves in the abdomen and pelvis.

teries. They receive fibres from the lumbar splanchnic nerves and small branches from the upper sacral ganglia (sacral splanchnic) of the sympathetic trunk. Superiorly, they are continuous with the superior hypogastric plexus (the presacral nerve) which lies below the bifurcation of the aorta. Distally, the main plexus divides into subsidiary plexuses along the visceral branches of the internal iliac artery. These plexuses communicate with each other and receive branches from the **pelvic splanchnic nerves**. (The pelvic splanchnic are preganglionic parasympathetic fibres from the third and fourth segments of the spinal cord.) Small ganglia are found in these plexuses and their extensions [Fig. 18.5].

Visceral autonomic plexuses in the pelvis

These are extensions of the inferior hypogastric plexuses on the walls of the pelvic viscera. (1) The **rectal plexus** receives a contribution from the inferior mesenteric plexus. It sends **parasympathetic fibres** back into the inferior mesenteric plexus and the sigmoid and descending colons. (2) The **vesical plexus** is continuous with that over the vas deferens, seminal vesicles, and prostate. (3) The **prostatic plexus** sends **cavernous nerves** along the membranous urethra to the penis. (4) The **uterine** and **vaginal plexuses** accompany the corresponding arteries. The vaginal plexus supplies the urethra and sends **cavernous nerves** to the bulbs of the vestibule and to the clitoris [Fig. 18.5].

Muscles of the lesser pelvis

Dissection 18.4 explores the muscles of the pelvis.

Piriformis

The piriformis muscle is conical in shape. It takes origin on the pelvic surface of the sacrum [Fig. 18.6] and passes inferolaterally. It enters the gluteal region through the greater sciatic foramen (below the sacro-iliac joint), crosses the posterior surface of the hip joint, and is inserted into the tip of the greater trochanter of the femur. **Nerve supply**: small branches from the ventral rami of the first and second sacral nerves. **Actions**: it helps to stabilize the hip joint. It can act as a lateral rotator of the extended femur or an abductor when it is flexed.

DISSECTION 18.4 Muscles of the pelvis

Objective

I. To clean and display the piriformis, coccygeus, and levator ani.

Instructions

1. Define the attachment of the piriformis to the sacrum. Follow it to the greater sciatic foramen or to the greater trochanter of the femur if the gluteal region has been dissected.

2. Identify the **ischial spine** [see Fig. 15.4] and the fibres of the coccygeus and levator ani that are attached to it [see Fig. 17.8].

3. Move the pelvic organs (bladder, prostate or uterus and vagina, and rectum) medially, and expose the superior surface of the **levator ani**. Take particular care posteriorly where the muscle is thin. Trace its fibres inferomedially to the insertion.

4. With a finger in the ischioanal fossa, determine the origin of the levator ani muscle from the ischial spine, the pelvic surface of the body of the pubis, and the fascia covering the obturator internus. Identify the free medial border of the muscle by removing the lateral attachment of the puboprostatic or pubovesical ligament from the fascia covering the levator ani.

Coccygeus

This is the muscular anterior part of the sacrospinous ligament. It is attached to the ischial spine and to the lateral margins of the coccyx and the last piece of the sacrum. It is parallel to the inferior margin of the piriformis and is edge to edge with the posterior border of the levator ani. It forms the lowest part of the posterior wall of the lesser pelvis. The coccygeus also forms the posterior part of the floor of the pelvis or the **pelvic diaphragm** [Fig. 18.7]. (The pelvic diaphragm is formed mainly by the levator ani.) **Nerve supply**: the lower sacral ventral rami. **Actions**: it may assist the sacrospinous ligament in supporting the pelvic contents. It can only produce minor movements of the coccyx.

Levator ani

The two thin sheets of the levator ani muscles together form the floor of the lesser pelvis and separate the pelvis from the ischioanal fossae. Each muscle has a

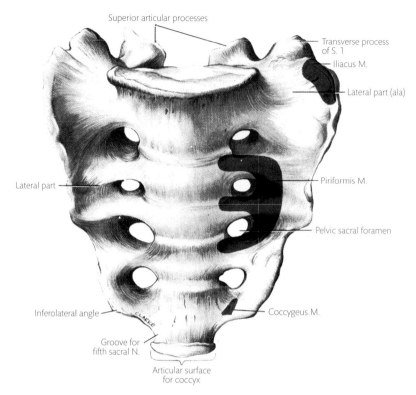

Fig. 18.6 The pelvic surface of the sacrum.

long, linear origin from: (1) the pelvic surface of the body of the pubis; (2) the **tendinous arch** or thickening of the fascia covering the obturator internus; and (3) the ischial spine. The right and left muscles converge and are inserted together into the central perineal tendon, the anal canal, the anococcygeal ligament, and the coccyx [Fig. 18.7]. The anterior fibres of both muscles pass horizontally backwards to the central perineal tendon. In the male, they pass below the prostate, forming the **levator prostatae**, and below the bladder [see Fig. 16.13; Fig. 18.7]. In the female, the anterior fibres pass on either side of the vagina and form the **pubovaginalis** [see Fig. 17.18]. The anterior fibres are separated from each other by a gap which transmits the urethra and vagina. The posterior fibres run inferomedially. Those that join the **anal canal** pass between the internal and external anal sphincters, merge with the longitudinal smooth muscle layer, and pass to the perianal skin [see Fig. 17.20]. Those that pass to the

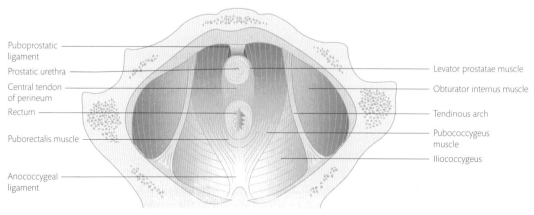

Fig. 18.7 Levator ani muscles viewed from above.

anococcygeal ligament and coccyx lie inferior to the terminal part of the rectum and support it.

The **puborectalis part** of the muscle arises from the pubis and passes posteriorly, inferior to the other fibres. It curves around and fuses with fibres of the opposite side on the posterior surface of the anorectal junction, forming a U-shaped sling on the anorectal junction.

Nerve supply: the pelvic surface of the levator ani is supplied by the ventral rami of the lower sacral and coccygeal nerves. The perineal surface is supplied by fibres from the inferior rectal nerve.

Actions: the two levator ani muscles act together to raise the pelvic diaphragm. This assists the muscles of the abdominal wall to compress the abdominal contents in forced expiration, coughing, vomiting, and urination and in fixing the trunk for strong movements of the upper limbs. The fibres that are inserted into the central perineal tendon support the prostate in the male and the posterior wall of the vagina in the female. In the female, the fibres inserted into the central perineal tendon, together with the bulbospongiosus muscles, act as an incomplete **sphincter of the vagina**. The fibres that are inserted into the anal canal and central perineal tendon pull the anal canal over the descending mass of faeces. The **puborectalis** pulls the anorectal junction forwards and increases the angulation between the rectum and the anal canal. In childbirth, the whole muscle supports the head of the fetus during dilatation of the cervix. ➲ The anterior part of the levator ani may be torn during childbirth as the head passes through the vagina. Such a tear reduces the support of the posterior vaginal wall.

Use instructions in Dissection 18.5 to study the obturator internus.

Obturator internus

This thick, fan-shaped muscle covers most of the side wall of the lesser pelvis. It arises from the obturator membrane, the margins of the obturator foramen (except at the obturator sulcus), and a wide area between the obturator foramen and the greater sciatic notch [see Fig. 17.8], medial to the acetabulum. The fibres converge postero-inferiorly on a strong tendon. The obturator tendon turns around the lesser sciatic notch and runs laterally over the posterior surface of the hip joint to the medial aspect of the greater trochanter of the femur. **Nerve supply**: nerve from the sacral plexus. **Actions**: it stabilizes the hip joint and laterally rotates the femur in the erect position, but abducts it when the hip is flexed.

DISSECTION 18.5 Obturator internus

Objective

I. To identify and clean the obturator internus.

Instructions

1. When the levator ani muscles have been fully dissected, separate them from their origins to expose the obturator fascia.

2. Remove the fascia from the obturator internus, and identify the pudendal canal and its contents.

3. Follow the fibres of the obturator internus to the lesser sciatic notch.

4. Lift the tendon of the obturator internus from the notch, and identify the bursa between it and the bone.

Obturator fascia

The dense obturator fascia covers the pelvic surface of the obturator internus. It fuses with the periosteum at the margins of the muscle, except: (1) at the obturator sulcus where it forms the floor of the obturator canal; and (2) postero-inferiorly where it unites with the falciform process of the sacrotuberous ligament [see Fig. 15.5].

Most of the levator ani muscle arises from the thickened **tendinous arch** of the obturator fascia which stretches between the body of the pubis and the ischial spine. Inferior to the tendinous arch, the fascia forms the lateral wall of the ischioanal fossa and splits to form the pudendal canal.

Joints of the lesser pelvis

The bony pelvis articulates with the rest of the axial skeleton at the **lumbosacral joints**, between the fifth lumbar vertebra and the sacrum. On each side, the lateral part of the sacrum articulates with the ilium at a **sacro-iliac joint**. These synovial joints are maintained by strong **interosseous** and **dorsal sacro-iliac ligaments**. In addition to the ligaments holding them together, the sacrum (and coccyx with it) are held in position relative to the hip bones by the **sacrotuberous** and **sacrospinous ligaments** [Fig. 18.8]. Anteriorly, the hip bones are united in the **pubic symphysis** which is described in Chapter 17. Inferiorly, the sacrum is joined to the coccyx by the **sacrococcygeal joint**.

Dissection 18.6 gives instructions for dissecting the sacro-iliac joints.

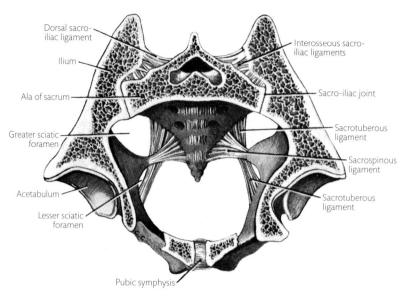

Dorsal sacro-iliac ligament

Ilium

Ala of sacrum

Greater sciatic foramen

Acetabulum

Lesser sciatic foramen

Pubic symphysis

Interosseous sacro-iliac ligaments

Sacro-iliac joint

Sacrotuberous ligament

Sacrospinous ligament

Sacrotuberous ligament

290

Fig. 18.8 An oblique section through the lesser pelvis to show the ligaments and sacro-iliac joints.

DISSECTION 18.6 Sacro-iliac joints

Objective

I. To study the ligaments and articulating surfaces of the sacro-iliac joint.

Instructions

1. Remove the remnants of the thoracolumbar fascia and the erector spinae muscles from the dorsal surface of the sacrum and the fifth lumbar vertebra. Complete the exposure of the iliolumbar and dorsal sacro-iliac ligaments.

2. Identify the **ventral sacro-iliac ligament** on the pelvic surface of the sacro-iliac joint.

3. If fusion between the lateral part of the sacrum and the ilium has not occurred, cut through the ligament

and open the joint by bending the sacrum backwards against the ilium. Note the thinness of the ventral sacro-iliac ligament.

4. Note that the cartilage-covered joint surfaces are irregular and fitted closely to leave very little possibility of movement.

5. Strip off the dorsal sacro-iliac ligaments to expose the interosseous sacro-iliac ligaments which lie deep to them. Divide the interosseous ligaments and separate the sacrum from the ilium.

6. Examine the joint surfaces again.

Lumbosacral joints

The lumbosacral joint is similar to joints between the lumbar vertebrae. However, the lumbosacral **intervertebral disc** is wedge-shaped, with a greater height anteriorly. This wedge shape helps to compensate for the considerable angulation between the adjacent surfaces of the fifth lumbar vertebra and the sacrum [see Fig. 1.2A]. The stability of the articulation between the fifth lumbar vertebra and the sacrum is increased by: (1) the widely

spaced articular processes; and (2) the strong iliolumbar ligaments.

➲A number of variations are commonly seen at this joint. The fifth lumbar vertebra or its transverse processes may be fused with the sacrum on one or both sides. This is known as sacralization of the fifth lumbar vertebra. The first sacral vertebra may be partly or completely separated from the remainder of the sacrum—a condition known as lumbarization of the first sacral vertebra. The normal sacral hiatus may extend superiorly into the upper part of the sacrum or lumbar region. This would result in spina bifida. Rarely, the spine, laminae, and inferior articular processes of the fifth lumbar vertebra are separate from the remainder of the vertebra. This condition allows the body of the fifth lumbar vertebra to slide forwards on the sloping superior surface of the sacrum—spondylolisthesis.

Sacrococcygeal joint

The sacrococcygeal joint between the sacrum and coccyx has a thin intervertebral disc and ligaments corresponding to the anterior and posterior longitudinal ligaments of other intervertebral discs. The sacral and coccygeal cornua and transverse processes are also linked by ligaments which may ossify. Coccygeal joints (between the individual coccygeal vertebra) are present in young subjects, but ossify early.

Sacro-iliac joint

The sacro-iliac joint is a very strong synovial joint responsible for transmitting the weight of the body to the hip bones. It allows little movement. The sacrum is wedged between the iliac bones so that the cartilage on the uneven **auricular surfaces** of both bones are firmly fitted to each other and held in position by powerful **interosseous** and **dorsal sacro-iliac ligaments**.

The weight of the body tends to drive the base of the sacrum downwards between the hip bones. This movement tightens the sacro-iliac ligaments and draws the articular surfaces closer together. The same force tends to tilt the apex of the sacrum upwards, moving the sacrum around a transverse axis. This tendency of the sacrum to tilt is resisted by the sacrotuberous and sacrospinous ligaments.

The **ventral sacro-iliac ligament** is composed of thin transverse fibres between the convex margins of the articular surfaces. The **interosseous sacro-iliac ligaments** are very strong. They unite the wide, rough areas that adjoin the concave margins of the auricular surfaces [see Figs. 7.4, 7.5, 15.4, 17.8] and close the sacro-iliac joints dorsally. The **dorsal sacro-iliac ligaments** are immediately superficial to the interosseous ligaments and are fused with them. They consist of: (1) short transverse fibres that pass from the ilium to the upper part of the lateral crest of the sacrum; and (2) a longer, more vertical band from the posterior superior iliac spine of the ilium to the upper part of the lateral sacral crest.

Posteriorly, the joint is covered by the erector spinae and gluteus maximus muscles. The skin dimple marking the position of the posterior superior iliac spine lies at the level of the middle of the joint.

The abdominal surface of the joint is covered by the psoas and iliacus, with the **obturator** and **femoral nerves** close to it. The pelvic surface is crossed by the **lumbosacral trunk** and the **first sacral ventral ramus**. ⊃ Any of these nerves may be involved in disease of the joint and may give rise to pain in their cutaneous distribution [see Fig. 19.1, Vol. 1]. The internal iliac vein and the superior gluteal vessels are also in contact with the pelvic surface of the joint. ⊃ The joint may become partly ossified with increasing age.

Movement at the joint is limited to a slight rotation around a horizontal axis towards the end of full flexion of the trunk on the hip joints (like in touching the toes with the knees straight). The main function of the joint is to absorb some of the forces suddenly applied to the feet, e.g. when landing from a height. The resilience of the sacrotuberous ligament cushions the shock [see Fig. 7.6]. The sacro-iliac ligaments, the pubic symphysis, and sacrococcygeal ligaments become softer and more yielding in the later stages of pregnancy, producing a combined effect which facilitates the passage of the fetus through the pelvis at term.

CHAPTER 19
MCQs for part 4:
The pelvis and perineum

The following questions have four options each. You are required to choose the most correct answer.

1. **The inferior layer of the urogenital diaphragm is the**

    A. central perineal tendon
    B. perineal membrane
    C. Colles' fascia
    D. Scarpa's fascia

2. **In the female, the base of the urinary bladder is directly related to the**

    A. cervix of the uterus
    B. body of the uterus
    C. rectum
    D. anal canal

3. **Which one of the following is NOT true of the ejaculatory duct?**

    A. is formed by the union of the duct of the seminal vesicle and the vas deferens
    B. is formed posterior to the neck of the bladder
    C. opens into the prostatic urethra
    D. passes between the anterior and median lobes of the prostate

4. **The inferior aperture of the pelvis is bounded by the following, EXCEPT the**

    A. ischiopubic ramus
    B. sacrotuberous ligament
    C. coccyx
    D. pecten pubis

5. **All the following statements are true regarding the iliolumbar ligament, EXCEPT that it**

    A. unites the transverse process of the fifth lumbar vertebra and the iliac crest
    B. plays an important part in maintaining the fifth lumbar vertebra in position
    C. gives attachment to the psoas major
    D. is related to the erector spinae muscle posteriorly

6. **The pelvic floor is formed by the**

   A. piriformis
   B. obturator internus
   C. obturator externus
   D. levator ani

7. **The root value of the lumbosacral trunk is**

   A. L. 4, L. 5, S. 1
   B. L. 5, S. 1, S. 2
   C. L. 4, L. 5
   D. L. 5, S. 1

8. **Which part of the male urethra is surrounded by sphincter urethrae?**

   A. bulbous urethra
   B. prostatic urethra
   C. membranous urethra
   D. spongy urethra

9. **Which one of the following is NOT a content of the deep perineal pouch?**

   A. sphincter urethrae
   B. deep transverse perineal muscles
   C. bulbospongiosus
   D. bulbo-urethral glands

10. **The lymph vessels from the testis drain into the**

    A. superficial inguinal lymph nodes
    B. deep inguinal lymph nodes
    C. sacral lymph nodes
    D. lumbar lymph nodes

11. **The left ovarian vein drains into the**

    A. inferior vena cava
    B. left renal vein
    C. internal iliac vein
    D. external iliac vein

12. **The medial umbilical ligament is the fibrous remnant of the intra-abdominal part of the**

    A. vitelline duct
    B. allantois
    C. umbilical vein
    D. umbilical artery

13. The uvula of the urinary bladder is produced by the

A. median lobe of the prostate
B. posterior lobe of the prostate
C. anterior lobe of the prostate
D. lateral lobe of the prostate

14. Which one of the following arteries is a branch of the posterior division of the internal iliac artery?

A. superior gluteal
B. inferior gluteal
C. obturator
D. internal pudendal

15. Which of the following statements is true regarding the internal anal sphincter?

A. it is present around the lower two-thirds of the anal canal
B. it is formed by the circular smooth muscle of the intestine
C. it is innervated by the inferior rectal nerve
D. it is voluntary in nature

Please go to the back of the book for the answers.

PART 5

The trunk

297

CHAPTER 20

Movements of the trunk and muscles involved in bodily functions

Introduction

The muscles, joints, and movement possible in the joints of the trunk have been described in the preceding section of the book. The muscles acting to move the trunk and in respiration and other functions, such as coughing, vomiting, voiding, and straining, are described in Tables 20.1, 20.2, and 20.3.

Table 20.1 Movements of the trunk

Movement		Muscles acting
Flexion	Without resistance, as in bending forwards while standing	Erector spinae acting excentrically
	Against resistance, as in raising the head and shoulders from the supine position	Rectus abdominis Psoas major External oblique Internal oblique
Extension	–	Erector spinae
Lateral flexion	Against resistance	Oblique muscles of the abdomen of the same side Quadratus lumborum of the same side Psoas of the same side Erector spinae of the same side Latissimus dorsi if arm fixed
	No resistance (with gravity)	Same muscles of the opposite side acting excentrically
Rotation to right	–	Left external oblique acting with the right internal oblique
Rotation to left	–	Right external oblique acting with the left internal oblique

Table 20.2 Respiratory movements

Movement		Muscles acting
Inspiration	In quiet respiration	Diaphragm increases the vertical extent of the thorax by lowering its dome (see accessory muscles) Scalene muscles of the neck raise the first and second ribs [Vol. 3] External intercostal muscles slide the upper ribs forwards on the lower ribs of each space. This raises the ribs and increases the space between them (only upper muscles involved in forced respiration) **Accessory muscles** Vertical posterior fibres of the internal and external oblique muscles and the quadratus lumborum hold down the lowest ribs and help in lowering the dome of the diaphragm

Table 20.2 Respiratory movements (*Continued*)

Movement		Muscles acting
	In forced respiration	Sternocleidomastoid raises the sternum Pectoralis major and minor help to raise the ribs, especially when the scapula and arm are elevated by the levator scapulae and trapezius Serratus anterior may also assist Erector spinae extends the trunk. This separates the ribs anteriorly and increases the distance between the first rib and the pubic symphysis, thereby enlarging both the thorax and abdomen
Expiration	In quiet respiration	Ribs are lowered by gravity and elastic recoil of the lungs Relaxed diaphragm is raised by elastic recoil of the lungs
	In moderate respiration and in other types of controlled expiration, e.g. singing	The diaphragm and external intercostal muscles are active in the early phases of expiration, to prevent too rapid expulsion of air by elastic recoil of the lungs
	In forced expiration	External oblique, internal oblique, and quadratus lumborum act from the hip to pull down the ribs Internal and innermost intercostals and subcostals act from below to slide the upper ribs backwards on the lower ribs, to lower and approximate the ribs (although the rectus abdominis is capable of lowering the sternum and costal cartilages, it is not so used, except in violent expiratory effort associated with trunk flexion)
	In more forced respiration or when it is necessary to maintain a steady flow of expiratory air as the elastic recoil of the lung diminishes	Abdominal compression by the external oblique, internal oblique, and transversus abdominis muscles. In forced expiration against resistance, e.g. in asthma, this may raise the intra-abdominal pressure sufficiently to cause discharge of urine from an incontinent bladder (in all cases where contraction of the abdominal muscles causes raised intra-abdominal pressure, it is accompanied by contraction of the perineal muscles)

Table 20.3 Muscles involved in other bodily functions

Activity	Muscles involved
In coughing and sneezing	These sudden, violent expirations use the same muscles as in forced expiration (with the addition of the latissimus dorsi). Air passages are closed by approximation of the vocal folds in the larynx (closure of the glottis) till the intrathoracic and intra-abdominal pressures have reached a high level. The vocal folds are then separated (opening the glottis) so that air is discharged through the mouth (coughing) or nose (sneezing)
In vomiting	Muscles used in this action are those used in coughing, except that there is no build-up of intrathoracic pressure since it is the diaphragm and abdominal muscles that contract. The stomach does not contract but is rhythmically compressed. The airway is normally closed during vomiting. Perineal muscles also contract
In urination against resistance, defecation, and parturition	In all of these actions, the expulsion of luminal contents is assisted by the contraction of the abdominal muscles. When these contractions are mild, they are associated with diaphragmatic contraction so that costal respiration can continue. When powerful, they are always associated with closure of the glottis and a build-up of intrathoracic as well as intra-abdominal pressures by contraction of the expiratory muscles without expulsion of air from the lungs. The end of the expulsive activity is marked by expiration of air previously held under pressure in the lungs
In any strenuous activity, e.g. lifting, pushing, and pulling heavy weights	Expiratory muscles of the thorax and abdomen are powerfully contracted against a closed glottis, together with perineal muscles and the flexor and extensor muscles of the trunk. This turns the trunk into a rigid structure on which the limbs can work, but also produces very high pressures within it. As in all other actions which raise intra-abdominal pressure, the lower fibres of the internal oblique and transversus abdominis which arch over the inguinal canal to fuse in the conjoint tendon close down on the spermatic cord In this action, as in powerful extension of the flexed vertebral column, the compressive force applied to the vertebral column is large and the pressure within the intervertebral disc rises accordingly. Any weakness of the annulus fibrosus may result in protrusion of the nucleus through it. Disc prolapse is made more likely if the vertebral column is flexed when the compression forces are applied, because the posterior part of the annulus is then stretched

CHAPTER 21
Cross-sectional anatomy of the trunk

This chapter describes the vertebral levels of important organs and provides an introduction to cross-sectional anatomy through the study of serial cross-sectional images, MRIs, and CTs.

Approximate levels of structures in the trunk

Prior to looking at images of cross-sectional anatomy, it is useful to recall the vertebral level of internal organs. It should be appreciated that all the horizontal levels given in this table are subject to considerable variation on account of various factors. (1) Certain organs, such as the heart, lungs, liver, stomach, spleen, and kidneys, are mobile. They move with respiration and with changes in body position (erect or recumbent, flexed or extended). (2) Organs are placed slightly differently in normal individuals of different physical types. In the cadaver, the recumbent position of the body, combined with relaxation of the diaphragm and the elastic recoil of the lungs, leads to abnormally high levels. Table 21.1 describes the vertebral spine and body levels as landmarks of internal organs.

Table 21.1 Vertebral spine and body levels as landmarks of internal organs

Vertebral body	Vertebral spine	Viscera	Surface landmarks (where available)
T. 1	C. 7	Apex of lung	1–3 cm superior to the medial one-third of clavicle
T. 3	T. 2	Upper limit of aortic arch	–
T. 4	T. 3	Formation of superior vena cava	Right first costal cartilage
T. 4 (lower border)	T. 3	Tracheal bifurcation	Sternal angle
T. 5 (upper border)	T. 4	Aortic arch begins and ends	Sternal angle
T. 5 (upper border)	T. 4	Upper border of heart	Sternal angle
	T. 8	Lower border of heart	–
T. 8	T. 8	Vena caval orifice in diaphragm	–
T. 10	T. 9	Oesophageal orifice in diaphragm	–
T. 10	T. 10	Gastro-oesophageal junction	–
T. 10	T. 10	Lower limit of lung	–
T. 11	T. 10	Upper limit of kidney	–
T. 12	T. 11	Aortic orifice in diaphragm	–
T. 12	T. 12	Lowest level of pleura	–
L. 1 (lower border)	T. 12	Pylorus	Transpyloric plane
L. 1 (lower border)	T. 12	Portal vein formation	Transpyloric plane
L. 1 (lower border)	T. 12	Hilum of kidney	Transpyloric plane

Table 21.1 Vertebral spine and body levels as landmarks of internal organs (*Continued*)

Vertebral body	Vertebral spine	Viscera	Surface landmarks (where available)
L. 1 (lower border)	T. 12	Superior mesenteric artery	Transpyloric plane
L. 1 (lower border)	L. 1	Fundus of gallbladder	Transpyloric plane, right ninth costal cartilage
L. 1 (lower border)	L. 2	Spinal cord terminates	–
L. 2	L. 2	Duodenojejunal flexure	–
L. 3	L. 3	Lower border of kidney	–
L. 3	L. 3	Inferior mesenteric artery	–
L. 3	L. 3	Third part of duodenum	–
L. 4	L. 4	Bifurcation of aorta	Highest point of iliac crest
L. 5	L. 5	Inferior vena cava begins	Transtubercular plane
S. 2	S. 2	End of dural sac	Posterior superior iliac spine

Serial sections through the trunk as seen in gross anatomy, CTs, and MRIs

Cross-sections through the trunk at different levels show the relationship of the viscera to each other and the body wall. In the series of figures presented in this chapter (Figs. 21.2–21.17), the first section [Fig. 21.2] is through the upper part of the superior mediastinum. The subsequent sections are taken one below the other, until the last sections which are taken through the pelvis. (Fig. 21.1 serves as a quick guide to show the level at which the horizontal sections are made.)

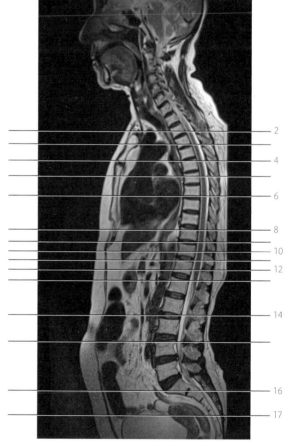

Fig. 21.1 Horizontal lines on the longitudinal section of the trunk indicating the approximate level of sections shown in Figs. 21.2 to 21.17.

(A)

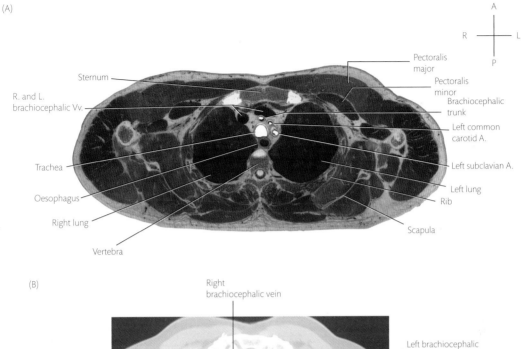

Sternum

R. and L.
brachiocephalic Vv.

Trachea

Oesophagus

Right lung

Vertebra

A
R ——|—— L
P

Pectoralis
major

Pectoralis
minor

Brachiocephalic
trunk

Left common
carotid A.

Left subclavian A.

Left lung

Rib

Scapula

(B)

Right
brachiocephalic vein

Brachiocephalic
trunk

Trachea

Left brachiocephalic
vein

Left common
carotid artery

Left subclavian artery

(C)

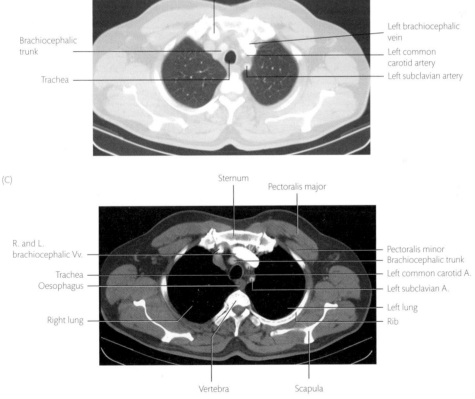

Sternum

Pectoralis major

R. and L.
brachiocephalic Vv.

Trachea

Oesophagus

Right lung

Pectoralis minor

Brachiocephalic trunk

Left common carotid A.

Left subclavian A.

Left lung

Rib

Vertebra

Scapula

Fig. 21.2 (A) A transverse section through the superior mediastinum. The skeletal elements seen are the sternum and costal cartilages (anteriorly), the vertebra (posteriorly), and the ribs. The scapula and humerus are also seen, as are the muscles of the upper limb. The upper lobes of the right and left lungs are seen on either side of the mediastinum. In the mediastinum, start by identifying the oesophagus and trachea in the midline. The three branches of the arch of the aorta—the brachiocephalic trunk, and left common carotid and left subclavian arteries—are seen in front of, and on the left of, the trachea. Further anteriorly, just behind the sternum are the right and left brachiocephalic veins. (B) An axial CT section of the superior mediastinum showing the brachiocephalic veins, branches of the arch of the aorta, the trachea, and the oesophagus. (C) A contrast-enhanced axial CT section showing the left and right brachiocephalic veins, the aortic arch branches, the trachea, and the oesophagus.

(A) courtesy of the Visible Human Project of the US National Library of Medicine. (B) and (C) courtesy of the Radiology Department, Christian Medical College, Vellore, India.

(A)

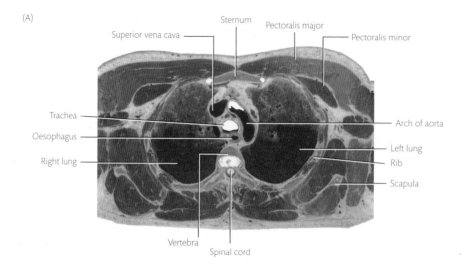

(B)

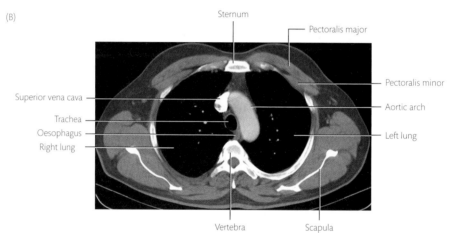

Fig. 21.3 (A) A section through the lower superior mediastinum showing the arch of the aorta, trachea, and oesophagus. The right and left brachiocephalic veins, seen in Fig. 21.2, have united at this level to form the superior vena cava. The right and left lungs are seen on either side of the mediastinum. Note the position of the spinal cord in the vertebral canal. (B) A contrast-enhanced axial CT scan inferior to the section in Fig. 21.2C, showing the aortic arch, superior vena cava, trachea, and oesophagus.

(A) courtesy of the Visible Human Project of the US National Library of Medicine. (B) courtesy of the Radiology Department, Christian Medical College, Vellore, India.

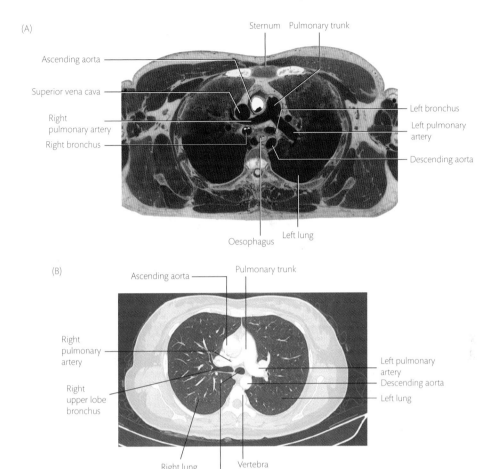

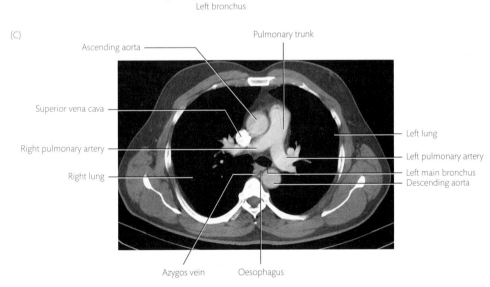

Fig. 21.4 (A) A section through the middle mediastinum at the upper border of the heart. The ascending aorta and pulmonary trunk lie side by side in the anterior part. The right and left pulmonary arteries are seen arising from the pulmonary trunk and entering the hilum of the lung. The terminal part of the superior vena cava lies to the right of the ascending aorta. The trachea, seen in more cranial sections, has bifurcated at this level, and the right and left principal bronchi are seen. The oesophagus lies immediately in front of the vertebral column, and the descending aorta to the left of it. The right and left lungs are seen on either side of the mediastinum. (B) An axial CT image and (C) a contrast-enhanced axial CT section (inferior to the section in Fig. 21.3B) showing the ascending and descending aorta, main pulmonary artery, right and left pulmonary arteries, superior vena cava, oesophagus, and azygos vein.

(A) courtesy of the Visible Human Project of the US National Library of Medicine. (B) and (C) courtesy of the Radiology Department, Christian Medical College, Vellore, India.

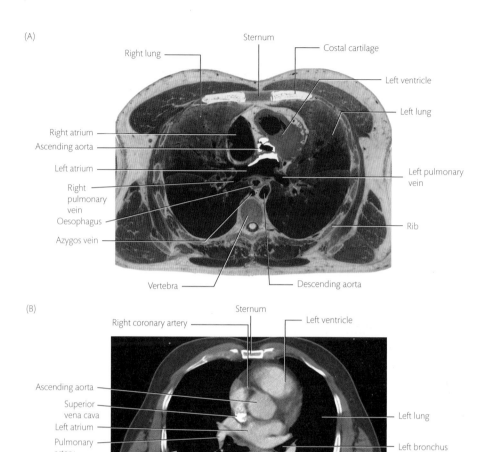

(A)

Right lung

Sternum

Costal cartilage

Left ventricle

Left lung

Right atrium

Ascending aorta

Left atrium

Right pulmonary vein

Oesophagus

Azygos vein

Left pulmonary vein

Rib

Vertebra

Descending aorta

(B)

Right coronary artery

Sternum

Left ventricle

Ascending aorta

Superior vena cava

Left atrium

Pulmonary artery

Right lung

Oesophagus

Azygos vein

Left lung

Left bronchus

Pulmonary artery

Decending aorta

Costovertebral joint

Fig. 21.5 (A) A section through the middle mediastinum at the level of the atria, inferior to the previous section. The right atrium is seen indenting the right lung. The beginning of the ascending aorta is seen between the right atrium and the left ventricle. The left atrium lies posteriorly, immediately in front of the oesophagus. The pulmonary veins from the hilus of the lung are seen entering the left atrium. The descending aorta on the left and the azygos vein on the right are seen on the vertebral body. The right and left lungs are seen on either side of the mediastinum. (B) A contrast-enhanced axial CT section at the level of the atria (inferior to the section in Fig. 21.4C). The superior vena cava is seen entering the right atrium. The right coronary artery is seen arising from the ascending aorta.

(A) courtesy of the Visible Human Project of the US National Library of Medicine. (B) courtesy of the Radiology Department, Christian Medical College, Vellore, India.

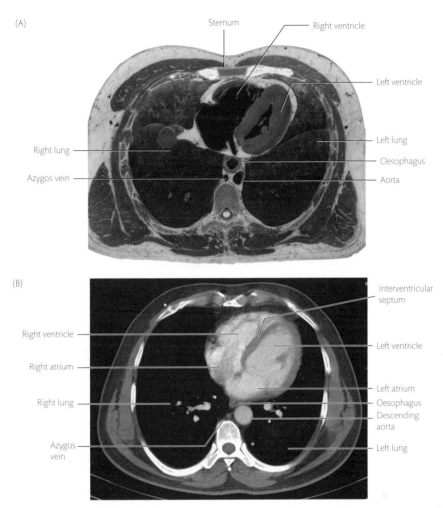

Fig. 21.6 (A) A section through the middle mediastinum inferior to the previous section, at the level of the ventricles. Note the difference in thickness of the walls of the right and left ventricles. The oesophagus, descending aorta, and azygos vein are seen in the posterior mediastinum. The right and left lungs are seen on either side of the mediastinum. (B) A contrast-enhanced axial CT section at the same level (inferior to the section in Fig. 21.5B). The interventricular septum is clearly seen.

(A) courtesy of the Visible Human Project of the US National Library of Medicine. (B) courtesy of the Radiology Department, Christian Medical College, Vellore, India.

(A)

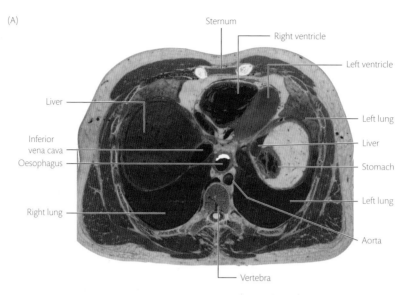

(B)

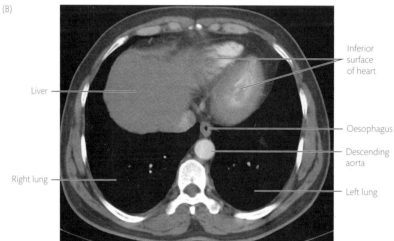

Fig. 21.7 (A) A section through the lower thorax and upper part of the abdomen, inferior to the section in Fig. 21.6A. Part of the right and left lungs, the right and left ventricles of the heart, the descending aorta, and the oesophagus are seen. On the right side, the upper part of the right lobe of the liver and the abdominal part of the inferior vena cava are seen. On the left are seen the stomach and a small segment of the left lobe of the liver. (B) A contrast-enhanced axial CT section at the level of the lower thorax and upper abdomen (inferior to the section in Fig. 21.6B).

(A) courtesy of the Visible Human Project of the US National Library of Medicine. (B) courtesy of the Radiology Department, Christian Medical College, Vellore, India.

(A)

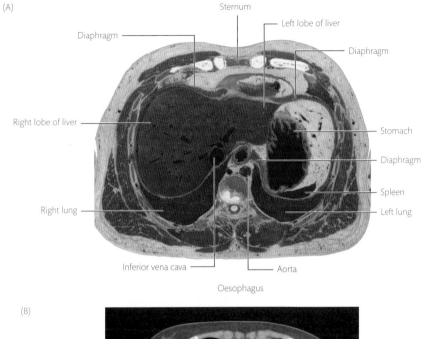

Sternum

Left lobe of liver

Diaphragm

Diaphragm

Right lobe of liver

Stomach

Diaphragm

Spleen

Right lung

Left lung

Inferior vena cava

Aorta

Oesophagus

(B)

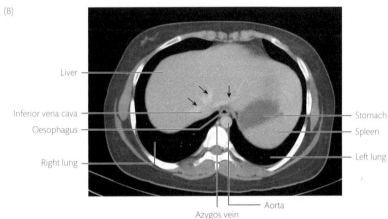

Liver

Inferior vena cava

Oesophagus

Stomach

Spleen

Right lung

Left lung

Aorta

Azygos vein

Fig. 21.8 (A) A section through the upper part of the abdomen, inferior to the previous section. The lower lobes of the right and left lungs are seen. The right lobe of the liver fills the entire right side of the abdomen. The inferior vena cava is seen buried in the groove on the liver. The fundus of the stomach and a small part of the spleen are seen on the left. The oesophagus, thoracic aorta, and azygos vein are seen in the posterior mediastinum, behind the diaphragm. (B) A contrast-enhanced (venous phase) axial CT section through the upper abdomen at the level of the upper liver, showing the hepatic veins (arrows), inferior vena cava, aorta, oesophagus, azygos vein, stomach, spleen, and lung bases.

(A) courtesy of the Visible Human Project of the US National Library of Medicine. (B) courtesy of the Radiology Department, Christian Medical College, Vellore, India.

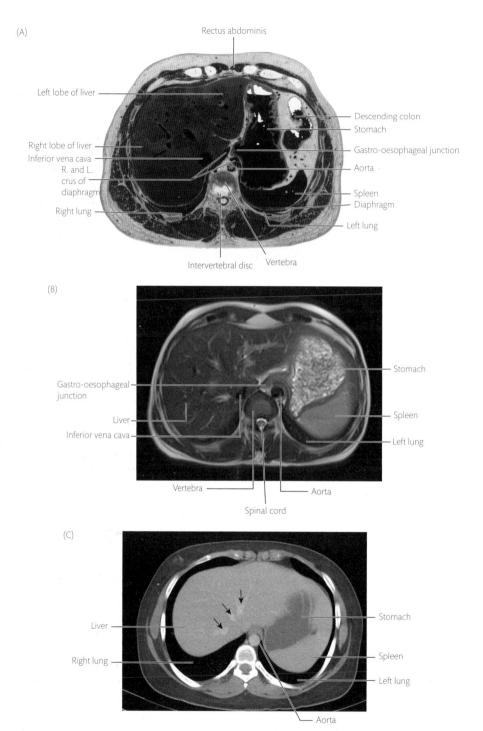

Fig. 21.9 (A) A section through the upper part of the abdomen, inferior to the previous section. The sternum is no longer seen and upper parts of the rectus abdominis are seen close to the midline. The right lobe of liver fills almost the entire right side of the image, except for a small sliver of the right lung that is still seen. The inferior vena cava appears to be embedded in the liver tissue. The oesophagus is seen entering the abdomen through the crus of the diaphragm and opening into the stomach at the gastro-oesophageal junction. The aorta lies immediately posterior at this point. Behind the stomach is seen the spleen, and to the left, parts of the descending colon. The section has gone through parts of the vertebra and the intervertebral disc posteriorly. (B) A T2W axial MRI section through the upper abdomen showing the liver, spleen, stomach, aorta, gastro-oesophageal junction, vertebra, and spinal cord. (C) A contrast-enhanced (venous phase) axial CT section through the upper abdomen, inferior to the section in Fig. 21.8B, showing the hepatic veins (arrows), inferior vena cava, aorta, stomach, spleen, and lung bases.

(A) courtesy of the Visible Human Project of the US National Library of Medicine. (B) and (C) courtesy of the Radiology Department, Christian Medical College, Vellore, India.

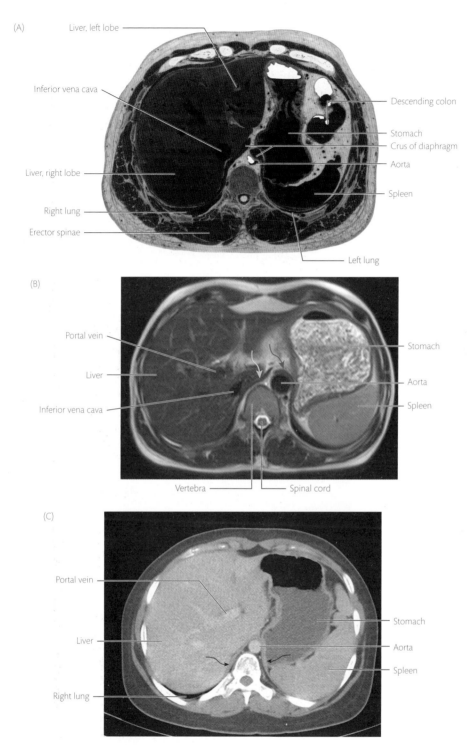

(A) Liver, left lobe

Inferior vena cava

Descending colon

Stomach

Crus of diaphragm

Aorta

Liver, right lobe

Spleen

Right lung

Erector spinae

Left lung

(B)

Portal vein

Stomach

Liver

Aorta

Inferior vena cava

Spleen

Vertebra

Spinal cord

(C)

Portal vein

Stomach

Liver

Aorta

Spleen

Right lung

Fig. 21.10 (A) A section through the upper part of the abdomen, just 5 mm inferior to the section in Fig. 21.9A, showing most of the same structures. Note that the sections through the lung are smaller and that the section through the spleen is bigger than in the previous image. The right and left crura of the diaphragm are clearly seen on either side and overlapping the anterior aspect of the descending aorta. (The intervertebral disc is not seen in this section.) (B) A T2W axial MRI section through the upper abdomen (inferior to the section in Fig. 21.9B), showing the liver, portal vein, spleen, stomach, aorta, inferior vena cava, vertebra and spinal cord, and right and left diaphragmatic crura (yellow and green arrows). (C) A contrast-enhanced (venous phase) axial CT section through the upper abdomen, just inferior to the section in Fig. 21.9C, showing the portal vein, aorta, diaphragmatic crura (black arrows), stomach, and spleen.

(A) courtesy of the Visible Human Project of the US National Library of Medicine. (B) and (C) courtesy of the Radiology Department, Christian Medical College, Vellore, India.

(A)

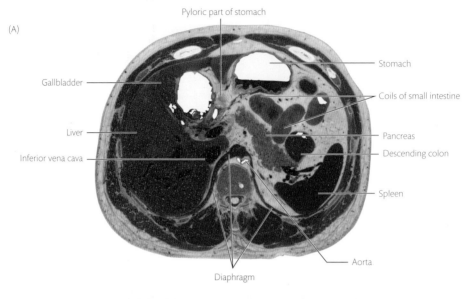

Pyloric part of stomach

Gallbladder

Liver

Inferior vena cava

Stomach

Coils of small intestine

Pancreas

Descending colon

Spleen

Aorta

Diaphragm

(B)

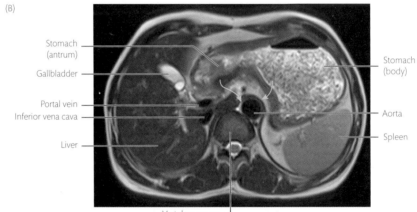

Stomach (antrum)

Gallbladder

Portal vein

Inferior vena cava

Liver

Stomach (body)

Aorta

Spleen

Vertebra

Fig. 21.11 (A) A section through the upper part of the abdomen, inferior to the section in Fig. 21.10A (at approximately T. 12 level). The pyloric part of the stomach is seen lying across the midline. The gallbladder is seen at this level, lying against the visceral surface of the liver. Coils of the small intestine (jejunum) and the descending colon are seen on the left side. The pancreas is seen anterior to the vertebral column and stretching towards the left (towards the hilum of the spleen). The right and left crura of the diaphragm unite in front of the aorta. At this level, the lungs are no longer in the section. (B) A T2W axial MRI section through the upper abdomen (inferior to the section in Fig. 21.10B), showing the liver, spleen, body and pylorus of the stomach, aorta, inferior vena cava, portal vein, right and left diaphragmatic crura (arrows), and vertebra.

(A) courtesy of the Visible Human Project of the US National Library of Medicine. (B) courtesy of the Radiology Department, Christian Medical College, Vellore, India.

(A)

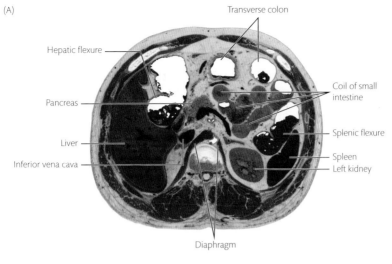

Transverse colon

Hepatic flexure

Pancreas

Liver

Inferior vena cava

Coil of small intestine

Splenic flexure

Spleen

Left kidney

Diaphragm

(B)

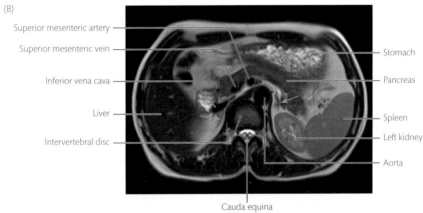

Superior mesenteric artery

Superior mesenteric vein

Inferior vena cava

Liver

Intervertebral disc

Stomach

Pancreas

Spleen

Left kidney

Aorta

Cauda equina

(C)

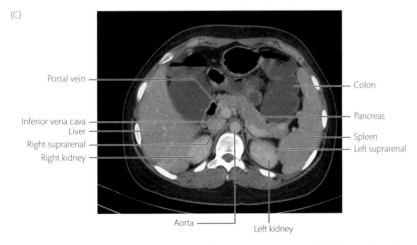

Portal vein

Inferior vena cava
Liver
Right suprarenal
Right kidney

Colon

Pancreas

Spleen
Left suprarenal

Aorta

Left kidney

Fig. 21.12 (A) A section through the upper part of the abdomen, inferior to the section in Fig. 21.11A. The liver, the second part of the duodenum, and the inferior vena cava are seen on the right. The spleen, descending colon, and coils of the small intestines are seen on the left. Multiple sections through the transverse colon are seen anteriorly and in proximity to the liver. More posteriorly, part of the pancreas is seen in front of the vertebra, and the left kidney is seen in the left paravertebral region. The aorta is seen between the two crura. (B) A T2W axial MRI section through the upper abdomen (inferior to the section in Fig. 21.11B), showing the liver, spleen, stomach, superior mesenteric artery and vein, aorta, inferior vena cava, right and left adrenal glands (green arrows), and left kidney. The intervertebral disc is seen in the midline posteriorly, and the cauda equina is seen in the vertebral foramen. (C) A contrast-enhanced (venous phase) axial CT section through the upper abdomen, inferior to the section in Fig. 21.10C, showing the portal vein confluence, pancreas, colon, spleen, aorta, inferior vena cava, suprarenal glands, and right and left kidneys.

(A) courtesy of the Visible Human Project of the US National Library of Medicine. (B) and (C) courtesy of the Radiology Department, Christian Medical College, Vellore, India.

(A)

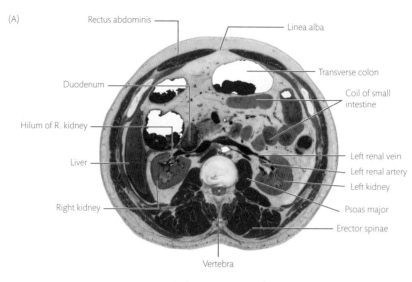

Rectus abdominis

Linea alba

Transverse colon

Duodenum

Coil of small intestine

Hilum of R. kidney

Left renal vein

Left renal artery

Liver

Left kidney

Psoas major

Right kidney

Erector spinae

Vertebra

(B)

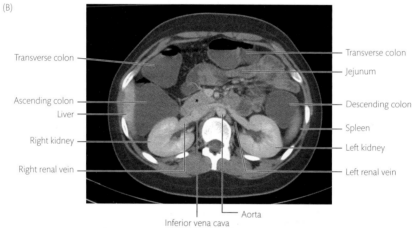

Transverse colon

Transverse colon

Jejunum

Ascending colon

Descending colon

Liver

Right kidney

Spleen

Left kidney

Right renal vein

Left renal vein

Inferior vena cava

Aorta

(C)

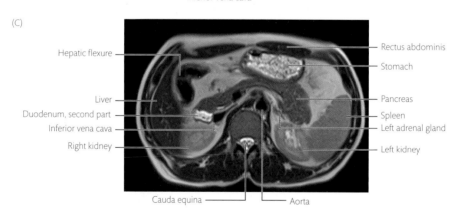

Hepatic flexure

Rectus abdominis

Stomach

Liver

Pancreas

Duodenum, second part

Spleen

Inferior vena cava

Left adrenal gland

Right kidney

Left kidney

Cauda equina

Aorta

Fig. 21.13 (A) A section through the abdomen (inferior to the section in Fig. 21.12A). The rectus abdominis on both sides and the linea alba in the midline are clearly seen. A smaller portion of the liver is seen on the right, in relation to the colon and right kidney. The transverse colon is seen anteriorly. The second part of the duodenum and head of the pancreas are seen to the right of the midline. Coils of the small intestine are seen on the left. This section shows the hilus of the kidneys, with the renal vessels entering it, and the cortex and medulla of the kidneys. The psoas and quadratus lumborum are seen on the posterior abdominal wall. (B) A contrast-enhanced (venous phase) axial CT section through the mid abdomen, inferior to the section in Fig. 21.12C, showing the right and left kidneys, right and left renal veins, aorta, inferior vena cava, jejunal loops, and ascending, transverse, and descending colons. The superior mesenteric vein (blue arrow) and superior mesenteric artery (red arrow) are seen in front of the uncinate process of the pancreas (asterisk). (C) A T2W axial MRI section through the upper abdomen (inferior to the section in Fig. 21.12B), showing the rectus abdominis, liver, spleen, stomach, hepatic flexure, second part of the duodenum, pancreas, left adrenal gland, right and left kidneys, aorta, inferior vena cava, and cauda equina.

(A) courtesy of the Visible Human Project of the US National Library of Medicine. (B) and (C) courtesy of the Radiology Department, Christian Medical College, Vellore, India.

(A)

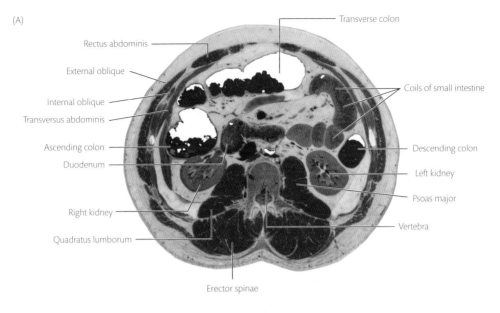

(B)

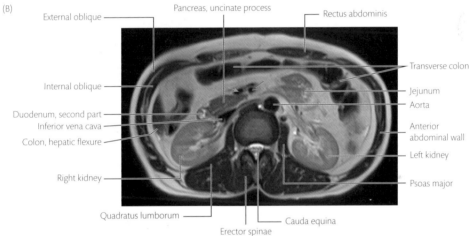

Fig. 21.14 (A) A section through the abdomen, inferior to the section in Fig. 21.13A. The anterior abdominal muscles—the external oblique, internal oblique, and transversus abdominis—are seen on the lateral side and contributing to the formation of the rectus sheath around the rectus abdominis. The posterior abdominal wall muscles—the psoas major and quadratus lumborum—are seen, as is the erector spinae. The transverse colon is seen across the abdomen anteriorly; the ascending and descending colons are seen on the right and left sides. The duodenum near the right kidney and coils of the jejunum in front of the left kidney are seen. Blue arrow: inferior vena cava. Red arrow: aorta. (B) A T2W axial MRI section through the mid abdomen, inferior to the section in Fig. 21.13B, showing the inferior tip of the liver, colon, aorta, inferior vena cava, right and left kidneys, uncinate process of the pancreas, superior mesenteric artery (red arrow), superior mesenteric vein (blue arrow), second part of the duodenum, hepatic flexure, rectus abdominis, external oblique, internal oblique, psoas major, quadratus lumborum, erector spinae, and cauda equina.

(A) courtesy of the Visible Human Project of the US National Library of Medicine. (B) courtesy of the Radiology Department, Christian Medical College, Vellore, India.

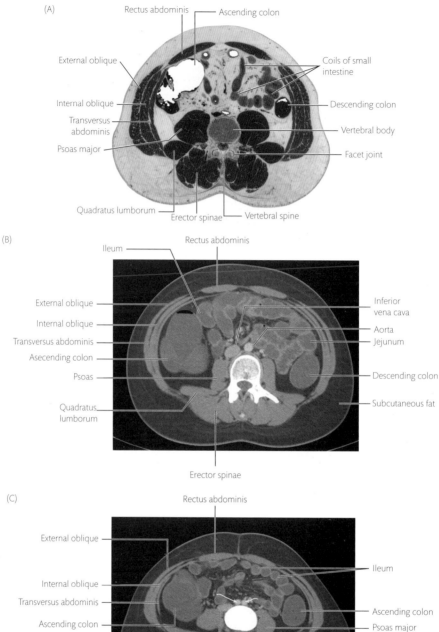

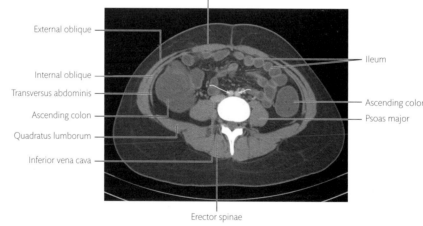

Fig. 21.15 (A) A section through the lower part of the abdomen, inferior to the section in Fig. 21.14A. The muscles of the anterior and posterior abdominal walls are well seen. The formation of rectus sheath is especially well visualized. The ascending and descending colons are seen, as well as coils of the small intestine. The kidneys are no longer seen as the section passes inferior to the inferior pole. The facet joints are clearly seen. (B) A contrast-enhanced (venous phase) axial CT section through the mid abdomen, inferior to the section in Fig. 21.14B, showing the small bowel loops, the ascending and descending colons, and muscles of the abdominal wall. (C) A contrast-enhanced (venous phase) axial CT section through the lower abdomen, just inferior to the section in Fig. 21.15B, showing almost the same structures, with the exception of the aorta. The aorta is no longer seen, but the two terminal branches—the right and left common iliac arteries—are seen (arrows).

(A) courtesy of the Visible Human Project of the US National Library of Medicine. (B) and (C) courtesy of the Radiology Department, Christian Medical College, Vellore, India.

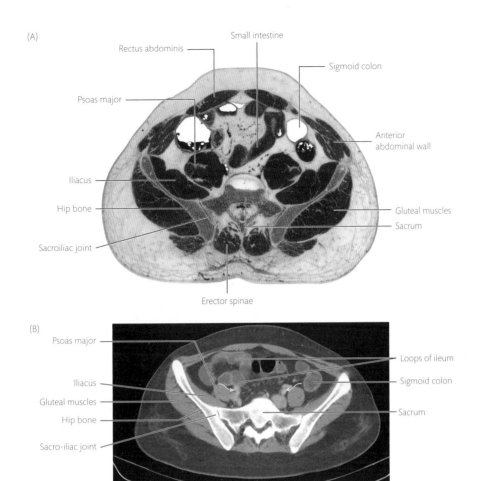

Fig. 21.16 (A) A section through the lower part of the abdomen, through the sacro-iliac joint, inferior to the section in Fig. 21.15A. The ascending and sigmoid colons and coils of the ileum are seen. The psoas major and iliacus are seen anterior to the ilium (hip bone), and the gluteal muscles are seen posteriorly. (B) A contrast-enhanced (venous phase) axial CT section through the upper pelvis, just inferior to the section in Fig. 21.15C, showing the small bowel loops, sigmoid colon, psoas, iliacus, and gluteal muscles. The common iliac vessels are shown by arrows.

(A) courtesy of the Visible Human Project of the US National Library of Medicine. (B) courtesy of the Radiology Department, Christian Medical College, Vellore, India.

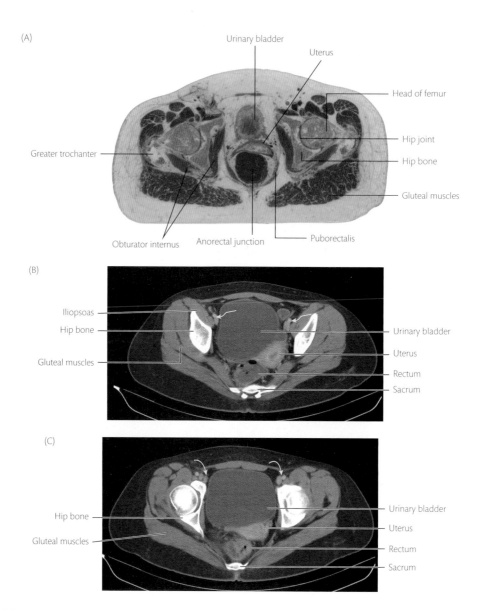

(A)

Urinary bladder

Uterus

Head of femur

Hip joint

Hip bone

Gluteal muscles

Greater trochanter

Obturator internus   Anorectal junction   Puborectalis

(B)

Iliopsoas

Hip bone

Gluteal muscles

Urinary bladder

Uterus

Rectum

Sacrum

(C)

Hip bone

Gluteal muscles

Urinary bladder

Uterus

Rectum

Sacrum

Fig. 21.17 (A) A section through the pelvis at the level of the hip joint (inferior to the section in Fig. 21.16A). The obturator internus is seen on the lateral wall of the pelvis, curving around the ischium and running towards the greater trochanter of the femur. Within the pelvic cavity, the urinary bladder lies anteriorly, followed by the uterus and the anorectal junction more posteriorly. The puborectalis is seen looping around the posterior aspect of the anorectal junction. (B) A contrast-enhanced (venous phase) axial CT section through the mid pelvis, just inferior to the section in Fig. 21.16B, showing the urinary bladder, uterus, rectum, iliopsoas muscles, gluteal muscles, external iliac vessels (arrows), sacrum, and roof of the acetabulum. (C) A contrast-enhanced (venous phase) axial CT section through the lower pelvis, just inferior to the section in Fig. 21.17B, showing the urinary bladder, uterus, rectum, gluteal muscles, external iliac vessels (arrows), sacrum, and hip joints.

(A) courtesy of the Visible Human Project of the US National Library of Medicine. (B) and (C) courtesy of the Radiology Department, Christian Medical College, Vellore, India.

Answers to MCQs

Answers for part 2:
The thorax

1. A
2. D
3. D
4. A
5. C
6. B
7. C
8. A
9. B
10. B
11. C
12. D
13. B
14. C
15. A

Answers for part 3:
The abdomen

1. B
2. B
3. D
4. B
5. C
6. A
7. C
8. B
9. A
10. B
11. B
12. D
13. D
14. B
15. A

Answers for part 4:
The pelvis and perineum

1. B
2. A
3. D
4. D
5. C
6. D
7. C
8. C
9. C
10. D
11. B
12. D
13. A
14. A
15. B

Index

321

Index

324